Advance Care Planning

Leah Rogne, PhD, is a professor of sociology at Minnesota State University, Mankato, where she teaches courses in aging, death and dying, and human services. She is the coordinator of Minnesota State's Applied Sociology program and former interim director of its Gerontology Program and Center on Aging. She is the coeditor of *Social Insurance and Social Justice: Social Security, Medicare, and the Campaign Against Entitlements* (2009).

Susana Lauraine McCune, MA, CT, is a doctoral student of clinical psychology at Antioch University Seattle, specializing in health psychology and art therapy. She has served as a hospice volunteer and employee. She is a member of the Washington State Psychological Association End-of-Life Special Interest Group. She brings an interdisciplinary perspective to education, research, and support for professional caregivers as they facilitate advance care planning and provide end-of-life care. Her published works include *Living Beyond the Other* (2012) and *Engaging A/r/tography to Reveal Countertransference: Enhancing Self-Awareness in Caregiving Professionals.*

Advance Care Planning

Communicating About Matters of Life and Death

Leah Rogne, PhD
Susana Lauraine McCune, MA, CT

Editors

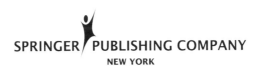

SPRINGER PUBLISHING COMPANY
NEW YORK

Copyright © 2014 Springer Publishing Company, LLC

Springer Publishing Company, LLC
11 West 42nd Street
New York, NY 10036
www.springerpub.com

Acquisitions Editor: Sheri W. Sussman
Production Editor: Dana Bigelow
Composition: Newgen Imaging

ISBN: 978-0-8261-1021-3
e-book ISBN: 978-0-8261-1022-0

13 14 15 16 17 / 5 4 3 2 1

The author and the publisher of this Work have made every effort to use sources believed to be reliable to provide information that is accurate and compatible with the standards generally accepted at the time of publication. The author and publisher shall not be liable for any special, consequential, or exemplary damages resulting, in whole or in part, from the readers' use of, or reliance on, the information contained in this book. The publisher has no responsibility for the persistence or accuracy of URLs for external or third-party Internet websites referred to in this publication and does not guarantee that any content on such websites is, or will remain, accurate or appropriate.

Library of Congress Cataloging-in-Publication Data
CIP data is available from the Library of Congress.

Special discounts on bulk quantities of our books are available to corporations, professional associations, pharmaceutical companies, health care organizations, and other qualifying groups. If you are interested in a custom book, including chapters from more than one of our titles, we can provide that service as well.

For details, please contact:
Special Sales Department, Springer Publishing Company, LLC
11 West 42nd Street, 15th Floor, New York, NY 10036-8002
Phone: 877-687-7476 or 212-431-4370; Fax: 212-941-7842
E-mail: sales@springerpub.com

Printed in the United States of America by Maple Press.

Contents

v

Contributors

Mercedes Bern-Klug, PhD, MSW
Associate Professor
University of Iowa School of Social Work
Director, Aging Studies Program
John A. Hartford Geriatric Social Work
 Faculty Scholar
Iowa City, Iowa

Kathy Black, PhD, MPH, MAQ, MSG
Hartford Geriatric Social Work Faculty
 Scholar
Professor
Social Work and Gerontology
College of Arts and Sciences
University of South Florida at Sarasota-
 Manatee
Sarasota, Florida

Linda A. Briggs, MS, MA, RN
Associate Director
Respecting Choices and Ethics Consultant
Gundersen Health System
La Crosse, Wisconsin

Judy Citko, JD
Executive Director
Coalition for Compassionate Care of
 California
Sacramento, California

Joe Jack Davis, MD
Retired General Surgeon
Bremerton, Washington

Jane Dohrmann, LISW, ACHP-SW
Director, Honoring Your Wishes
Iowa City Hospice
Iowa City, Iowa

Patrick A. Dolan Jr., PhD
Lecturer
Department of Rhetoric
University of Iowa
Iowa City, Iowa

Annalu Farber MBA, MATS
Consultant
Tyler Associates
Tacoma, Washington

Stu Farber, MD
Professor
Department of Family Medicine
University of Washington School of
 Medicine
Director
Palliative Care Service
University of Washington Medical Center
Seattle, Washington

Jolene Formaini, RN, MA, CT
Educator/Consultant on Issues of
  Dying, Death and Bereavement
Healing Hearts Grief Education and
  Support Services
Kittanning, Pennsylvania

Ana Tuya Fulton, MD, FACP
Chief of Internal Medicine, Butler
  Hospital
Assistant Professor of Medicine
Division of Geriatrics
Warren Alpert Medical School of
  Medicine Brown University
Providence, Rhode Island

Jill Harrison, PhD
Research Consultation Specialist
Planetree, a Non-Profit Dedicated to
  Patient-Centered Care
Derby, Connecticut

**Cari Borenko Hoffmann, BA,
  BSW, RSW**
Project Implementation Coordinator
Fraser Health
Surrey, British Columbia
Canada

Cory Ingram, MD
Assistant Professor of Family and
  Palliative Medicine
Mayo Clinic, College of Medicine
Medical Director, Palliative Medicine
Mayo Clinic Health System
Mankato, Minnesota

Nancy S. Jecker, PhD
Professor
Department of Bioethics and
  Humanities
University of Washington School of
  Medicine
Seattle, Washington

Marshall B. Kapp, JD, MPH
Director and Professor
Center for Innovative Collaboration in
  Medicine and Law
Florida State University
Tallahassee, Florida

Allan Kellehear, PhD, AcSS
Professor of Community Health
Mental Health, Social Work, and
  Inter-professional Learning
Middlesex University
London, United Kingdom

Dr. Ben Lobo, FRCP (UK)
Executive Medical Director
Derbyshire Community Health Services
  NHS Trust
United Kingdom

Beverly Lunsford, PhD, RN, CNS-BC
Assistant Professor, School of Nursing
George Washington University
Director
GW Center for Aging, Health and
  Humanities
Director
The Washington DC Area Geriatric
  Education Center Consortium
Washington, DC

Susana Lauraine McCune, MA, CT
Doctoral Student
Antioch University Seattle
Seattle, Washington

Cynthia Pearson, BA
Author and Caregiver
Founding Member and Board Secretary
Take Charge of Your Life Partnership
Co-Project Director of "Just Talk About It"
Pittsburgh, Pennsylvania

Katherine Irene Pettus, PhD
Political Science and International
  Relations
University of Pécs
Pécs, Hungary

Leah Rogne, PhD
Professor
Department of Sociology and
    Corrections
Minnesota State University, Mankato
Mankato, Minnesota

John Ryan, PhD
Professor and Chair
Department of Sociology
Virginia Polytechnic Institute and State
    University
Blacksburg, Virginia

**Helen Stanton Chapple, PhD, RN,
    MA, MSN, CT**
Nurse Ethicist, Assistant Professor
Center for Health Policy and Ethics,
    School of Nursing
Creighton University
Omaha, Nebraska

Margaret L. Stubbs, PhD
Professor
Department of Psychology
Chatham University
Pittsburgh, Pennsylvania

**Dena Jean Sutermaster, RN, MSN,
    CHPN**
Director of Education Products
Hospice and Palliative Nurses
    Association
Pittsburgh, Pennsylvania

Joan M. Teno, MD, MS
Professor of Health Services, Policy
    and Practice
Professor of Medicine
Associate Director of the Center for
    Gerontology and Health Care
    Research
Warren Alpert Medical School of Brown
    University
Providence, Rhode Island

Ben Wolfe, MEd, LICSW
Former Program Manager/Grief
    Therapist
Essentia Health–St. Mary's Medical
    Center's Grief Support Services
Adjunct Instructor
University of Minnesota, Duluth School
    of Medicine
Duluth, Minnesota

Preface

This book is intended to help facilitate meaningful communication and effective decision making about medical care at end of life (EOL). With an aging population and rapidly expanding life-saving technologies that transform how we deal with life-threatening illness at any age or stage of life, concerns about how we want to live at the end of our days become more and more crucial for a growing number of people in our communities. However, research on EOL decision making shows that people have difficulty both asking and answering important questions about EOL care for themselves and for their loved ones. Many people are overwhelmed by the complexity of the health care system and do not know that they have the right to decide what kind of care they would like to have when they are critically ill or how to indicate their desires to their health care providers.

Advance directives (ADs) (living wills and health care proxies) have received great attention in recent decades as tools for providing for self-determination and quality of life near the EOL. Yet, despite years of enthusiastic advocacy by major health care organizations, they have not been as widely used as hoped. Due to complexities involved in making and documenting EOL care choices, lack of understanding of how they should document their choices, and discomfort about talking about dying, a majority of Americans face life-threatening illness without having a plan in place. Also, due to communication problems among patients, families, and health care providers and lack of awareness of how advance care planning (ACP) can best be done, people who have planned ahead and have ADs in place often do not get the care they had hoped for during the dying process. Furthermore, it has become more and more apparent that the focus on autonomy and self-determination at the expense of any other ethical principles or human motivations may not take into consideration the variety of ways that people approach, with their loved ones, the profound and complicated challenges presented as we face our mortality.

Featuring the voices of scholars and practitioners from a variety of disciplines, this volume provides a history of ADs and describes barriers to effective ACP. Contributors share effective communication strategies that address some of the shortcomings of a forms-completion approach to EOL planning and show how a focus on facilitating meaningful conversations between patients and their families and among patients, families, and their health care providers can provide for better outcomes at the EOL. Authors describe innovative regional or statewide initiatives for promoting effective ACP and present some "big ideas" for how we as communities and as a society could be charting a new course for how we deal with life-threatening illness, dying, loss, and death. Those who are seeking guidance for their own ACP or who want to be a part of initiatives to help communities address these important issues will find a wide range of contacts and resources.

At the heart, this project is intended to provide individuals with the awareness of the need to plan ahead for their EOL and the tools to be effective in doing so, and to provide professionals with key strategies to be successful in facilitating communication with patients and families. Too often, after experiencing the death of a loved one, people will say "if I had only known..." or "if we had only talked...." Meaningful conversations with one another about what we value and what is important to us in life are the basis for an effective ACP process. We hope that readers—professionals, educators, and members of the general public—will find the perspectives, strategies, and tools (as well as the vision) the authors present in this volume to be helpful in providing a path to a dying process without regret.

Leah Rogne
Susana Lauraine McCune

Acknowledgments

I would like to thank the many elders I served as a nursing home social worker for the wisdom they offered on how to live well until we die. I am forever grateful to my mentor Michelle Matchie for introducing me to the heart and soul of dying and for her many lessons about the meaning of life and death. I would like to dedicate my work on this book to my parents, Katherine and Leslie Rogne, who gave their children the gift of planning well for their end of life.

—*Leah Rogne*

I would like to thank Mary Wieneke, PhD, and Philip Cushman, PhD, for giving me the wind I needed to fill my sails when they sagged so I could do what I believed needed to be done, even though at times on this journey land was far from sight. I thank the hospice patients and families and the grieving young people with whom I have been honored to work for their courage and honesty. They continue to inspire me. I would like to dedicate this book to my mother, Elizabeth Louise Hudson McCune, who gave me the gift of understanding the necessity of preparing for dying and showed me how to live and die courageously. My work on this book is dedicated to her. I would like to express my deepest gratitude to Dr. Leah Rogne for trusting me enough to embark on this project together and for mentoring me as a budding editor and author. Thank you, Steve, for traveling with me on this journey. Thank you, Dad, for believing in me.

—*Susana Lauraine McCune*

In addition, we thank our editor, Sheri W. Sussman, and all the staff at Springer Publishing Company for their encouragement and support in making this project a reality. Most importantly we thank the authors who contributed to this volume for their dedication to research and practice on EOL care. Working with them has been a great pleasure, and we have learned so much from them in the process.

Finally, in memory of those who have gone before, and for those who will come after, we encourage you to communicate with loved ones and professional caregivers about advance care planning. We encourage you to communicate about matters of life and death.

CHAPTER 1

Introduction: A Matter of Life and Death

Leah Rogne
Susana Lauraine McCune

The principle of respect for autonomy, captured in ideas of negative liberty and noninterference, has a particular appeal in the United States, which is founded on the belief that all people have the right to live as they choose. Autonomy is a formative notion on which U.S. culture and our system of health care is largely based. Such a preoccupation with autonomy obscures the fact that we ultimately lack control over aging, illness, disability, suffering, and death. To admit this lack of autonomy is to admit that the human condition is beyond our control; to relinquish autonomy is to acknowledge our deep vulnerability....

Martha B. Holstein, Jennifer B. Parks,
and Mark H. Waymack, 2011, pp. 11–12

At the end of the day, an advance directive is just a piece of paper. But an effective program for advance care planning is an opportunity to help people grow, create meaning, and make their lives (and deaths) better.

Benjamin H. Levi and Michael J. Green, 2010, pp. 8–9

To advocate human conversation as the means to restore hope to the future is as simple as I can get. But I have seen there is no more powerful way to initiate significant change than to convene conversation....

1

It is always like this. Real change begins with the simple act of people talking about what they care about.

Margaret Wheatley, 2009, p. 22

PLANNING FOR ENDINGS

One of the most difficult, terrifying, and confusing moments of life is when a life-threatening accident or illness strikes you or a loved one. Among the most challenging aspects of these events is that people are faced with decisions about accepting or foregoing, initiating or withdrawing aggressive medical care. These options require complex decisions.

In the midst of such confusion, patients and their loved ones are not only confronted with a life-threatening illness and complex decisions about care; they are also forced to deal with a medical system that they often experience as unfamiliar and impersonal. At these times, a myriad of perspectives and needs converge. Yet, if plans are not made in advance, patients, their loved ones, advocates, and clinicians are forced to make decisions about medical care quickly, under less-than-desirable circumstances.

The growing availability of sophisticated life-support technology only increases the likelihood of such tough decision making. These evermore regularly occurring situations call for Americans to face end-of-life (EOL) decisions before an emergency—to acknowledge their mortality and begin thinking about and planning for medical care through life and death in advance. The optimal time to make these decisions is not during a crisis, as these critical care choices can result in irrevocable consequences.

Our current conceptions in the United States about how health care is given, along with the consequences of our lack of communicating about considering medical care in advance, have implications not just for individuals, but also for society as a whole. Due to these conditions, both individuals and communities bear the costs—both emotional and physical, as well as financial—of not planning in advance for the medical care one would desire to receive at EOL.

THE PROMISE OF ADVANCE DIRECTIVES

Heralded as the Miranda warning for persons considering the EOL (Sloane, 1990), the Patient Self-Determination Act (PSDA) was passed by the U.S. Congress in 1990 with high expectations for what many thought would be a new day in which people would be able to exercise personal control of the dying process.

The PSDA required hospitals and nursing homes to ask people at the time of admission if they had advance directives (ADs) (a living will specifying which procedures or treatments they wanted or did not want at EOL and a durable power of attorney for health care matters or proxy, in which they would name someone to make decisions on their behalf if the patient could no longer speak for himself/herself). The act requires admitting personnel to provide forms for patients to fill out and document that these procedures had been followed.

The hope was that completing living wills and appointing proxies would lead to a better dying in which individuals' preferences would be granted in their final days. Guided by a strong commitment to the ethical principle of autonomy and the deeply held ideology of individualism so embedded in U.S. culture (see, e.g., Chapple, 2010; Holstein, Parks, & Waymack, 2011; Kaufman, 2005), ADs were seen as an extension of personal control on unto death, after the individual could no longer speak for himself/herself.

By the mid-1990s the rosy glow only half a decade old had begun to dim, and scholars and practitioners began to question whether this initiative had had the results it had intended. The comprehensive intervention project and research report, the Study to Understand Prognoses and Preferences for Outcomes and Risks of Treatments (SUPPORT), found that the PSDA had made little difference in whether patients' preferences were upheld at the time of death (Teno et al., 1997). Surgeon Tonelli (1996) argued that it was "time to pull the plug" on living wills, as studies began to indicate that the documents had not fulfilled their promise and that dying patients did not experience a better death for having completed them. Fagerlin and Schneider (2004) asserted:

> A crescendoing empirical literature and persistent clinical disappointments reveal that the rewards of the campaign to promote living wills do not justify its costs. Nor can any degree of tinkering ever make the living will an effective instrument of social policy. (p. 30)

At the same time, Fagerlin and Schneider did not call for the elimination of living wills. Living wills are appropriate, they said, for some patients; persons who have a high need for control should be informed about living wills and proxies. But the PSDA was bad policy, they argued, and we should "abjure programs intended to cajole everyone into signing living wills" (Fagerlin & Schneider, 2004, p. 39).

In an editorial in the prestigious *Annals of Internal Medicine*, Harvard professor and physician Joan Teno said it was "time to move on," citing the empirical literature showing that having a living will had not reduced hospital costs at EOL. Nevertheless, Teno stated she didn't "mean to imply that advance directives are unimportant" (Teno, 2004, p. 59).

Proxies, by which persons give someone else the legal authority to make health care decisions for them if they cannot speak for themselves, have fared somewhat better. The body of research shows, however, that too often the surrogates chosen by the individual either do not know they have been given this responsibility, are poor predictors of what their family member or friend would want, or refuse to act when difficult decisions are required (Covinsky, Fuller, & Yaffe, 2000; Emanuel, 1995; Tonelli, 1996).

So, 20 years after the PDSA, where are we now and where are we going?

In the wake of strong concerns on the part of practitioners and scholars about the effectiveness of ADs, conversations about EOL planning have shifted from product to process (Hammes, 2003; Wenger, Shugarman, & Wilkinson, 2008), from a focus on completion of documents to a focus on ADs as tools to stimulate communication between patients and families and their health care providers about EOL care. Advance care planning (ACP) has come to be seen part of a comprehensive and ongoing approach to educate ourselves and our communities about dying and death and to provide knowledge that can help us prepare ourselves, our families, and our society for a better way to die.

ORGANIZATION OF THIS BOOK

This volume brings together scholars and practitioners from various disciplines—social workers, sociologists, psychologists, physicians, ethicists, political scientists, nurses, and others—to assess the current state of efforts to plan in advance for dying and death and suggest paths toward a more effective approach to death education and EOL care.

The essays in the book are organized into five parts. Part I details the history and current status of ADs and their use in EOL planning and care, focusing on current challenges, including resistance to talking about death and dying, legal and ethical issues, the problem of overtreatment, and the cultural and spiritual considerations around EOL care. In Part II, authors discuss a variety of innovative ways or best practices to facilitate meaningful conversations about EOL, and Part III highlights successful initiatives in ACP. Part IV presents some big picture ideas about the kind of ethical view, leadership philosophy, and community development orientation it will take to undertake the kind of cultural transformation necessary to create a new way to deal with dying, death, loss, and care. Finally, Part V presents selected resources on death and dying, ACP, and palliative care.

Increasingly in the coming decades, the aging of the population in combination with rapidly advancing medical technologies will force an unparalleled number of people and their loved ones to make unprecedented decisions about life and death in an age of simultaneously abundant technology, economic disparity, and strained resources. No forms or legal documents, no matter how carefully crafted, can automatically guarantee us the death we want for ourselves or our loved ones. But we can prepare ourselves by having the courage to convene conversations about dying, death, and loss within our families and communities and with our health care practitioners, as well as by raising the awareness of the entire community—of any age, any health status, in any venue—of the centrality of issues related to death and caring for the dying as a universal human experience.

REFERENCES

Chapple, H. S. (2010). *No place for dying: American hospitals and the ideology of rescue*. Walnut Creek, CA: Left Coast Press.

Covinsky, K. E., Fuller, J. D., & Yaffe, K. (2000). Communication and decision-making in seriously ill patients: Findings of the SUPPORT Project. *Journal of the American Geriatrics Society, 48*(5), 187–193.

Emanuel, L. L. (1995). Advance directives: do they work? *Journal of the American College of Cardiology, 25*(1), 35–38.

Fagerlin, A., & Schneider, C. E. (2004). Enough: The failure of the living will. *The Hastings Center Report, 34*(2), 30–42.

Hammes, B. J. (2003). Update on *respecting choices*: Four years on. *Innovations in End-of-Life Care, 5*(2), 1–18.

Holstein, M. B., Parks, J. A., & Waymack, M. H. (2011). *Ethics, aging, and society: The critical turn*. New York, NY: Springer.

Kaufman, S. R. (2005)....*and a time to die: How American hospitals shape the end of life*. Chicago, IL: University of Chicago Press.

Levi, B. H., & Green, M. J. (2010). Too soon to give up: Re-examining the value of advance directives. *The American Journal of Bioethics: AJOB, 10*(4), 3–22.

Sloane, L. (1990, December 8). *91 law says failing patients must be told of their options*. *New York Times*. Retrieved from http://search.proquest.com.ezproxy.mnsu.edu/docview/427916511/fulltext/13B5CAF3F3E78FCD134/1?accountid=12259

Teno, J. M. (2004). Advance directives: Time to move on. *Annals of Internal Medicine, 141*(2), 159–160.

Teno, J., Lynn, J., Wenger, N., Phillips, R. S., Murphy, D. P., Connors, A. F., Knaus, W. A. (1997). Advance directives for seriously ill hospitalized patients: Effectiveness with the patient self-determination act and the SUPPORT intervention. SUPPORT Investigators. Study to Understand Prognoses and Preferences for Outcomes and Risks of Treatment. *Journal of the American Geriatrics Society, 45*(4), 500–507.

Tonelli, M. R. (1996). Pulling the plug on living wills: A critical analysis of advance directives. *Chest, 110*(3), 816–822.

Wenger, N. S., Shugarman, L. R., & Wilkinson, A. (2008). *Advance directives and advance care planning: Report to Congress*. RAND Corporation Report to U.S. Department of Health and Human Services. Retrieved from aspe.hhs.gov/daltcp/reports/2008/ADCongRpt-B.pdf

Wheatley, M. (2009). *Turning to one another: Simple conversations to restore hope to the future*. San Francisco, CA: Berrett-Koehler.

PART I

Advance Care Planning: Promise and Challenge

Introduction

Susana Lauraine McCune

Advance directives (ADs) (living wills, health care proxies, etc.) and Physician Orders for Life-Sustaining Treatment (POLST) can help ensure self-determination and quality of life near the end of life (EOL). Yet, despite years of enthusiastic advocacy by major health care organizations, they have not been as widely used as hoped. Due to complexities involved in making and documenting EOL care choices, lack of understanding of the role of ADs, and discomfort about talking about dying, a majority of Americans face life-threatening illness without having completed and documented their advance care plan (ACP). Moreover, at times people who do have ADs often do not get the care they had hoped for during the dying process.

The following chapters in Part I review the history and discuss the challenges and the current status of ADs. The authors address common barriers to effective ACP, call attention to legal and ethical issues involved in ACP, and present religious, spiritual, and cultural considerations for ACP.

In Chapter 1 Susana Lauraine McCune and Leah Rogne discuss the promise of ADs and the challenges that proponents of planning have faced in their attempts to create widespread change in how we plan for EOL. They review the ethical foundations of ADs and outline the potential benefits of and challenges in using ADs to provide for satisfactory EOL decision making. The authors end with a discussion of the new focus on ACP and ongoing communication and community involvement as key mechanisms to transform how we plan for EOL care.

In Chapter 3, physicians Ana Tuya Fulton and Joan M. Teno (whose previous work has been instrumental in calling for a new look at living wills and proxies) review existing research on ACP, noting the lack of clear evidence that ADs, on their own, make a difference in the care patients receive at the EOL. Arguing that too much emphasis has been on "finding the perfect form," they call instead for a multifaceted approach that invites varied conversations with patients depending on the stage of life and their health status. They call attention to the current lack of a financial reimbursement system to encourage and compensate health care providers for having these important conversations, and they provide a useful case study that shows how conversations about ACP should evolve in response to the specific changing health status of the individual.

In Chapter 4, sociologists John Ryan and Jill Harrison apply the sociological concepts of rationalization, specialization, and professionalization to help explain why Americans, who are otherwise great planners—saving and planning ahead for future activities such as higher education, weddings, and vacations—are so overwhelmingly averse to planning for death, an event that is universally inevitable. They argue that the growth of a society that privileges technical expertise and specialized knowledge has led to the dependence of the average person on the expert knowledge of the professional, as lay people cede control of the situation and become "clients" rather than exercise their own agency.

Chapter 5 outlines the contemporary American legal environment pertaining to EOL medical decision making. Attorney and professor of geriatrics Marshall B. Kapp identifies and analyzes the various ways the legal environment either facilitates or impedes particular forms of ACP, and most importantly how health care providers' legal anxieties impact the likelihood that ADs actually assure that patients' wishes about EOL care get honored in practice. In light of identified deficiencies in the ACP status quo, Kapp suggests legal alternatives to existing planning mechanisms, with special emphasis on the POLST paradigm.

In Chapter 6, medical ethicist Nancy S. Jecker draws on philosophical and ethical considerations, using a Kantian analysis, to examine the problem of overtreatment and dilemmas of "moral distress" that emerge for providers when providing EOL care. While Jecker emphasizes the principle of autonomy in her discussion of the need for ACP, she raises the alternative framework of "easing burden" as a guideline for decision making that does not necessarily privilege autonomy over every other ethical principle. Further, she argues that futility may in essence veto patient or family autonomy and choice when there is empirical evidence and consensus among providers that a treatment is in vain.

Finally, in Chapter 7, Beverly Lunsford, professor of geriatric nursing, makes a compelling case for the important role of religion, spirituality, values, and culture when working with patients and their loved ones in relation to ACP and EOL care decision making. Lunsford tackles the ineffable topics of religion and spirituality and existential aspects of ACP decision making, including the human search for meaning in living, dying, illness, and the experience of pain.

CHAPTER 2

Planning for End-of-Life Care: Where Are We and How Did We Get Here?

Susana Lauraine McCune
Leah Rogne

SETTING THE STAGE

Scenario 1

Unsteady on his feet but determined to water a young tree on a day in early summer, a 93-year-old North Dakota farmer with mild to moderate dementia tripped and fell in his garden. He managed to pull himself up and, with his wife's help, got back to the house. The next day he was driving his golf cart around the farm, making plans with his wife and daughter for how to cut back on the large garden, telling his family which irises and lilies to keep and which he could no longer care for. The next day he began a sharp decline in his motor abilities and soon could no longer dress himself.

After being hospitalized overnight for observation and a brain scan, he and his daughter shared a soda while waiting for the test results. The neurologist came in and told them that there was a subdural hematoma—a bleed in his brain—that was causing his sharp decline, perhaps caused by the fall. By this time, the farmer could no longer talk.

(continued)

Scenario 1   (*continued*)

The doctor told the daughter that they could bore a hole in his skull and suck out the blood or, if that did not work, they could open up his cranium and remove the clot. The daughter told him her father was clear about his wishes, and he would not want this kind of procedure.

When the daughter brought her father to the hospital, she had a large manila envelope containing information on his wishes about his dying and death. The envelope was kept by the front door of the house on a bookshelf, and all the family knew what it was and where it was. One of the documents had been signed in 1963—46 years before the accident. There was a form donating his body to the state medical school. One form was his living will. Another document gave his daughter the right to make decisions for him if he could no longer speak for himself. The documents were the result of numerous conversations over the years between the farmer, his wife, and their children over the years about their desires about end of life (EOL).

Though grieving at the news that her father's death would come sooner than she'd expected, the daughter had complete confidence in what he would have wanted and complete confidence in her right—and her responsibility—to act on his behalf. The farmer went home to the farm and died 9 days later under the care of hospice, 30 feet from the spot where he had been born.

Scenario 2

A woman in her mid-50s experienced symptoms that indicated a possible serious illness. Her symptoms included severe, unrelenting vertigo, nausea, vomiting, disorientation, diminished vision and cognition, and shortness of breath. Her primary care physician referred her to several specialists. Since a hospital admission had been discussed as a possibility, to each doctor appointment she brought with her a file folder labeled "Advance Directives."

When she checked in for her doctor appointments she said, "I brought my advance directives with me, and I'd like to have them added to my chart." Receptionists looked at her with a blank stare and responded, "I don't deal with that. You'll have to take that up with the nurse or the doctor."

When called from the waiting room to the examining room, she said to the medical professional, "I brought with me my advance directives. I'd like to have them added to my chart." They gave her either a quizzical look or a blank stare and replied, "I don't know what that is." Or asked, "What is that?"

(*continued*)

Scenario 2   *(continued)*

She explained, "They are documents I have completed to direct my medical care in case I am not able to advocate for myself. They include naming a health care proxy to make medical care decisions for me if I can't make them myself. I'd like to have a copy added to my chart." The medical professionals typically responded, "I don't deal with that. You should talk about it with the doctor."

When the physician entered the exam room, the patient said, "I brought a copy of my advance directives. I'd like to have them added to my chart." One physician said, "Oh, that is a good idea. I am so glad you have thought about that. I wish more people would do this. It is so important." Three other physicians paused and said, "Give those to the nurse."

None of the physicians initiated a discussion with her about the specifics of her advance directives (ADs) or her treatment goals for EOL care.

During her appointment with one of the physicians, she initiated a conversation about her ADs. She said, "You have come highly recommended to me and I would like to discuss designating you as my primary physician of record, so I'd like to discuss my advance directives with you."

The physician replied, "Let me take a look at your paperwork." The physician flipped through the directives, which included a health care proxy, and specific directions in a living will, including instructions to allow natural death (AND), do not resuscitate (DNR), and do not intubate (DNI).

The physician said, "I cannot honor these requests. They are against my moral and ethical beliefs, and against my duty as a physician. I believe life is sacred and is to be preserved." At this point the visit ended and she left.

Scenario 3

Working on a presentation to her fellow students on EOL planning and taking seriously what she had read about the failure of ADs to satisfy the need that had been identified 20 years earlier, a graduate student passed out a copy of the new Physician Orders for Life-Sustaining Treatment (POLST) form to her Sociology of Death class. She asked that all the students in the class—most of them in their early twenties—fill them out on the spot and get them signed by their physicians. Puzzled, her young classmates hesitated.

(continued)

Scenario 3 *(continued)*

POLST is a doctor's order that is designed for someone who has a life-threatening illness and for whom it would not be surprising if they were dead within a year—entirely inappropriate for a healthy 20-something college student. But in light of the sharp criticism ADs have received in recent years, this earnest graduate student saw the new POLST as the solution for all.

ADVANCE DIRECTIVES AND ADVANCE CARE PLANNING: WHERE ARE WE NOW?

Twenty years after the passage of the federal Patient Self-Determination Act (PSDA), intended to provide persons with a way to express their wishes about the care they would want at EOL, we are faced with EOL care situations such as those reported in the three scenarios above. Some EOL scenarios go well, with families, patients, and their physicians having been in continuous conversation with one another to share their values about how the patients see the EOL unfolding for them and making sure that their desires are documented. At the same time, some patients find it difficult to engage their providers in having a conversation or even understanding the purpose of a request to address EOL, decision making, and care. There is also widespread misunderstanding of how to document one's wishes and what is the appropriate path to protect oneself from unwanted treatment in a life-threatening situation.

Despite decades of institutional mandates such as the PSDA, only a minority of adults have expressed their wishes about EOL care in writing. Wenger, Shugarman, and Wilkinson (2008) reported only 18% to 36% of adults have completed ADs. Members of the public receive contradictory and confusing information—if they receive any information at all—about how to document their wishes. Those who do prepare documents often do not share them with their families or tell their families or closest friends that they even have the documents. EOL planning documents may be stored in a safety deposit box and remain unknown to health care providers or families who would need to access the information at the time of crisis. People do not want to talk about death.

In this chapter, we discuss the promise of ADs and the challenges that proponents of planning have faced in their attempts to create widespread change in how we plan for EOL care. We start with a definition of ADs and ACP and follow with a brief history of the social currents that led to and shaped the development of ADs. We discuss the ethical foundations of ADs and outline some of the benefits of and challenges in using ADs to provide for satisfactory EOL decision making. We end with a discussion of the new focus on ACP and on ongoing communication and community involvement as key mechanisms to transform how we plan for EOL care.

Defining Advance Directives and Advance Care Planning

Advance Directives

ADs or advance health care directives are documents that "formally convey an individual's wishes about medical decisions to be made in the event that he or she loses decision-making capacity" (Levi & Green, 2010, p. 4). They are written in advance of serious illness to state health care choices and name someone to make those choices when one can no longer speak for oneself (American Hospital Association, 2005, p. 2). These documents include living wills, a durable power of attorney for health care that names health care advocates (also known as proxies, surrogates, and agents), and the most recent innovation, POLST, which is a doctor's order specifying treatment desires for those with life-threatening conditions. The instructions in ADs can be very specific or very general. More general instructions provide directions that any and all life-prolonging care be delivered, or that such care be refused, withheld, or withdrawn. Instructions can convey an individual's wishes about pain relief, antibiotics, artificial nutrition and hydration, and the use of CPR and mechanical ventilation. ADs can include instructions for care such as Do Not Resuscitate (DNR), Do Not Intubate (DNI), and Allow Natural Death (AND).

Advance Care Planning

ACP refers to "a process that involves preparing for future medical decisions in the hypothetical event that individuals are no longer able to speak for themselves when those decisions need to be made" (Levi & Green, 2010, p. 4). Levi and Green explained that ACP includes communication among patients, their loved ones and advocates, and clinicians about patients' values, beliefs, desires, and quality of life, along with care goals. The process of ACP often culminates in the creation of ADs.

How Did We Get Here: A Brief History of Advance Care Planning

Advance care planning documents have developed in the context of increasing longevity, advances in medical technology, and the expanding consumer rights movement (Lamers, 2005). In addition, major court cases involving EOL decision making and increasing litigation on health care matters have shaped how ADs and ACP have evolved (Meisel & Jennings, 2005; Sabatino, 2010).

The Longevity Revolution

The global population is undergoing what Butler (2008) called the "longevity revolution." The population of older adults in the United States is expected to grow from approximately 12% to 20% by the middle of the century. From 2010 to 2050 the elder population will more than double, from a little over 40 million to more than 88 million (U.S. Census Bureau, 2012). No society in history has had such a high proportion of elders.

Upon her retirement, noted journalist Ellen Goodman (2011) called attention to the challenge facing us:

> As 2011 opens, the first of the baby boomers will turn 65 at the rate of 10,000 a day for the next 19 years. We are the leading edge of what is optimistically called the Longevity Revolution. In little more than a century, Americans have gone from a life expectancy of 47 to one of 78.... The decisions that we make individually and collectively about how to spend this gift of time will reshape the country.

One of the fastest-growing age cohorts is those 85 years of age or older, expected to number almost 20 million, or 20% of older adults, by 2050 (U.S. Census Bureau, 2012). These elders are naturally prone to multiple degenerative illnesses occurring over the later years of life. As the population ages and baby boomers reach later life, we can expect even higher rates of disability, especially related to obesity and the sedentary lifestyles of this age cohort (Butler, 2008). This, combined with rapidly rising rates of dementia, results in a troubling prospect for the coming generation of elders. These conditions have emerged in the United States during the last 50 years and they will become more frequent and more widespread going forward (e.g., Lamers, 2005; Lynn & Adamson, 2003; Lynn, 2004). These trends, in combination with continually advancing medical technology, mean that complex EOL care considerations are taking place among an increasing number of individuals and over an extended duration of their lives.

Expanding Medical Technology

It is impossible to deny that all living beings ultimately will die. However, dying is different today. Technological developments in medicine that began to be developed during the 1960s and 1970s, as Sabatino (2010) has noted, "Thrust medicine into a new world where for the first time, it often became difficult to distinguish saving life from prolonging suffering and death" (p. 213). During the past 50 years in the United States, progress in medical care facilitated by technology has blurred the lines between rescue and long-term suffering before death (e.g., Chapple, 2010; Colby, 2006; Shen, 1999). To put it plainly, prolonging life through care can often mean prolonging suffering before death.

Due to the availability of advanced medical technology and the general compulsion to use this technology at all times, individuals, families, and clinicians regularly face demanding plan-of-care decisions concerning when advanced technological treatments (such as CPR, mechanical ventilation, and supplying artificial nutrition and hydration) should be initiated or withheld, and if initiated, when treatments are no longer beneficial for the patient and should be stopped (e.g., Colby, 2006; Lynn, 2004). Concerns about overtreatment and undertreatment, along with anxieties about initiating and withdrawing treatment, can engender ethical dilemmas that can cause moral distress for patients, their advocates, and clinicians (e.g., Austin, 2012; Epstein & Delgado, 2010; Pauly, Varcoe, & Storch, 2012).

The Consumer Movement and Advent of Advance Directives

ADs came on the scene in the wake of the social movements of the 1960s and the developing consumer rights movement (Lamers, 2005; Wilkinson, 2011), along with several pivotal events focused specifically on death and dying. According to Lamers (2005), consumers became increasingly aware of their rights to disclosure and control over decision making in relation to a wide range of aspects of their lives. "The power of informed consumers began to have an impact on providers of services as well as on producers of goods" (Lamers, 2005, p. 107).

Dame Cicely Saunders founded St. Christopher's Hospice in the UK in 1967, and hospice came to the United States in 1971 with the establishment of Hospice Inc. in New Haven, Connecticut, and the opening of the first hospice home care service there in 1973 (Conner, 2009). The publication of Elizabeth Kübler-Ross's groundbreaking book *On Death and Dying* (1969) helped spark community initiatives to encourage people to talk with one another about death and dying. The popularity of Kübler-Ross's ideas and the new innovation of hospice care helped spark an explosion of conversations about death and dying, with public education programs taking place in church basements, service clubs, and other community venues throughout the country. Hospice volunteers were trained and family caregivers were educated about a new way of dealing with death—accepting, open, and out in public.

However, as is often the case when a social movement is "successful" and becomes institutionalized, the community conversations that had brought discussions of death to the grassroots faded in the 1980s as hospice programs became more established. Hospice became a benefit through the

Medicare program, and communities began to depend on hospice as the entity that "handled" death and dying.

The Legal Environment of Advance Care Planning

ADs are legal documents that meet requirements of federal and state laws, statutes, and regulations. This legal approach to documenting desires regarding one's future medical care emerged in 1969 when Luis Kutner, an Illinois attorney writing for a law journal, proposed the first living will that, by being modeled after an estate will, allowed individuals to express their health care desires should they lose their capacity to do so (Kutner, 1969). As the document was in the form of a "will" but conveyed instructions relevant to the person's life while they were still alive, it came to be known as the "living will." Similar to the power of attorney that authorizes another person to handle financial and business matters, the power of attorney for health care authorizes a person to handle health care matters on another's behalf if he or she should become physically or mentally incapacitated and unable to speak for himself or herself.

Legal scholars have referred to this approach of modeling health care documents after legal documents as the legal-transactional approach to ADs and ACP (e.g., Castillo et al., 2011; Sabatino, 2010). This became the paradigm we have lived with for decades in the United States. Today, all 50 states have their own statutes and laws that speak to ADs, with approved documents or forms varying by state.

Legal documents were created in response to increasing sophistication and prevalence of medical technology and in response to highly publicized legal cases about withdrawing life support in cases of "persistent vegetative state" and "brain death" (e.g., Colby, 2006), legal cases in which the extension and withdrawal of life-support technology is a point of contention. Thus, in conjunction with technological developments, legal cases "exert a powerful influence on the provision of medical services to patients in end-of-life (EOL) situations" (Kapp, Chapter 5, in this volume).

Ethical Foundations of Advance Care Planning

Initiatives around planning for EOL have been guided by the central principles of autonomy and self-determination (Holstein, Parks, & Waymack, 2011; Seymour & Horne, 2011; Wilkinson, 2011). The hospice philosophy was rooted in humanism (Conner, 2009), which holds that individuals have the right to pursue their individual potential and thus the right to determine how they will be treated by the medical establishment, including at EOL. The legal framework that has guided the framing of living wills and health care proxies has been founded on the principles of informed consent and the right to refuse treatment, either directly (when one is competent) or indirectly (through a living will and/or a proxy decision maker) (Tiano & Beyer, 2005).

The first living will was developed in California in 1969, and in 1975 California gave living wills the force of law as it passed the Natural Death Act (Wilkinson, 2011). Other states followed in recognizing the living will, with Pennsylvania in 1983, the first to recognize a durable power of attorney for health care matters, giving the right to designate a surrogate or proxy to make health care decisions when one is no longer able to speak for oneself (Wilkinson, 2011).

Potential Benefits of Advance Care Planning

Research has indicated that planning for medical care in advance can help in managing the emotional conflict engendered in decisions about care near the EOL. ACP can help patients ensure self-determination and quality of life near the EOL by making sure that patients receive the care they desire, thereby bringing peace of mind, comfort, and certainty to patients, their loved ones, and clinicians.

As Halpern and Emanuel (2012) observed, documenting care preferences can "assuage guilt, doubts, or lingering uncertainty" (p. 267) over care decisions made on behalf of another. Importantly, the authors acknowledge that making health care decisions in these situations without benefit of the patient's clearly expressed—and understood—desires for care can cause remorse, anxiety, and doubt in clinicians, patients' loved ones, and patients' surrogate decision makers. Therefore, in addition to other benefits, using ADs to facilitate communication about ACP can reduce stress, anxiety, and depression in surviving relatives and advocates, and protect patients' loved ones, their advocates, and clinicians from "the burdens of surrogate decision making" (p. 266).

Challenges to Effective Advance Care Planning

Taken together, the legal, medical, and cultural problems with ADs exist in no small part because the forms emphasize delineation of care, and obscure the need for ongoing communication about ACP. The forms approach to documenting and communicating about desired health care was perpetuated and shaped by legislation such as the PSDA of 1990. The PSDA served as an information and education mandate to Medicare and Medicaid laws requiring hospitals to inform patients about the opportunity to provide ADs. The act, however, did not require completion of or communication about ADs nor reimburse clinicians for communicating with patients and their loved ones about their wishes for EOL.

Despite the high hopes there had been about passage of the PSDA, research soon began to show that the legislation had had little effect. The findings of the Study to Understand Prognoses and Preferences for Outcomes and Risks of Treatments (SUPPORT), a comprehensive intervention and research project looking at provider–patient communication about EOL care preferences (Teno et al., 1997), found that "neither the legislation nor the SUPPORT intervention had major impacts on the documentation of patients' preferences regarding end-of-life care" (Garas & Pantilat, 2001).

The SUPPORT researchers and other studies have found a number of problems with ADs. They are as follows:

Underutilization

ADs are disappointingly underused. Kass-Bartelmes and Hughes (2003) and Sabatino (2010) observed that despite years of enthusiastic advocacy by major health care organizations, ADs have not been as widely used as hoped. Consequently, many patients transition into physical and mental incapacity and enter EOL care without a health care advocate and without having ADs in place. Without ADs and an advocate, patients may receive unwanted aggressive medical care. Such care may be burdensome and costly and may prolong suffering in a degraded quality of life.

Reluctance to Talk About Death and Dying

Research on EOL decision making reveals that people have difficulty both asking and answering important questions about EOL care planning for themselves and for their loved ones. In addition, physicians themselves may not take the initiative to talk about dying and EOL decision making with their patients. In a report to the U.S. Department of Health and Human Services, researchers for the RAND Corporation (Wenger et al., 2008) reported that physicians cite "lack of time, lack of formal training in and knowledge of palliative measures, belief that patients and families do not want to engage in such discussions, association of palliative care with death, and lack of belief that such discussions are needed" (p. xi).

Lack of Awareness About Advance Directives and Advance Care Planning

Among members of the general public and, even more alarmingly, among clinicians, there is a lack of awareness of how the ACP process can best be conceived, documented, and used (e.g., Fagerlin & Schneider, 2004; Levi & Green, 2010; Sabatino, 2010). Even when ADs have been completed, they may not be available at the time of a health care crisis. Physicians may not know their patients have completed ADs. One study showed that 66% of people who had completed ADs had not discussed their treatment wishes with their physician (Porensky & Carpenter, 2008).

Difficulties in Deciding on Specific Treatments

Critics of living wills have argued that it is difficult for people to choose their preferences for specific medical treatments or procedures they would or wouldn't want at some unknown time in the future. Medical jargon is intimidating and off-putting, and according to Tonelli (1996), it is difficult for patients to evaluate the risks or benefits of various options at some time in the future. Standard living wills tend to state treatment options as cut-and-dried choices with little attention to the real-life complexities involved in what may be the reality of the future situation the patient is likely to encounter (Winter, Parks, & Diamond, 2010). Further, Tonelli argued, the patient will still be reliant on the judgment of the physician, who will determine whether the patient is competent to make decisions.

Inability of Surrogates to Predict Patient Preferences

The SUPPORT Intervention (Teno et al., 1997) and other studies have shown that surrogates or proxies, those who have been given the responsibility to make decisions for another, are often not able to accurately report the patient's preferences. According to Covinsky, Fuller, and Yaffe (2000), the SUPPORT study showed that many surrogates could not accurately report whether the patient valued comfort or maximum life expectancy; surrogates were inaccurate in predicting whether the patient wanted to receive resuscitation or live permanently in a nursing home. Emanuel (1995) found spouses (and physicians) had a "surprising inability" (p. 36) to accurately predict a patient's prior wishes. She found that patients frequently did not discuss their wishes with their proxies, with only 16% to 55% of patients having talked with their proxy about their EOL concerns. Tonelli (1996) stated that "the poor concordance between patients and their surrogates makes proxy decisions based on the presumed wishes of the patient the practical and moral equivalent of an educated guess or, at worst, the flip of a coin" (pp. 818–819).

Lack of Health Care Provider Skills in Communication

As Parker et al. (2007) observed, clinicians are frequently not trained to facilitate communication with patients and their loved ones about ADs, ACP, EOL care, and death. This lack of training is due, in part, to reliance on previous models used by clinicians to conceptualize the patient–clinician relationship based on paternalism and autonomy (see, e.g., Schermer, 2003;

Smith & Newton, 1984). Tulsky, Fischer, Rose, and Arnold (1998) found physicians used vague language in talking with patients about ADs and rarely explored "patients' values and attitudes toward uncertainty" (p. 441; also see Prommer, 2010).

Focus on Autonomy and Control

ADs arose as a way for individuals to exert control over their own dying process, even after they could no longer speak for themselves. According to Holstein, Parks, and Waymack (2011), this has led to an "individualistic, treatment-specific, and decontextualized approach to the dying process that somehow erases the vulnerable, hurting self in favor of the rational, cognitive self" (p. 234). The focus on autonomy and control and the legalistic approach to documenting individual preferences—as one would pass on his or her estate—led to the devaluation of other principles central to life and death, such as community, relationship, and interdependence (Holstein et al., 2011). In addition, cross-cultural studies of EOL decision-making processes show that some people do not want to talk about death and dying or have control over care decisions at EOL, and would rather trust medical professionals and/or relatives to make their own decisions on their behalf. Grudzen et al. (2011), for example, found that few Latino patients had talked with their physicians about their preferences and most derived comfort from their belief in God, who they believed controlled their fate. Language or literacy barriers also create barriers for members of racial or ethnic minorities (Wilkinson, 2011).

The Ideology of Rescue

As Chapple (2010) has pointed out, there is a prominent ideology of rescue in the U.S. health care system. The virtually unquestioned devotion to saving life at all costs is compelling for clinicians, patients, and their loved ones. Led by this ideology, providers apply advanced medical care during advanced stages of disease as well as in emergency situations as an unconscious reflex—and most patients and families unquestionably accept it. Our current medical culture and health care system appear driven by the heroic use of all available medical care to rescue all patients, and prevent, or at least delay, deaths in all situations and at all costs (e.g., Chapple, 2010; Kaufman, 2005). As a result, "death seems distant from everyday life, bolstered by the 'mythology' of CPR" (Chapple, 2010, p. 3). Accompanying this rescue paradigm is the pervasive view that a patient's death is the clinician's defeat, leaving little room for asserting the necessity of ACP (e.g., Beckstrand, Callister, & Kirchhoff, 2006; Colby, 2006; Seravalli, 1988; Lynn, 2004).

THE COMMUNICATION REVOLUTION IN ADVANCE CARE PLANNING: A NEW PATH FORWARD

It is clear that neither simply enshrining in law the right for individuals to make decisions about EOL care through ADs nor concerted interventions to encourage people to complete ADs have been adequate to realize the benefits hoped for 20 years ago when the PSDA was passed. Early efforts to address the apparent shortcomings of the documents focused on trying to find the perfect form (e.g., Abbo, Sobotka, & Meltzer, 2008). In the manner of Goldilocks, the forms were variously said to be either too specific or too vague, and early advocates attempted to find the document that was "just right." This is perhaps best reflected in the wide variety of documents adopted by the various states as official living will or proxy forms. The plethora of documents in itself has helped create a sense of overwhelm and confusion on the part of the general public, contributing to the low rate of completion of directives.

However flawed or fraught with difficulty in implementation and application ADs might be, most scholars and practitioners have not given up on them. Realizing that ADs are not an end in themselves, the focus has shifted to the broader concept of ACP, with ADs as tools or vehicles to stimulate meaningful discussion about EOL care (Fagerlin, Ditto, Hawkins, Schneider, & Smucker, 2002; Levi & Green, 2010; Robb-Nicholson, 2010).

From Product to Process: From Advance Directives to Advance Care Planning

Increasingly, the focus of efforts to encourage planning for EOL care has shifted from product (the form) to process (the conversation) (Wenger et al., 2008), from a legal-transactional approach to a communications approach (Sabatino, 2010). Efforts to foster effective communication between individuals and their families, and among individual and families and their physicians, have taken center stage among practitioners working to increase quality of life at EOL and among scholars evaluating these initiatives. An AD is seen as just one piece—albeit, an important one—in a broader agenda to best assure quality of life at EOL.

Mature ACP involves not just the completion of legal documents, but rather a process of communication, a series of conversations, or a "developmental discussion process" (Wenger et al., 2008, p. xvii)—often over the course of years—about one's beliefs, values, fears, and wishes about EOL care. ACP is conceptualized not as a one-time event, but rather as an ongoing process of communication between the individual and his or her loved ones, advocates, health care providers, and others involved in his or her life (Hammes, 2003). Based on a meta-analysis of studies of interventions aimed at increasing the completion of ADs, Bravo, Dubois, and

Wagneur (2008) recommended "oral information over multiple sessions" and "repeated encounters with knowledgeable informants" so that individuals could be able to make informed decisions (p. 1131).

According to Detering, Hancock, Reade, and Silvester (2010), this kind of ACP encompasses a coordinated, systematic, patient-centered approach. ADs need to be revised whenever a person's circumstances, medical condition, and goals of care change; an ongoing communications approach allows for such revisions (Kayseer, 2010; Nevidjon & Mayer, 2012). These conversations are "sensitive and time-consuming" (Nevidjon & Mayer, 2012, p. 150), but necessary if individuals and their families are to be equipped with information to explore their options and desires related to EOL care.

Respecting Choices®, of Gundersen Lutheran Medical Foundation in LaCrosse, Wisconsin—one of the most well-known and widely emulated initiatives in ACP—has been a leader in the shift to a focus on ongoing communication about values and goals about EOL care. Instead of being solely guided by the principle of personal autonomy, the focus of *Respecting Choices* "is on helping persons, in the context of their relationships, to explore and to discuss what it would mean to care about each other if a life-changing medical problem occurred" (Hammes, 2003). The Gundersen model is an iterative one that engages community members in ongoing discussions within their families and with their health care providers at various points in their lives when their social circumstances and medical conditions may change. Rather than asking patients what are their individual preferences about EOL care, they ask, "How can you guide your loved ones to make the best decisions for you?", placing at center stage a process of ongoing communication among people in relationship with one another. Consultants from Gundersen have traveled throughout the country and abroad helping facilitate community-wide, communication-focused ACP initiatives, and many local, regional, and statewide programs aimed at fostering dialogues about EOL care are underway throughout the United States. (See Part III of this volume for examples of these successful initiatives as well as the chapter on Resources in Part V.)

Bringing the Community Back In

> Too often we do not name the activity that is most important to living and dying. It is not medicines and holy oils that make us want to live, or die, in peace, but the social relationships and meanings of a personal lifetime. It is important to realize that the history of travellers in the valley of the shadow of death is also a history of our community care and support for each other.
>
> Allan Kellehear, 2005, p. 2

Critical to the new path currently being charted in ACP is a shift from a provider-focused model to a community focus (Hammes, 2003), returning matters of life and death to the wider milieu of family and community, which from the beginning of human history has played the central role in death, dying, and loss (Kellehear, 2007). This shift also signals a move from a rights-driven process focusing on individual autonomy and control to a shared process that acknowledges that we live and die not alone, but fundamentally in relationship with others (see Briggs, 2003; Hammes, 2003; Holstein, et al., 2011; Kellehear, 2005, 2007).

Ethicists Holstein et al. (2011) assert that any change in how we deal with dying and death must start with "a consideration of what is special about dying people and those who love and care for them" (p. 246). Accepting our vulnerability and embracing relationship and mutual interdependence, not individual choice and self-control, they suggest, should be at the foundation of an approach to ACP that takes into account the wide variation in how people want to participate in decisions related to EOL care. Emphasizing the importance of the discussions that should precede the signing of documents, Holstein and her colleagues recommend the use of "interpreters" (p. 250) or advocates who help facilitate discussions among individuals, families, and health care professionals. Finally, they conclude:

> With our understanding of people as essentially relational, developing their identity and values from the contextual features of their lives, we take as essential the continuity of relationships and care as central to whatever chances for well-being remain for people nearing death (p. 251).

According to Seymour and Horne (2011), changing the way we plan for EOL care requires nothing short of a "sea change in attitudes to discussing and anticipating end-of-life care among the public" (p. 23). They argue that "the traditional autonomy-focused framework of ACP and emphasis on the completion of instructional directives is out of step with the perspectives and needs of patients" (p. 21). They point out that existing research on ACP indicates a need for broader initiatives that focus on discussions that identify persons' values and goals and, especially important, public education in schools and the wider community to raise awareness of issues related to EOL care prior to a life-threatening illness. They conclude: "Finally, in order for Advance Care Planning to be successful, it needs to be embedded in systems of care designed to provide support to those facing the end of life, in recognition that serious illness and dying are worthy of the same care and attention that we give to birth, acute illness, and injury" (p. 24).

The RAND Corporation's comprehensive report on ACP recommended a multi-component approach including not just education focusing on patients and providers and health behaviors but intensive and targeted community campaigns including innovations such as the use of social marketing; support of ACP models that focus on a developmental discussion process, not form completion; the development of health information systems to share care decisions across systems; and continued research on the effectiveness of these concerted efforts (Wenger et al., 2008). Likewise, nurse educators Nevidjon and Mayer (2012) called for members of the nursing profession to capitalize on the "unique trust relationship" (p. 151) nurses hold with the public and help stimulate community conversations (similar to those sparked 40 years ago by Kübler-Ross and Dame Cecily Saunders) in churches, service organizations, and other venues.

Community is also the central focus of sociologist Allan Kellehear's comprehensive recommendations for a public health approach to death education. Any effort toward ACP cannot be effective without what he calls a "whole community" model, moving from control by medical professionals and health care institutions to the development of community support systems in a wide variety of venues, including the workplace, churches, and other institutions (Kellehear, 2005, p. 24). Kellehear points out that the community has over time ceded control of dying and death to medical, legal, and religious professionals (Kellehear, 2007). He advocates for the democratization of EOL care, pointing out that community and family members don't need permission or reimbursement to talk to one another about EOL (Kellehear, 2005).

Kellehear calls for a participatory, community development approach to death education that includes the employment of community development workers by health care and government institutions and (even more important) the deployment of unpaid community activists—such as those who championed civil rights and other justice movements—who apply their organizing skills to build what he calls "compassionate cities" (Kellehear, 2005) that provide support to those experiencing dying, death, and loss—which is all of us.

CONCLUSION: WHERE DO WE GO FROM HERE?

We have made huge cultural changes before. A generation ago, Americans transformed birth. That didn't happen because doctors urged women out of stirrups; hospitals didn't put out the welcome mat for dads and their video cameras. No institution promoted soft lights and doulas. Instead women recognized that there was a better way and insisted on changing their own experience. Today we're recognizing how badly we are "doing death" and that we must change our experience with it, too.

Ellen Goodman, 2012, pp. 58–59

The power to change how we plan for death is in our hands. Clearly, legal or bureaucratic mandates such as the PSDA or health care provider-driven initiatives have not been enough to cause the cultural shift that brings conversations about death, dying, loss, and care to the kitchen table, as Pulitzer Prize-winning columnist Ellen Goodman called for as she launched her retirement mission, The Conversation Project (http://theconversation project.org/). The Conversation Project, with the collaboration of the Institute for Healthcare Improvement, is one of the groups in the country leading the effort to transform our culture around issues of EOL. Leaders in the medical professions, such as Dr. Ira Byock, author, past president of the American Academy of Hospice and Palliative Medicine, and advisor to the Conversation Project, place the focus of this transformation project in the hands of the community. Byock states:

> The medicalization of aging, dying, and grief ignores the innate, healthy human drive to care for one another. It erodes core cultural roles and suppresses latent caregiving skills that reside within families and communities. Even in a person's dying—*especially in a person's dying*—family and community comprise the proper context for a person's life. (Byock, 2012, p. 150)

Physicians, nurses, social workers, psychologists, and other professionals (such as those who have contributed their expertise in this volume) can share their wisdom on best practices for how we can better communicate about death and dying. Their voices are essential in helping us know how best to meet the needs of a variety of people as they face with their families the challenging passage from life to death. But as it took a grassroots movement of ordinary people working in their communities to realize the cultural and structural changes that resulted from the civil rights movement, the women's movement, the gay rights movement, and other social movements of the 20th century, so too will it take a community organizing and social movements orientation to fully realize the aims of a new way to deal with dying. The challenge is ours to take.

REFERENCES

Abbo, E. D., Sobotka, S., & Meltzer, D. O. (2008). Patient preferences in instructional advance directives. *Journal of Palliative Medicine, 11*(4), 555–562.

American Hospital Association. (2005). Put it in writing: Questions and answers on advance directives. In A. H. Association (Ed.), *American Hospital Association* (Vol. 166909): Author.

Austin, W. (2012). Moral distress and the contemporary plight of health professionals. *HEC Forum, 24*(1), 27–38.

Beckstrand, R. L., Callister, L. C., & Kirchhoff, K. T. (2006). Providing a "Good Death": Critical care nurses' suggestions for improving end-of-life care. *American Journal of Critical Care, 15*(1), 38–45.

Bravo, G., Dubois, M., & Wagneur, B. (2008). Assessing the effectiveness of interventions to promote advance directive among older adults: A systematic review and multi-level analysis. *Social Science and Medicine, 67*, 1122–1132.

Briggs, L. (2003). Shifting the focus of advance care planning: Using an in-depth interview to build and strengthen relationships. *Innovations in End-of-Life Care, 5*(2), 1–16.

Butler, R. N. (2008). *The longevity revolution: The benefits and challenges of living a long life.* New York, NY: Public Affairs Books.

Byock, I. (2012). *The best care possible: A physician's quest to transform care through the end of life.* New York, NY: The Penguin Group.

Castillo, L. S., Williams, B. A., Hooper, S. M., Sabatino, C. P., Weithorn, L. A., & Sudore, R. L. (2011). Lost in translation: The unintended consequences of advance directive law on clinical care. *Annals of Internal Medicine, 154*, 121–128.

Chapple, H. S. (2010). *No place for dying: American hospitals and the ideology of rescue.* Walnut Creek, CA: Left Coast Press.

Colby, W. H. (2006). *Unplugged: Reclaiming our right to die in America.* New York, NY: American Management Association.

Conner, S. (2009). *Hospice and palliative care: The essential guide.* New York, NY: Routledge.

Covinsky, K. E., Fuller, J. D., & Yaffe, K. (2000). Communication and decision-making in seriously ill patients: Findings of the SUPPORT Project. *Journal of the American Geriatrics Society, 48*(5), 187–193.

Detering, K. M., Hancock, A. D., Reade, M. C., & Silvester, W. (2010). The impact of advance care planning on end of life care in elderly patients: Randomised controlled trial. *BMJ: British Medical Journal, 340*:c1345, 1–9. Retrieved from http://www.ncbi.nlm.nih.gov/pmc/articles/PMC2844949/

Emanuel, L. L. (1995). Advance directives: Do they work? *Journal of the American College of Cardiology, 25*(1), 35–38.

Epstein, E. G., & Delgado, S. (2010). Understanding and addressing moral distress. *Online Journal of Issues in Nursing, 15*(3), manuscript 1. Retrieved from 10.3912/OJIN.Vol15No03Man01

Fagerlin, A., Ditto, P. H., Hawkins, N. A., Schneider, C. E., & Smucker, W. D. (2002). The use of advance directives in end-of-life decision-making: Problems and possibilities. *American Behavioral Scientist, 46*, 268–283.

Fagerlin, A., & Schneider, C. E. (2004). Enough: The failure of the living will. *Hastings Center Report, 34*(2), 30–42.

Garas, N., & Pantilat, S. Z. (2001). *Advance planning for end-of-life care.* Chapter 49 of Evidence report/technology assessment number 43, Making health safer: A crucial analysis of patient safety practices. U.S. Department of Health and Human Services. Retrieved from http://www.ahrq.gov/clinic/ptsafety/chap49.htm

Goodman, E. (2011). The baby boomers' longevity revolution. *Washington Post* January 2. Retrieved from http://www.washingtonpost.com/wp-dyn/content/article/2010/12/31/AR2010123102689.html

Goodman, E. (2012). Die the way you want to. *Harvard Business Review, 90*(1/2), 58–59.

Grudzen, C. R., Stone, S. C., Mohanty, S. A., Asch, S. M., Lorenz, K. A., Torres, J. M.,...Timmermans, S. (2011). "I want to be taking my own last breath": Patients' reflections on illness when presenting to the emergency department at the end of life. *Journal of Palliative Medicine, 14*(3), 293–296.

Halpern, S. D., & Emanuel, E. J. (2012). Advance directives and cost savings: Greater clarity and perpetual confusion. [Editorial]. *Archives of Internal Medicine, 172*(3), 266–267.

Hammes, B. J. (2003). Update on *Respecting Choices*: Four years on. *Innovations in End-of-Life Care, 5*(2), 1–18.

Holstein, M. B., Parks, J. A., & Waymack, M. H. (2011). *Ethics, aging, and society: The critical turn*. New York, NY: Springer.

Kapp, M. B. (2013). Advance medical care planning: The legal environment. In L. Rogne & S. L. McCune (Eds.), *Advance care planning: Talking about matters of life and death*. New York, NY: Springer.

Kass-Bartelmes, B. L., & Hughes, R. (2003). *Advance care planning: Preferences for care at the end of life* (Vol. Research in Action Issue #12). Rockville, MD: Agency for Healthcare Research and Quality.

Kaufman, S. R. (2005).... *And a time to die: How American hospitals shape the end of life*. New York, NY: Scribner.

Kayseer, J. R. (2010). Imagine my surprise: A controversial advance directive scenario. *Journal of Palliative Medicine, 13*(8), 1033–1034.

Kellehear, A. (2005). *Compassionate cities*. New York, NY: Routledge.

Kellehear, A. (2007). *A social history of death*. New York, NY: Cambridge University Press.

Kübler-Ross, E. (1969). *On death and dying*. New York, NY: Scribner.

Kutner, L. (1969). The living will: A proposal. *Indiana Law Journal, 44*(1), 539–554.

Lamers, W. M., Jr. (2005). Autonomy, consent, and advance directives. In K. J. Doka, B. Jennings, & C. A. Corr (Eds.), *Ethical dilemmas at the end of life* (pp. 105–123). Washington, DC: Hospice Foundation of America.

Levi, B. H., & Green, M. J. (2010). Too soon to give up: Re-examining the value of advance directives. *The American Journal of Bioethics, 10*(4), 3–22.

Lynn, J. (2004). *Sick to death and not going to take it any more: Reforming health care for the last years of life*. Berkley, CA: University of California Press.

Lynn, J., & Adamson, D. M. (2003). *Living well at the end of life: Adapting health care to serious chronic illness in old age*. Santa Monica, CA: Rand Health.

Meisel, A., & Jennings, B. (2005). Ethics, end-of-life care, and the law: Overview and recent trends. In K. J. Doka, B. Jennings, & C. A. Corr (Eds.), *Ethical dilemmas at the end of life* (pp. 105–123). Washington, DC: Hospice Foundation of America.

Nevidjon, B. M., & Mayer, D. K. (2012). Death is not an option, how you die is—reflections from a career in oncology nursing. *Nursing Economics, 30*(3), 148–52.

Parker, S. M., Clayton, J. M., Hancock, K., Walder, S., Butow, P. N., Carrick, S.,…Tattersall, M. H. N. (2007). A systematic review of prognostic/end-of-life communication with adults in the advanced stages of life-limiting illness: Patient/caregiver preferences for the content, style, and timing of information. *Journal of Pain and Symptom Management, 34*(1), 81–93. doi: 10.1016/j.painsymman.20609.035

Pauly, B. M., Varcoe, C., & Storch, J. (2012). Framing the issues: Moral distress in health care. *HED Forum, 24*(1), 1–11.

Porensky, E. K., & Carpenter, B. D. (2008). Knowledge and perceptions in advance care planning. *Journal of Aging and Health, 20*(1), 89–106.

Prommer, E. E. (2010). Using the values-based history to fine-tune advance care planning for oncology patients. *Journal of Cancer Education, 25*(1), 66–69.

Robb-Nicholson, C. (2010). A doctor talks about advance care directives. *Harvard Women's Health Watch, 17*(12), 5.

Sabatino, C. P. (2010). The evolution of health care advance planning law and policy. *Milbank Quarterly, 88*(2), 211–239. doi: 10.1111/j.1468–0009.2010.00596.x

Schermer, M. (2003). *The different faces of autonomy: patient autonomy in ethical theory and hospital practice* (Vol. 13). New York, NY: Springer.

Seravalli, E. P. (1988). The dying patient, the physician, and the fear of death. *New England Journal of Medicine, 319*(26), 1728–1730.

Seymour, J., & Horne, G. (2011). Advance care planning for the end of life: An overview. In K. Thomas & B. Lobo (Eds.), *Advance care planning in end of life care* (pp. 16–27). New York, NY: Oxford University Press.

Shen, B. (1999). Forward. *Sudden death and the myth of CPR* (pp. xi–xiii). Philadelphia, PA: Temple University Press.

Smith, D. G., & Newton, L. H. (1984). Physician and patient: Respect for mutuality. *Theoretical Medicine and Bioethics, 5*(1), 43–60. doi: 10.1007/bf00489245

Teno, J., Wenger, L. J., Phillips, R. S., Murphy, D. P., Connors, A. F. Jr., Desbiens, N.,…Knaus, W. A. (1997). Advance directives for seriously ill hospitalized patients: Effectiveness with the patient self-determination act and the SUPPORT intervention. SUPPORT Investigators. Study to Understand Prognoses and Preferences for Outcomes and Risks of Treatment. *Journal of the American Geriatrics Society, 45*(4), 500–507.

Tiano, N., & Beyer, E. (2005). Cultural and religious views on nonbeneficial treatment. In K. J. Doka, B. Jennings, & C. A. Corr (Eds.), *Ethical dilemmas at the end of life* (pp. 41–59). Washington, DC: Hospice Foundation of America.

Tonelli, M. R. (1996). Pulling the plug on living wills: A critical analysis of advance directives. *Chest, 110*, 816–822.

Tulsky, J. A., Fischer, G. S., Rose, M. R., & Arnold, R. M. (1998). Opening the black box: How do physicians communicate about advance directives. *Annals of Internal Medicine, 129,* 441–449.

U.S. Census Bureau. (2012). *Table 9: Resident population projections by sex and age: 2010 to 2050.* Retrieved from www.census.gov/compendia/statab/2012/tables/12s0009.pdf

Wenger, N. S., Shugarman, L. R., & Wilkinson, A. (2008). *Advance directives and advance care planning: Report to Congress.* RAND Corporation Report to U.S. Department of Health and Human Services. Retrieved from aspe.hhs.gov/daltcp/reports/2008/ADCongRpt-B.pdf

Wilkinson, A. M. (2011). Advance directives and advance care planning: The US experience. In K. Thomas & B. Lobo (Eds.), *Advance care planning in end of life care* (pp. 189–204). New York, NY: Oxford University Press.

Winter, L., Parks, S. M., & Diamond, J. J. (2010). Ask different questions, get a different answer: Why living wills are poor guides to care preferences at the end of life. *Journal of Palliative Medicine, 13*(5), 567–572.

CHAPTER 3

Advance Care Planning: Focus on Communication and Care Planning Rather Than on Building the Perfect Form

Ana Tuya Fulton
Joan M. Teno

BACKGROUND

The living will movement was given force in 1976 with the passage of the Natural Death Act in California. This followed the case of Karen Ann Quinlan, who in 1975 was left in a persistent vegetative state at the age of 21 after suffering cardiac arrest. The New Jersey Supreme Court granted her parents' wishes to stop life-sustaining treatments. This case marked the movement endorsing that patients can refuse medical treatment, even if life sustaining, in certain situations. The next landmark case was that of Nancy Cruzan in 1983. Cruzan was a 32-year-old woman who was left in a persistent vegetative state after a car accident. After years of no change, her parents determined that their daughter would not want to be kept alive in her current state; the hospital disagreed, and the courts became involved. Ultimately, the U.S. Supreme Court upheld her right to refuse life-sustaining treatment, but ruled that states can impose safeguards to ensure that there is convincing evidence to support patient wishes (Polaniaszek & Peres, 2008).

The debate surrounding living wills and patients' rights to refuse treatment have largely been marked by cases such as those above. In everyday medical practice, the patients who face these situations are very different. They are not young adults who suffered tragic circumstances and are left in clear persistent vegetative states. Typically, they are older adults or patients with multiple chronic illnesses who have been on a gradual trajectory of decline. For these patients, the decision is often one of choosing quality of life over quantity of time. This decision is never an easy one. To the extent of persons' desire, such decisions should be guided by their goals and values. Often, these decisions are made for persons who lack decision-making capacity.

INTRODUCTION

Some four decades after the creation of the living will, a major area of focus is on creating the perfect form rather than on creating a set of multifaceted interventions and tools that support and encourage communication over time. Advance directives (ADs) should be a product of a larger, more complex process—advance care planning (ACP)—and are one of many communication tools to accomplish this process and not the be all and end all. ACP can be defined as a "structured dialogue with the ultimate goal that clinical care is shaped by a patient's preferences when the patient is unable to participate in decision making" (Teno & Lynn, 1996). This process will help persons formulate goals of care and clarify value sets and wishes, and ultimately design a detailed care plan to honor those wishes and values. The health care provider working with the patient with decision-making capacity or a surrogate decision maker helps to develop care plans that meet those goals and formulates treatment plans for expected events while the patient is dying (e.g., opiates on hand for shortness of breath if the person does not want intubation).

The extent of specification of preference in advance as opposed to the naming of proxy decision maker will depend on the patient's values, prognosis, and where he or she is in the disease trajectory. We propose that for ACP to achieve its goals, multifaceted interventions that are able to deal with many different situations and the many varying types of patients are needed. These will support ACP while recognizing that not every patient or person will be interested in participating. ADs are one of those tools. Family dynamics, patient values, and cultural factors will all affect which tools and what sorts of tailored communication geared to the needs of the patient are required. In some situations, the clinician may need to be paternalistic while in another situation the role of the health care provider is to educate the patient and family about the likely prognosis and treatment options.

In this chapter, we will review the previous research and evidence regarding ACP, noting that many studies have overly focused on the completion of an AD, rather than on a more complex set of multifaceted interventions designed to ensure targeted interventions based on the disease trajectory and needs of the patient. We will also discuss how to incorporate ACP into medical practice, discussing some of the challenges and pitfalls to doing so with some potential solutions.

DISCUSSION: THE PROBLEM

The process of ACP is an ongoing one and should ideally begin long before the patient is terminally ill. Timing of discussions and evolving decisions based on changes in condition and prognosis are important, but even more important is what questions you ask. Asking the tried and true, "If your heart stops do you want us to try to resuscitate you?" may not be relevant for the older adult with long-standing, gradually progressive chronic illnesses such as dementia. The better questions are those focused around goals of care, and definition of quality of life. Each conversation will vary based on the person's decision-making style, level of understanding, and readiness to plan or even discuss the topic. Each health care provider must provide communication that meets the unique needs and expectations of the patient and family before him or her.

In 1991, the Patient Self-Determination Act (PSDA) was enacted by Congress. The law required health care facilities receiving Medicare and Medicaid funds to ask patients if they had an AD, to provide information about their rights to make one, and to make AD forms available to patients who wanted them (Polaniaszek & Peres, 2008). The goal was to increase completion and documentation of ADs to avoid patients and families being left to make decisions in vacuums. Requiring facilities to ask for them and obtain copies for records would assist in making care decisions with the appropriate documentation available. While there has been much progress in the realm of ADs and extensive research devoted to it, there is not a clear-cut body of evidence that increasing the creation of ADs is a clear success. There has been no definitive evidence of improved quality of care or of decreased utilization of resources at the end of life (EOL). Concerns have been raised over the utility and role of ADs because of the instability of patient preferences, on the ability of ADs to reduce health care utilization or costs, or their ability to ensure a better EOL experience (Teno, 2004). Many of the concerns raised center around the forms used to document and discuss ADs. A large portion of the research and publications surrounding ADs focus on increasing use and documentation of ADs or centers on creating a better or more useful form. However, there may be more to the story than just not having the right form or not getting enough people to fill it out. A review of some of the relevant literature does not provide evidence that merely increasing use of ADs leads to reduced health cost or improved quality of care while dying. One randomized prospective control trial performed by Schneiderman and colleagues demonstrated no significant differences in care received among patients who completed an AD or those who did not (Schneiderman, Kronick, Kaplan, Anderson, & Langer, 1992). There were no differences in type of care received, number of days receiving aggressive interventions, or in overall cost of care. This finding held true even when looking just at the last 30 days of life. However, it is important to note that in most of the patients included, ADs were not needed because patients retained their decision-making capacity and were able to participate in discussion.

In comparison, Chambers and colleagues demonstrated a cost reduction with discussion of ADs in their retrospective review (Chambers, Diamond, Perkel, & Lasch, 1994). The study demonstrated that patients without documentation of a discussion of ADs spent up to three times more than similar patients who did have a discussion documented. However, the study did not account for selection bias of which patients complete an AD. Persons who complete an AD are very different from those who do not. An additional retrospective cohort study by Weeks and colleagues also demonstrated cost reduction during the terminal hospitalization with the existence of previously completed ADs, but again, did not control for selection bias (Weeks, Kofoed, Wallace, & Welch, 1994).

In contrast, Teno and colleagues replicated analysis done by previously published studies in their 1997 prospective cohort study and block randomized controlled trial (Teno et al., 1997). The study results are contrary to those studies that noted cost reductions. By not just performing a secondary retrospective analysis, their prospective design allowed the inclusion of multiple potential confounders. In the control group of patients, an increase in the documentation of ADs was noted, and a reduction in resource use was also found. However, in the intervention group (SUPPORT intervention) (Murphy, Knaus, & Lynn, 1990; The SUPPORT Investigators, 1995) there was a higher rate of AD documentation, yet there was not a similar association with cost reduction.

The study demonstrated that despite the PSDA-related increase in documentation of ADs and further increase with SUPPORT trial intervention there was not an associated reduction in resource utilization. In addition, many times physicians were unaware of the existence of the document in the chart and had not had a discussion with the patient or family. When physicians were aware, and documented do not resuscitate (DNR) orders as a result, it tended to be in a biased group of patients who were much sicker and clearly preferred a palliative approach. Without evidence of communication and discussion around the ADs, it seems unlikely that they are guiding care.

This evidence leads us to the conclusion that focusing on the completion of ADs or any singular focus is not working to improve quality of care and reduce utilization at the EOL. The creation of a perfect form that works for everyone is not only unlikely, but also impossible, and will not be the end of the pursuit to improve quality of care. More widespread use of ACP, with ADs being incorporated as a tool for discussion and product of this process, will better work toward obtaining the information needed to create detailed care plans to care for persons at the EOL, or those who have lost the capacity to participate in decision making.

There are many potential reasons for the failure of a public policy that focuses on the AD's movement and process. The goal of ADs is to encourage planning and decision making, ideally, at a time when a person has no acute illness or chronic disease. Hypothetical scenarios are used to have a person delineate what he or she would want to have done, or how he or she would want their decision maker to act. Not everyone is comfortable thinking in this way or is able to envision these scenarios in a realistic fashion to allow meaningful decisions. The forms typically focus on extraordinary measures and not the more commonly encountered situations of hospitalizations, IV antibiotics, and such that come up with chronic diseases such as advanced cognitive impairment. As the research demonstrates, some people are more able to abstract and be future oriented, and these will be the people who are more likely to complete AD forms. This difference among people contributes to the selection bias and variation in results noted in the studies.

A health care provider needs to adapt his or her communication styles to the person's particular needs—age, comorbidity, diagnosis, prognosis, decision-making style, and needs for information and level of detail. In addition, the product of ACP, though it will often include an AD, will also have more details as to wishes, goals of care, and contingency plans to carry out those wishes. If a patient has a specific set of wishes (e.g., no further hospitalizations), it is important that the health care provider develop a care plan that ensures those wishes are honored. ACP is an ongoing conversation that evolves over time and can better incorporate prognosis and current health status. When the patient has specific wishes, the care plan should incorporate contingency planning. For example, outlining a person's wishes to avoid hospitalization or aggressive care is not enough alone; documenting how to manage EOL symptoms such as pain or shortness of breath and including orders for such will avoid the middle of the night ER visit when the primary provider cannot be reached.

Talking to each patient will vary according to the patient's age, disease, prognosis, and level of understanding and desire for information. For some people simply outlining information about what their options are is enough. They will then determine if they want to use tools such as AD, living will, or designate decision makers. For others, a more paternalistic approach might be needed. They might desire the more direct approach: "Given your advanced age and underlying issues, the likelihood of CPR being successful in restoring you to your current level of function is very low." A person's personality and decision-making style as well as the stage of readiness for change will play a major role in the ACP process.

[handwritten: Models for Figuring out who is ready for ACP or AD discussions]

This will require a multifaceted intervention approach to make sure it is successful for a range of patients with whom a clinician undertakes ACP. One-size-fits-all ACP will not reach each of these decision-making types. We must target each decision-making style with the approach that will maximize that person's ability to make an informed decision with which he or she is comfortable.

Many have proposed using the idea of behavioral change and the models such as the Transtheoretical Model (TTM) or the Prochaska stages of change, for example, to help understand whether a person is ready to consider or discuss ACP and to help determine the best approach to use in communication. For example, in the TTM the stages are as follows: precontemplation (no intention to change), contemplation (thinking about changing a behavior), preparation (commitment to change), and action (a recent change in behavior) (Prochaska & DiClemente, 2005). How a person is approached will vary based on his or her stage of readiness, and the way the discussion is approached and the tools used will vary based on stage as well. Using these models can ensure that the discussion and intervention is tailored to the individual's needs (Fried et al., 2010). In this same study by Fried and colleagues, 304 community-dwelling older adults (over 65) were recruited from physician offices and interviewed about their knowledge of and participation in ACP, their health status and their feeling of the quality of health, and various sociodemographic factors. They identified various discrete behaviors that comprised components of ACP—clarifying values, having conversations with a physician, family, and others, and completing written directives (Fried et al., 2010). When using the behavior change model, they found that most of the older adults were in the action stage for all but the communication with physician behavior. It brought to light that encouraging and supporting communication with providers should be a major focus of effort. Adults will discuss and complete paperwork with family and lawyers, but do not often discuss with their providers. Providers should start these conversations and work to help patients reach a care plan over time that evolves with changes in their status.

Another tool often used to help guide conversations and improve ACP is Buckman's six-step protocol (Baile et al., 2000). The steps are: (1) get started, (2) find out how much the patient knows, (3) find out how much the patient wants to know, (4) share information, (5) respond to the patient's feelings, and (6) plan and follow through. The getting started step includes finding the right setting and time for the patient to hear the news, and asking the patient who else should be in the room to hear the news. Step 2 should begin with an open-ended question such as, "What have you been told about your illness?" This will guide the physician on what the patient already knows and the level of understanding and the language with which to continue the conversation. Step 3 should elicit the level of detail the patient wants to hear—forest or trees. Step 4 is the main discussion of the disease process: what options there are for treatment, and what side effects and changes should be expected. It is useful here to offer prognostic information if available. This is an overwhelming part of the discussion and pieces will often need to be discussed again, or covered in more than one conversation. Having a second listener here is often helpful. Step 5 is a listening step; allow the patient to voice concerns, express emotions, and react to the knowledge. If they are not forthcoming, asking, "How are you feeling right now?" is appropriate. Finally, the last step involves coming up with a plan for the next steps—when will the next conversation be, follow-up appointment, and creating a concrete plan for care and future communication.

[handwritten: Incorporating the Advanced Care Planning into yearly doc. visits]

CONCLUSIONS: PROPOSED SOLUTIONS

Making ACP a part of routine care is important and necessary to incorporate into medical practice. The primary care physician is in the best position to discuss wishes and value set for care since he or she should know the patient best and have the most information about underlying conditions and level of function. Providers should incorporate it as part of their routine annual visits, and add it to the problem list and to-do list for all patients, just like eliciting vaccination and health maintenance information. This is the easiest and most effective way to incorporate ACP into medical practice. However, performing full ACP in every patient is time consuming and therefore targeted approaches based on age, illness, and prognosis can be used. For example, in a young patient coming in for an annual visit, the conversation may be as simple as asking, "If you are unable to speak for yourself, who would you want to do so?" Spending a great deal of time on more details would be of low yield and time would be better spent on other counseling like smoking cessation and health maintenance. With an adult with a terminal illness, one would have much more detailed conversations and would focus on prognosis, treatment options, EOL preferences for sedation, comfort, and ultimately place of death. More important would be outlining contingency planning around potential symptoms and complications. If the person signs a do not intubate order, for example, providing orders and planning for potential shortness of breath will be crucial to avoid an ER visit. An older adult with a chronic comorbidity but no terminal illness will have longer conversations, again focused on desired decision maker if they are unable to participate, but also some aspects of goals of care for any acute illness and some discussions of how they would like to die. There are some challenges that need to be met to make the broad incorporation of ACP a reality, but it can be done.

Mrs. G is a 69-year-old woman who is fully independent, lives in her own home, and volunteers at her church daily. She is an avid golfer and plays almost daily. A passion of hers is eating out and enjoying different types of foods—she was always one of the first to visit a new restaurant. She has three children and six grandchildren. She presents to her primary care doctor yearly for annual physicals and over time has discussed her wishes for future care. She has completed an AD and states she doesn't want extraordinary measures in the setting of terminal or advanced illness. Her eldest daughter is her designated power of attorney in case she cannot speak for herself. Since she is healthy and independent, the conversations are brief and straightforward.

The current health care system financial reimbursements do not support ACP. Reimbursement structure instead encourages higher level of care, interventions, and doesn't reimburse the primary care provider for prolonged counseling sessions on ACP and prognosis. To encourage careful ACP, over time, with the primary care physician, there needs to be a reimbursement structure in place to pay for the physician's time and for quality ACP. The process should be reimbursed as a routine service or the system should incentivize providers for the time spent to do it right. In that vein, we need to have better measures of "doing it right."

An additional challenge to ACP resides in physician comfort and education. Most medical school curricula do not have detailed training on discussing prognosis, EOL issues, or ACP. It is something that most medical students and residents pick up while doing clinical rotations, generally by modeling what their senior residents and attendings say and do. There is inconsistency among training programs and variable curricula. This leads to varying levels of comfort and ability and leaves most physicians at a disadvantage, which hurts the patients who would like to talk to them about these issues. Research supports that some of the most effective interventions involve incorporating direct patient and provider interactions over multiple visits (Ramsaroop, Reid, & Adelman, 2007); there needs to be a way to make providers more comfortable and skilled at having these difficult conversations. As outlined by Feudtner in a perspective piece, physicians are often uncomfortable discussing prognosis for fear of taking away patients' hope (Feudtner, 2009). However, as he points out, giving news helps patients define new hopes and clarify values and wishes for care such as relief of pain, suffering, and the hopes around the kind of death they would want. Physicians need help to deliver the news, carefully outline choices and prognosis, and continually carry on a conversation about patients' hopes and fears around their disease or condition. Doing this over time, and with each change in condition, can ensure that an accurate and useful care plan is the result of ACP.

Mrs. G. returns at the age of 75, this time with her daughter, who has noted gradual changes in her mother. She has been doing less of her typical activities—golfing, volunteering, and staying at home more. When pressed, she reported difficulty with driving and getting lost one day on her way to the church. Her family has been keeping closer tabs on her and noted gradual decline in her housekeeping, cooking, and self-care skills as well. She was seen by a neurologist and memory testing indicated early stages of dementia of the Alzheimer's type. Today the daughter, who is the designated decision maker, joins the visit to discuss additional ACP. Mrs. G expresses a desire to stay in her home as long as possible, and agrees to stop driving and accept home help. A brief discussion of the trajectory of dementia is begun, but the primary care doctor schedules another visit in one month to discuss further and in more detail.

Readdressing her wishes at this visit is crucial, as a person's preference changes dramatically over time, and with the development of chronic illness, one's desired quality of life might change as well. What wasn't acceptable as a state of living to a healthy 40-year-old might be more acceptable to a 70-year-old with multiple chronic issues who is now used to some level of disability (Messinger-Rapport, Baum, & Smith, 2009). It has been demonstrated that individuals have trouble predicting what they would really want in future situations because the predictions lack the context of what their social, medical, and financial situations will be (Sudore & Fried, 2010). A person's treatment values and decisions will change over time based on situation and definition of quality of life at the time. *This is why ADs are problematic*

Mrs. G, when in her sixties, might have stated to family that she would not want to live without her independence and the ability to do the things she loved such as golfing and volunteering. However, now in the early stages of her dementia, she might voice other wishes—enjoying family visits and smaller outings to restaurants might be pleasurable enough to make her enjoy her life as it is. Other instances that are often cited as examples include the patient with chronic lung disease who does not want intubation but develops an infection—how do the ADs apply there? A short-term intubation with a return to previous quality of life might be acceptable as opposed to the idea of long-term intubation without return to previous level of function. This is the major reason why ACP is an ongoing series of conversations and incorporates more than just the one-time completion of an AD. Wishes change over time, and without the current context of quality of life and prognosis—they are often incorrect.

Mrs. G returns with her daughter one year later and is now living in a locked dementia unit at assisted living after having wandered out of her home twice. Her daughter provides most of the history during this visit. Mrs. G has started to lose weight and is having trouble eating regularly. Her memory loss has progressed, she requires assistance with several activities of daily living, and her family is managing all financial and health care decisions. She can still walk and joins family for outings on weekends, but given trouble with eating is no longer enjoying the restaurant outings. Her family wants to plan for her continued decline. The physician discusses feeding problems as a prognostic indicator of the decline of her dementia and that decisions about treating aspiration events, weight loss, and continued functional decline are around the corner. Her daughter expresses her mother's wishes to avoid heroic, extraordinary measures as outlined in her AD. The decision is made to sign a DNR and a do not hospitalize order. The family moves her to a nursing home. Mrs. G's family was aware of her wishes as she discussed them with her doctor over time. The family had the information and knowledge of her wishes and sits down with the nursing staff and the nursing home administration to sign paperwork for making their mother a do not hospitalize patient and ask that comfort be the focus of her care. They hire a companion to help her eat her meals and focus on comfort feeding as the goal. Her lifelong love for food helps them make this decision; they know if she had the capacity to make her own decision she would never agree to a feeding tube. She maintains her weight for a few months, but then develops aspiration pneumonia. She is treated at the nursing home with oral antibiotics but does not improve. Hospice is involved in her care, and she has a comfortable death in the nursing home surrounded by family.

While there are many inherent challenges to supporting good quality ACP and excellent EOL care, there are some potential solutions. The first step toward this is to accept that the completion of an AD does not equal good quality ACP. It is only a step, and usually a beginning to the discussion. Nor does finding the perfect form mean the problems are over. We must find a better way to convey a patient's wishes, value set, and highest priority goals—quality of life, freedom from pain, being alert at the EOL, preserving functional status, and so on. We should continually work to perform formal ACP, the structured dialogue to define the person's value set, life plan, and goals for treatment. This should be a series of conversations over time. The result of the process should provide not only a person's wishes and goals for care, but also contingency plans with details to make sure that even in the middle of the night with a covering doctor, their wishes can be honored. We should work to engage all patients in at least the basic conversations and advance the discussion over time as the patient ages, accumulates comorbidity, or faces a terminal diagnosis. The nature of these conversations will vary greatly by patient, based on decision- making style, age, comorbidities, and preferences. The discussion should happen with all patients, but should vary accordingly and should be targeted by their needs, decision-making style, and disease burden. As with anything in life, everyone is different in their approach to making decisions, in their philosophy on life, and in their definition of a good death or quality of life. Therefore, most important is to put the focus on increasing the use of ACP, and working toward linking ADs to a comprehensive care plan that describes wishes, values, preferences, and instructions for honoring those. We should aim to create a toolbox of interventions and communication styles that when put together are tailored to the individual patient and his or her care plan. As discussed, each person is different in the ability to plan ahead and to visualize hypothetical scenarios, and preferences will change over time based on the social, financial, and health situation. Stages of behavior change will also affect a person's ability to participate in ACP. Finally, we must also recognize that despite creating a toolbox of interventions, there may still be patients who are not interested in participating.

REFERENCES

Baile, W. F., Buckman, R., Lenzi, R., Glober, G., Beale, E. A., & Kudelka, A. P. (2000). SPIKES-A six-step protocol for delivering bad news: Application to the patient with cancer. *The Oncologist, 5*(4), 302–311.

Chambers, C. V., Diamond, J. J., Perkel, R. L., & Lasch, L. A. (1994). Relationship of advance directives to hospital charges in a Medicare population. *Archives of Internal Medicine, 154*(5), 541–547.

Feudtner, C. (2009). The breadth of hopes. *The New England Journal of Medicine, 361*(24), 2306–2307.

Fried, T. R., Redding, C. A., Robbins, M. L., Paiva, A., O'Leary, J. R., & Iannone, L. (2010). Stages of change for the component behaviors of advance care planning. *Journal of the American Geriatrics Society, 58*(12), 2329–2336.

Messinger-Rapport, B. J., Baum, E. E., & Smith, M. L. (2009). Advance care planning: Beyond the living will. *Cleveland Clinic Journal of Medicine, 76*(5), 276–285.

Murphy, D. J., Knaus, W. A., & Lynn. J. (1990). Study population in SUPPORT: Patients (as defined by disease categories and mortality projections), surrogates and physicians. *Journal of Clinical Epidemiology, 43*, 11S–28S.

Polaniaszek, S., & Peres, J. (2008). *Historical perspective and ethical issues in advance directives and advance care planning: Report to Congress* (pp. 1–48). U.S. Department of Health and Human Services: Office of the Assistant Secretary for

Planning and Evaluation. Retrieved from aspe.hhs.gov/daltcp/reports/2008/ADCongRpt-B.pdf

Prochaska, J. O., & DiClemente, C. C. (2005). The transtheoretical approach. In J. Norcross & M. Goldfried (Eds.). *Handbook of psychotherapy integration* (2nd ed., pp. 147–171). New York, NY: Oxford University Press.

Ramsaroop, S. D., Reid, M. C., & Adelman, R. D. (2007). Completing an advance directive in the primary care setting: What do we need for success? *Journal of the American Geriatrics Society, 55*(2), 277–283.

Schneiderman, L. J., Kronick, R., Kaplan, R. M., Anderson, J. P., & Langer, R. D. (1992). Effects of offering advance directives on medical treatments and costs. *Annals of Internal Medicine, 117*(7), 599–606.

The SUPPORT Investigators. (1995). A controlled trial to improve outcomes for seriously ill hospitalized patients: The study to Understand Prognoses and Preferences for Outcomes and Risks of Treatment (SUPPORT). *Journal of the American Medical Association, 274,* 1591–1598.

Sudore, R. L. & Fried, T. R. (2010). Redefining the "Planning" in Advance Care Planning: Preparing for End-of-Life Decision Making. *Annals of Internal Medicine, 153,* 256–261.

Teno, J. M., & Lynn, J. (1996). Putting advance-care planning into action. *The Journal of Clinical Ethics, 7*(3), 205–213.

Teno, J. M. (2004). Advance directives: time to move on. *Annals of Internal Medicine, 141*(2), 159–160.

Teno, J., Lynn, J., Connors, A. F., Wenger, N., Phillips, R. S., Alzola, C., Knaus, W. A. (1997). The illusion of end-of-life resource savings with advance directives. SUPPORT Investigators. Study to Understand Prognoses and Preferences for Outcomes and Risks of Treatment. *Journal of the American Geriatrics Society, 45*(4), 513–518.

Weeks, W. B., Kofoed, L. L., Wallace, A. E., & Welch, H. G. (1994). Advance directives and the cost of terminal hospitalization. *Archives of Internal Medicine, 154*(18), 2077–2083.

CHAPTER 4

Barriers to Advance Care Planning: A Sociological Perspective

John Ryan
Jill Harrison

People plan for things. Certainly not everyone and maybe not all the time, but people plan for the future in various ways. They plan for weddings, they plan for college, they buy health insurance, they open savings accounts, they buy car insurance, they start retirement mutual funds, and a few buy long-term care insurance. It's an uncertain world and one way of reducing uncertainty is planning. People plan for death. There is no uncertainty that death will come, but when, where, and in what form is uncertain. So people buy life insurance and they buy burial plots. What people don't do, at least most of them don't, is plan for the type of medical care they will receive at the end of their lives (Black, 2010; Fagerlin & Schneider, 2004). Despite efforts to promote and educate, advance care planning (ACP) is in place for only a relatively small fraction of adults in the United States (see, e.g., Barnes et al., 2011; Gallo et al., 2002). Despite well-intentioned and expertly developed education programs, and a conducive legislative environment, efforts to empower patients to engage in ACP do not appear to be working (Jezewski, Meeker, Sessanna, & Finnell, 2007). So the question is, what is it about ACP that seems to make it a particularly problematic form of planning for the future?

In this chapter, we argue that ACP poses a particular set of dilemmas for the public that are either absent or less salient in planning for other life events. We argue further that these dilemmas, while being enacted at the microlevel of social interaction (e.g., between patients and doctors, among family members and friends), are embedded in broad cultural themes that leave many people feeling ill equipped to do what we are being asked to do—decide on future medical interventions. Our purpose here is to examine some of those cultural themes and the ways in which they may impact decision making using a sociological perspective. This chapter is organized in the following way: First, we place ACP in the context of cultural themes that we believe problematize its use for both physicians and the public. Second, we use Parsons's (1959) conceptualization of the sick role to frame the dynamics of end-of-life (EOL) care.

THE KNOWLEDGE SOCIETY AND THE CULTURE OF DECISION MAKING

Rational Knowledge

We know that most people do not engage in ACP. Numerous explanations have been offered for this phenomenon, across a wide range of studies (see, e.g., Field & Cassel, 1997; Fischer, Arnold, & Tulsky, 2000), including: confusion, procrastination, avoidance, anxiety related to death, denial of needing to complete ACP, lack of time, no one to name as a health care proxy, suspicion, and lack of trust. While these studies are important in explaining the lack of ACPs, in this section we explain this reluctance in the context of a broader cultural force that, we will argue, makes the decision to engage in ACP extremely problematic. This cultural force is the rationalization of knowledge (Weber, 1978). By the rationalization of knowledge we mean an increased emphasis on technical expertise, empirical knowledge, cost–benefit analysis, and efficiency over traditional forms of knowledge and moral judgment. The aim of rationalization is both efficiency and a reduction in uncertainty. Both are thought to be aided by developing knowledge through careful, objective, and methodical observation with the scientific method as the prototypical model. This knowledge is codified, certified, and placed in the hands of credentialed experts who are able to apply it in appropriately designated areas of social life.

The roots of rationalization can be traced through the Renaissance, the Protestant Reformation, and the Enlightenment, leading to the flowering of science in the 19th century (Gellner, 1988; Illich, 1975). The rationalization of knowledge is both a cause and consequence of the increasing size and complexity of societies. In a mutually reinforcing cycle, size and complexity go hand-in-hand with more knowledge production and an increased division of labor. In the process, jobs become more specialized and knowledge becomes detached from the everyday experience of the average person. While less complex societies are held together by the shared experience of their members, large complex societies are held together by this specialization and the interdependencies it produces (Durkheim, 1947). In the process, the pursuit and economic exploitation of knowledge became a defining feature of modernism and what is often referred to as the "knowledge society" (Böhme & Stehr, 1986; Gellner, 1988; Kirkpatrick, 2008).

Professionalization

A notable indication of this phenomenon is in the growth of professions (Cheetham & Chivers, 2005). Professions are a way of asserting control over some body of knowledge. Typical tactics of control include drawing boundaries around a particular body of knowledge and skills, and then requiring certification, typically through a designated educational experience, building group identification, requiring membership in professional associations, and so on. Through these means, entry into the profession is tightly controlled. Often these efforts are supported by the state in the form of licensure requirements with negative legal sanctions applied to those who violate those requirements.

Once a profession is established, it typically results in professional autonomy and financial gain for its members, who are able to use the entry requirements as a way of controlling competition and increasing monetary rewards and prestige (McDonald, 1995). At the same time, the gain for society is that there is some guarantee that practitioners are qualified to do what the general public is unable to do for itself. It is not surprising then that members of occupations struggle for the legitimacy associated with having their work defined as a profession. The expansion of occupations defined as such is well documented (see, e.g., Freidson, 1986; McDonald, 1995). Professions then control certain spheres of social life not only by expertise but by also by law. To cite just two of the most stringent examples, practicing law or medicine without a license carries criminal penalties in every U.S. state.

Reliance on Experts

As Bauman (1992) has pointed out, the expansion of professions is just part of a wider phenomenon of reliance on experts that characterizes the knowledge society. Experts, whether carrying full professional status or not, mediate between various forms of knowledge and the average person. Bauman refers to the fact that experts mediate and interpret "supra-personal" knowledge, meaning knowledge that individuals are unable or unwilling to acquire on their own. He writes:

> The expert is a person capable, simultaneously, of interrogating the fund of trustworthy and supra-personal knowledge and of understanding the innermost thoughts and cravings of a single person. As an *interpreter* and a *mediator*, the expert spans the

otherwise distant worlds of the *objective* and the *subjective*. He bridges the gap between the guarantees of being in the right (which can only be social) and making the choices one wants (which can only be personal) (p. 82).

All of this is to say that the individual in modern society is confronted with a large number of tasks to accomplish that require skills and knowledge beyond his or her own experience. The system upon which we depend for our survival: the electrical grid, transportation, food production and distribution, the water supply, and waste removal, are beyond control or even understanding for most. At the more personal level, the inner workings of our automobiles, the plumbing and wiring of our homes, and the appliances we rely on, all increasingly require Bauman's (1992) "supra-individual" knowledge. We rely on experts to make use of this knowledge on our behalf, usually in return for financial compensation.

Experts and Routine Activities

The expansion of expertise into daily life is pervasive and taken for granted. This is most obvious in areas such as medicine and law where reliance on experts is not only preferred but also, as noted earlier, legislatively mandated. More routine activities are affected as well, from "checking the weather" to purchasing healthy food. Take clothing as an example. Not only are most incapable of making their clothing, but the importance of "style" as a social resource leads to reliance on magazines, electronic media, the Internet, and, if one can afford it, consultants to guide an adequate presentation of one's identity (Meares, 2011). Likewise, normative grooming expectations have spawned an industry of licensed hair stylists who in a variety of complex and hierarchical organizational settings provide an array of products and services that many are compelled to make use of to make what they perceive to be an adequate presentation of self (Campbell, 1996; Goffman, 1959; Kleine, Kleine, & Kernan, 1993).

As noted by Andrew (1981) the expansion of reliance on experts and rationalized knowledge has spread from work to leisure. An entire industry has grown around providing expertise for nearly any leisure activity including biking, hiking, running, knitting, gardening, bird watching, photography, and so on. At the same time, book shelves are stocked with expert advice on how to get into relationships, get out of relationships, get pregnant (or not), how to raise a child (with specializations on every stage of development), and further specialization on subissues within stages, for example sleep issues among infants, sex issues among teens, and so on (see, e.g., Ryan, Wentworth, & Chapman, 1994). Such books cover virtually every aspect of the human experience, and what is common to all of them is that the reader is seeking expert advice, even if the goal of that advice is to "do it yourself."

The Attack on Professions

There is some irony in this. The self-help movement is in part an outgrowth of the attack on professionals beginning in the 1970s (e.g., Abbott, 1988; Freidson, 1970; Johnson, 1972; Larson, 1977). This attack focused on the monopoly power of professionals as well as conflicts of interest between professionals and other interest groups. These conflicts of interest were shown to result in financial gain for professions, while at the same time disadvantaging consumer clients (Evetts, 2006). An example is the federal investigation into the orthopedic device industry's alleged kickbacks to doctors and hip and knee surgeons (Feder, 2008).

This movement to demystify and regulate professions resulted in declining trust in professions, increased regulation, and expectations that clients and consumers be empowered in their relationships with experts (Pfadenhauer, 2006). In the health arena, people are expected to be empowered through healthy lifestyle behaviors, seeking out health information to engage more fully in dialogue with health care providers, seeking second opinions, and engaging with alternative providers (Lupton, 1997).

However, does the critique of the professions truly decrease reliance on experts? Or does it simply lead consumers to consult experts about experts? For example, before seeing their physician, many patients are now able to search the Internet for information they believe is relevant to their symptoms (Ferguson, 2002; Nettleton, 2004). Some of this is provided by nonexpert fellow health consumers, but as noted by Broom (2005), much is provided by reputable sources as well. What is key to our argument is that consumers are no less reliant than in the past on information from outside sources. While more information is available, it still largely comes from traditional experts. What is new is that consumers now have the added task of discerning which information comes from reliable sources and which does not. An indicator of this dilemma is that government and health agencies are devoting resources in an attempt to aid consumers in this task (see, e.g., the Food and Drug Administration [FDA] website: www.fda.gov/Drugs/ResourcesForYou/Consumers/BuyingUsingMedicineSafely/BuyingMedicinesOvertheInternet/ucm202863.htm).

The important point here is not that more information is available to and consumed by the public; this is well documented. For example, according to a poll conducted by the National Center for Health Statistics (2010), in 2009, 45.6% of adults aged 18 years or older said they had looked up health information on the Internet in the past 12 months. As noted above, our central point is that not only is most of this information created by experts, but also that locating, making sense out of, and utilizing this information still requires reliance on still more outside expertise. For example, Broom (2005) in his study of prostate cancer patients found that information gleaned from the Internet by patients did not result in the deprofessionalization or disempowerment of the physician, but did alter the nature of the discourse between patient and doctor. Patients who used the Internet brought more questions to the doctor but ultimately still relied on the doctor's expertise in making decisions.

So, despite the wealth of information available in the knowledge society, experts continue to mediate between that knowledge and consumers. Even if one chooses a path outside of traditional mainstream experts, other strata of experts take their place; for example, providers of supplements, acupuncture, homeopathy, and various other alternative health therapies may be sought out as an alternative to traditional health care. But here too knowledge is increasingly mediated by experts who are required to have some form of certification (Baer, 2001).

Our argument thus far has been that even in the knowledge society, much of the knowledge necessary for living is mediated through experts. Even the simplest decisions require reliance on some sort of "expert" knowledge, and this reliance is necessary for social life because—as sociologists Berger and Luckmann (1967) point out—we can't know everything. From this stock of common knowledge we develop personalized "knowledge recipes," choosing only the ingredients that are required for our existence. For example, we need to know how to use our computers to write this chapter, but we do not need to know how computers are made or where the parts come from. Therefore, this knowledge is excluded from our recipes (Berger & Luckmann, 1967). It is this knowing that we don't have to know everything because there are "experts" for each pocket of specialized knowledge that can potentially lead to an overreliance on the experts and less personal efficacy. As stated dramatically by Bauman (1992, p. 90), in modern society, "the living cannot sustain their own life." Meaning, taking all of this together, in modern society people often don't know how to do what they need or want to do to manage the problems of daily living. When it comes to daily living, the average person is, in a sense, deskilled.

Deskilling in the Knowledge Society

John McKnight (1984) draws a suitable analogy between our reliance on rational technical expertise and John Deere's 1837 invention of the steel plow. Prior to his invention, the great grass prairies of Wisconsin were not suitable for large-scale farming due to the impenetrability of the thick matted grasses and the wet earth. Conversely, Deere's steel plow (the "sod buster") was sharp enough to cut through the grasses and soil and enabled settlers to open the land to wheat farming. However, within just 30 years of intense farming, the soil was depleted and tens of thousands of farmers were driven off their land. In the same light, McKnight argues, the reliance on technical expertise has created a nation of "clients" whose own knowledge and capabilities have been depleted in the same way as the Wisconsin soil.

Using bereavement counseling as an example, McKnight (1984) argues that where once communities, families, and individuals had the capacity to deal adequately with the grieving process, after the professionalization of bereavement counseling, this capacity, or just as importantly the community's, the family's, and the individual's belief in this capacity, was eroded. In each case, the belief that there is a technically correct way of providing this comfort, and this technically correct knowledge lies in the hands of those with proper certification, creates insecurity about their own abilities and alienates them from the process. It becomes easy then, and, more importantly, *expected*, to turn the process over to the experts. Thus, reliance on technical expertise matters because it comes with a social cost (Weber, 1930); that cost is the deskilling of the population in an ever-expanding arena of social activities.

Following McKnight (1984) and Bauman (1992), our argument is that the modern individual lives in a world dominated by expert knowledge. In the medical arena, reliance on experts problematizes the notion of the empowered patient who feels confident in making decisions about his or her own health care. If the patient is empowered, it is only in the sense of having to locate and sort through competing expert opinions. As Bauman (1992, p. 90) writes:

> Modern society, in other words, is a site of *mediated action*. Few if any daily and mundane tasks may be accomplished without the assistance of supra-individual knowledge wrapped into a tool or mechanism, or delivered in a verbalized form of spoken or printed briefing. The skills needed for the effective performance of the tasks are enclosed in artifacts or step-by-step instructions. The skills the individuals deploy on their own serve the need of locating and getting access to artifacts or instructions adequate to the task they wish to perform. *depressing thought!*

If our argument is correct, we would expect that the greater one's medical expertise, the more likely one would be confident in making EOL decisions for themselves, and therefore the more likely one would have an ACP. As stated by Gallo et al. (2003, p. 961), "One of the key variables in discussions about the validity and stability of choices related to EOL care is the extent to which the individual has experience and knowledge with the health conditions that might be encountered in the future." The researchers hypothesized that, for these reasons, physicians would be more likely to have ACPs than would the general public. This is exactly what was found in their study of physicians' EOL decisions. In a survey of 765 physicians, the researchers found that 64% had some form of ACP. This compares with what they estimate as 20% of the general public.

Theme: uneducated + poor least likely to have ACP docs.

Thus far, we have been talking about a broad cultural theme, the rationalization of knowledge, the reliance on expert knowledge, and the resultant deskilling of the population in areas outside of their own expertise. In the next section, we examine how these culture dynamics play out at the interactional level among patients, family members, and medical caregivers as an individual approaches the EOL.

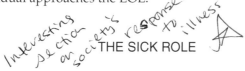

THE SICK ROLE

Being ill is more than a physical condition. Illness exists within a social context of societal norms and relationships. As Parsons (1951) pointed out in his classic work *The Social System*, being sick is a social role and like all social roles consists of both rights and obligations. Parsons argues further that being sick is a *deviant* status in the sense that an individual is unable to carry out the duties normally expected of someone in their social position. For example, a sick worker is unable to work, a sick parent is unable to parent, and a sick student is unable to attend class, and so on. Thus, while sickness may appear to be an individual problem, Parsons makes the connection between what he refers to as a form of personal disorganization and larger social disorganization. So, for example, the illness of a key worker, or a large number of workers (personal disorganization), can cripple the capacity of an organization (social disorganization). Similarly, the illness of a family member can upset the social organization of the family unit and the illness of a large number of students or teachers can disrupt the functioning of a school.

For Parsons (1951), then, being sick is deviant because of its implications for larger social systems. Due to its effects on group functioning, deviance in the form of failing to fulfill one's duties is normally negatively sanctioned in some way. For example, those who fail to contribute at work are likely to experience disapproval or even social banishment (being fired). Likewise, failure to fulfill the parenting role is likely to bring social disapproval or banishment as well (loss of custody).

But Parsons (1951) argues that there is a way to avoid such negative sanction. What he terms as the "sick role" (p. 436) serves as a form of protection against such disapproval. In essence, it exempts the individual, for a time, from some of the normal obligations of everyday life. For this to happen, this role must be endorsed by the social networks within which the individual is embedded and which are impacted by the illness. That is, one's story must be believable by key stakeholders. In the most concrete sense, one must have either tangibly or figuratively a "note from one's doctor." As an illness extends temporally, more proof may be required, particularly in secondary instrumental relationships. In other words, one's own family is likely to demand less in the way of proof than is one's employer. An employer, for example, may literally require a note from the doctor, but there is no guarantee that either the employer or coworkers will necessarily accept the diagnosis.

Performing Illness

so true!!

To increase the likelihood of believability the individual must develop a presentation of self (Goffman, 1959) that is consistent with the diagnosis. In other words, the sick person must "perform illness" in a satisfactory way. An acceptable performance, fulfilling the obligations of the "sick role," requires several elements. For example, as Parsons (1951) points out, performing illness often requires removing oneself from the normal flow of daily life. That is, a sick person is supposed to stay at home or in a medical facility until judged well enough to return to daily life. The expected duration of this absence varies according to the audience's perception of the seriousness of the condition. Note that our emphasis here is not on the time that is biologically required to recover sufficiently, but rather on the perceptions of others as to whether or not one has taken "too much" time, or, "too little" time.

At the same time, it is important that one should not be sick too often, as judged by the audience, or suffer the risk of overdrawing one's account in the "sympathy bank" (Clark, 1997). Another social rule might be that a person who has missed a few days of work with a cold or the flu should not arrive back at work looking well rested and full of energy. If the illness is chronic, say a back problem that allows one to work but not at the same level as fellow workers, then performing illness takes on a very public role. So, one must complain about one's back hurting (but not too much), perhaps wear a brace, and so on.

Advance Care Planning and Trying to Get Well

Being sick is, therefore, both a biological condition and a social role. Like other social roles, it entails rights and obligations. The right to remove oneself from normal responsibilities is attached to the fulfillment of a range of obligations. Most importantly for our discussion of ACPs and the reluctance of people to have them, is the expectation, as part of the sick role, that the individual try to get well. That is, the sick individual is expected to follow a socially accepted protocol for getting well, which often includes seeking appropriate medical attention. A patient, for example, who refuses to take his/her medicine is violating the norms of the sick role and thus is labeled as deviant. As Parsons (1951, p. 437) explains it, the individual occupying the sick role, in proportion to the severity of the condition, is under the obligation "to seek *technically competent* help, namely, in the most usual case, that of a physician and to *cooperate* with him in the process of trying to get well."

[handwritten marginal note at top: The role our social expectations re: "the sick role" play in one's decision to develop an ACP.]

Returning to our main focus, ACPs, where they emphasize limiting medical interventions near the EOL, such as choosing to not have a ventilator, feeding tube, or resuscitation, clearly run contrary to the norms of the sick role. The expectation of "trying to get well" is so powerful because it is embedded in a system of relationships. It falls not only on the patient to try to get well, but also on family, caregivers, and physicians alike. That is, while the patient is expected to "not give up," family members feel obligated to encourage the patient to not give up, and medical providers are expected to do all within their expertise to produce a cure. Thus, limiting care is a difficult decision for all involved and it is no wonder that the discussion of EOL care is so socially difficult. Frank (2005) writes about the cost of this to the patient. He writes that part of being a "good patient" is to at least appear cheerful and optimistic about recovery. He writes that family, friends, and medical staff play key roles in this performance:

> To be ill is to be dependent on medical staff, family, and friends. Since all of these people value cheerfulness, the ill must summon up their energies to be cheerful. Denial may not be what they want or need, but it is what they perceive those around them wanting and needing. This is not the sick person's own denial, but rather his accommodation to the denial of others. (p. 28)

[handwritten marginal note, left side: act cheerful]

Within this context, patients feel the obligation to play the sick role in such a way that they appear cheerful and desiring of getting well, family and friends feel the need to encourage the patient in getting well, and doctors feel obligated to bring whatever technical expertise they possess to make it happen (Edwards & Tolle, 1992), even if the likely outcome is dismal. At this stage, even the discussion of an ACP may appear to be "giving up" and thus violating the expectation of trying to get well.

Doctors too are trapped in their part of the interaction. The other side of the coin of reliance on experts is that experts must perform expertise even in the face of uncertainty (Groopman, 2007). Research shows (Gallo et al., 2003) that physicians, even those with ACPs, are unlikely to talk about their preferences with others. The researchers conclude: "If physicians do not discuss preferences or execute advance directives, others without direct experience or training related to the EOL care will be unlikely to do so" (Gallo et al., 2003, p. 961).

Given our argument about the rationalization of knowledge and the reliance on experts, only those in the role of the physician are likely to be able to give permission to let go. Not surprisingly, research shows that physicians' attitudes affect patient attitudes on appropriate care (Gramelspacher, Zhou, Hanna, & Tierney, 1997; Schneiderman, Kaplan, &

Rosenberg, 1997), including the decision to withdraw life support (Christakis & Asch, 1995).

DISCUSSION

All human decisions are inherently bound up in social relationships and cultural contexts in which beliefs and structures constrain action. Now that we have placed ACP in a sociocultural context, we argue that the context for ACP is to *not* plan. Why? As we have argued, we exist in a cultural context wherein we have given over our power to experts and technology, and as a result, we experience a loss of capacity to make independent decisions. At the same time, the sociocultural context of the sick role and its various rules and obligations is reinforced across all stages of the life course. The process of proactive ACP in the context of advancing old age works against the idea that the medical system has the ability to cure you, faith in technology, faith in expertise, and medicine; not to mention the cultural contexts of denying and avoiding old age. The process of ACP in the context of terminal illness, regardless of age, means that individuals must choose to not perform their roles adequately as sick people because they are supposed to try and get well and believe that experts and their technology will save them. We argue that these social contexts constrain ACP decisions much more than they support it. These sociocultural contexts and social norms are so embedded and important to human interactions that interventions at the individual level to increase ACP have not been successful. Focusing on the broad cultural themes that shape engagement and decision making could result in more nuanced understandings of ACP and the complexities of the social relationships and roles that constrain it. Although ACP is focused on death and dying, the process must be acted out against the sociocultural backdrop of life and living.

We believe that this perspective provides an important context for studies of ACP. For example, some research has found that a barrier to ACP is confusion about the treatment options (Sudore, Schillinger, Knight, & Fried, 2010). Our argument is that confusion is built into a system that emphasizes reliance on technical expertise while at the same time giving the illusion of patient choice. Other research (Barnes et al., 2011) has found that cancer patients had not spoken with health care professionals and close persons about ACP. A primary reason was fear of distressing family members. We argue that the concept of the sick role and its expectations help explain this phenomena.

In summary, our argument is that ACP is embedded in a larger cultural context that greatly hinders its implementation. Studies of the microlevel forces that influence the decision to engage in ACP are best understood by acknowledging these broad forces of the reliance on expert knowledge and sick-role expectations in a knowledge society.

REFERENCES

Abbott, A. (1988). *The system of professions: An essay on the division of expert labor.* Chicago, IL: Chicago University Press.

Andrew, E. (1981). *Closing the iron cage: The scientific management of work and leisure.* Montreal, ON: Black Rose Books.

Baer, H. A. (2001). The sociopolitical status of U.S. naturopathy at the dawn of the 21st century. *Medical Anthropology Quarterly, 15*(3), 329–346.

Barnes, K. A., Barlow, C. A., Harrington, J., Ornadel, K., Tookman, A., King, M., & Jones, L. (2011). Advance care planning discussions in advanced cancer: Analysis of dialogues between patients and care planning mediators. *Palliative & Supportive Care, 9*(1), 73–79.

Bauman, Z. (1992). Life world and expertise: Social production of dependency. In N. Stehr & R. V. Ericson (Eds.), *The culture and power of knowledge: Inquiries into contemporary societies* (pp. 81–105). New York, NY: Walter de Gruyter.

Berger, P., & Luckmann, T. (1967). *The social construction of reality: A treatise in the sociology of knowledge.* Garden City, NJ: Doubleday.

Black, K. (2010). Promoting advance care planning through the National Healthcare Decisions Day Initiative. *Journal of Social Work in End-of-Life & Palliative Care 6,* 11–26.

Böhme, G., & Stehr, N. (1986). *The knowledge society: The growing impact of scientific knowledge on social relations.* Boston, MA: D. Reidel.

Broom, A. (2005). Virtually he@lthy: the impact of internet use on disease experience and the doctor-patient relationship. *Qualitative Health Research, 15*(3), 325–345.

Campbell, C. (1996). The meaning of objects and the meaning of actions: A critical note on the sociology of consumption and theories of clothing. *Journal of Material Culture, 1*(1), 93–105.

Cheetham, G., & Chivers, G. E. (2005). *Professions, competence and informal learning.* Northampton, MA: Edward Elgar.

Christakis, N. A., & Asch, D. A. (1995). Physician characteristics associated with decisions to withdraw life support. *American Journal of Public Health, 85*(3), 367–372.

Clark, C. (1997). *Misery and company: Sympathy in everyday life.* Chicago, IL: The University of Chicago Press.

Durkheim, E. (1947). *The division of labor in society.* New York, NY: The Free Press. (Originally published in 1893.)

Edwards M. J., & Tolle S. W. (1992). Disconnecting a ventilator at the request of a patient who knows he will then die: The doctor's anguish. *Ann Intern Med* 117:254–256.

Evetts, J. (2006). Introduction: Trust and professionalism: Challenges and occupational changes. *Current Sociology, 54*, 515–529.

Fagerlin, A., & Schneider, C. E. (2004). Enough. The failure of the living will. *The Hastings Center Report, 34*(2), 30–42.

Feder, B. J. (2008). *New focus of inquiry into bribes: Doctors.* The New York Times. March 22, 2008. Retrieved from http://www.nytimes.com/2008/03/22/business/22device.html?_r=1&ref=strykercorporation.

Ferguson, T. (2002). From patients to end users. *BMJ (Clinical Research Ed.), 324*(7337), 555–556.

Field, M. J., & Cassel, C. K. (1977). Approaching death: improving care at the end of life. *Health Progress (Saint Louis, Mo.), 92*(1), 25.

Fischer, G. S., Arnold, R. M., & Tulsky, J. A. (2000). Talking to the older adult about advance directives. *Clinics in Geriatric Medicine, 16*(2), 239–254.

Frank, A. (2005). The cost of appearances. In N. King, R. Strauss, L. R. Churchill, S. E. Estroff, G. E. Henderson, & J. Oberlander (Eds.), *The social medicine reader* (Vol. 1, pp. 26–40). Durham, NC: Duke University Press.

Freidson, E. (1970). *Professional dominance: The social structure of medical care.* New York, NY: Atherton Press.

Freidson, E. (1986). *Professional powers: A study of the institutionalization of formal knowledge.* Chicago, IL: University of Chicago Press.

Gallo, J. J., Straton, J. B., Klag, M. J., Meoni, L. A., Sulmasy, D. P., Wang, N. Y., & Ford, D. E. (2003). Life-sustaining treatments: what do physicians want and do they express their wishes to others? *Journal of the American Geriatrics Society, 51*(7), 961–969.

Gellner, E. (1988). *Plough, sword and book.* London, UK: Collins Harvell.

Goffman, E. (1959). *The presentation of self in everyday life.* New York, NY: Anchor Books.

Gramelspacher, G. P., Zhou, X. H., Hanna, M. P., & Tierney, W. M. (1997). Preferences of physicians and their patients for end-of-life care. *Journal of General Internal Medicine, 12*(6), 346–351.

Groopman, J. (2007). *How doctor's think.* Boston, MA: Houghton Mifflin Company.

Illich, I. (1975). *Medical nemesis: The expropriation of health (open forum).* New York, NY: Pantheon Books.

Jezewski, M. A., Meeker, M. A., Sessanna, L., & Finnell, D. S. (2007). The effectiveness of interventions to increase advance directive completion rates. *Journal of Aging and Health, 19*(3), 519–536.

Johnson, T. (1972). *Professions and power.* London, UK: Macmillan.

Kirkpatrick, G. (2008). *Technology and social power.* New York, NY: Palgrave MacMillan.

Kleine, R. E., Kleine, S. S., & Kernan, J. B. (1993). Mundane consumption and the self: a social-identity perspective. *Journal of Consumer Psychology, 2*(3), 209–235.

Larson, M. S. (1977). *The rise of professionalism.* Berkeley, CA: University of California Press.

Lupton, D. (1997). Foucault and the medicalization critique. In A. Petersen & R. Bunton (Eds.), *Foucault, health and medicine* (pp. 94–110). London, UK: Routledge.

McDonald, K. M. (1995). *The sociology of the professions.* Thousand Oaks, CA: Sage.

McKnight, J. (1984). John Deere and the bereavement counselor: The fourth annual Schumacher Lecture, New Haven CT. In G. Morgan (Ed.), *Creative organizational theory: A resource book* (pp. 245–251). Newbury Park, CA: Sage.

Meares, A. (2011). *Pricing beauty: The making of a fashion model.* Berkeley, CA: University of California Press.

National Center for Health Statistics. (2010). *QuickStats: Percentage of adults aged ≥ 18 years who looked up health information on the internet, by age group and sex.* National Health Interview Survey, United States, January–September 2009. http://www.cdc.gov/mmwr/preview/mmwrhtml/mm5915a7.htm. Accessed April 27, 2011.

Nettleton, S. (2004). The emergence of e-scaped medicine? *Sociology, 38*(4), 661–679.

Parsons, T. (1951). *The social system.* New York, NY: The Free Press.

Pfadenhauer, M. (2006). Crisis or decline? Problems of legitimation and loss of trust in modern professionalism. *Current Sociology, 54,* 565–578.

Ryan, J., Wentworth W., & Chapman, G. (1994). Models of emotions in therapeutic self-help books. *Sociological Spectrum, 14*(3), 241–256.

Schneiderman, L. J., Kaplan, R. M., & Rosenberg E. (1997). Do physicians' own preferences for life-sustaining treatment influence their perceptions of patients' preferences? A second look. *Cambridge Quarterly of Healthcare Ethics, 6,* 131–137.

Sudore, R. L., Schillinger, D., Knight, S. J., & Fried, T. R. (2010). Uncertainty about advance care planning treatment preferences among diverse older adults. *Journal of Health Communication,* 15 Suppl 2, 159–171.

Weber, M. (1930). *The protestant ethic and the spirit of capitalism.* New York, NY: Charles Scribner's Sons.

Weber, M. (1978). *Economy and society.* Berkley, CA: University of California Press.

CHAPTER 5

Advance Medical Care Planning: The Legal Environment

Marshall B. Kapp

The actual and perceived legal environments (which are not always synonymous) in the United States exert a powerful influence on the provision of medical services to patients in end-of-life (EOL) situations. Legal rights and risks, both real and misunderstood, may either promote or inhibit the effective use of advance directives (ADs) as mechanisms of sustaining patients' personal autonomy.

This chapter first briefly outlines the contemporary American legal climate pertaining to EOL decision making. It then identifies and analyzes the various ways in which the legal environment facilitates or impedes particular forms of advance care planning (ACP), and most importantly how health care providers' legal anxieties impact the likelihood that ADs will have the effect of actually assuring that patients' wishes about EOL care get honored in practice. In light of identified deficiencies in the ACP status quo, the chapter concludes with suggestions for a legal alternative to existing planning mechanisms, specifically focusing on the Physician Orders for Life-Sustaining Treatment (POLST) Paradigm, which provides for a signed physician's order regarding EOL care for persons with serious, life-threatening illness.

THE CONTEMPORARY LEGAL ENVIRONMENT

The legal environment surrounding EOL decision making in the United States has been evolving since the 1976 Karen Anne Quinlan case (*Matter of Quinlan*, 1976) brought the matter clearly into the public consciousness. This legal environment is largely a product of statutes enacted by Congress and individual state legislatures, particularly regarding ADs. However, statutes must be consistent with principles contained in the federal and various state constitutions; these documents, as their provisions are interpreted and applied by the courts, are Americans' primary source of individual rights and constraints on government powers.

The 1990 case of Nancy Cruzan (*Cruzan v. Director, Missouri Department of Health*, 1990) is still the only U.S. Supreme Court decision that directly decides the issue of discontinuing life-prolonging medical treatment for a particular person. Cruzan was an automobile accident victim who was kept alive in a permanent vegetative state within a government (state of Missouri) long-term care facility through the use of feeding and hydration tubes. Her parents asked that this intervention be discontinued, a request they believed was consistent with the patient's previously expressed (although not formally documented) wishes. The attending physicians refused to honor this request, and the Missouri Supreme Court denied the parents' petition to discontinue treatment.

On appeal, the U.S. Supreme Court held that a mentally capable adult has a fundamental constitutional right, under the liberty provision of the Fourteenth Amendment's Due Process clause, to make personal medical decisions, even regarding refusal of artificial feeding and hydration. For patients with insufficient cognitive and emotional ability, however, the Court ruled that the state's legitimate interest in preserving life is strong enough to permit the state, if it so chooses, to require "clear and convincing" evidence—prior to following a surrogate's discontinuation instructions—that the patient would want that treatment withdrawn if the patient were currently able to make and express an autonomous choice. Ordinarily, a written declaration made by the patient while the patient was still cognitively and emotionally capable would provide sufficient evidence of the patient's treatment preference in the event of subsequent incapacity. Under the *Cruzan* decision, states also are free to set lower standards of proof than "clear and convincing" evidence for incapacitated patients, namely proof by a preponderance of the evidence (in other words, greater than a 50% likelihood), but not many states have chosen to avail themselves of this opportunity.

One form of treatment limitation around which there is substantial agreement is the do not resuscitate (DNR)—also known as do not attempt resuscitation (DNAR) or no code—order, which instructs caregivers not to initiate CPR for a patient who suffers a foreseeable cardiac arrest. There have been very few reported legal decisions regarding this topic. Nonetheless, the prevailing rule is that a decisionally capable patient has the right to refuse CPR, and that surrogates may choose to forego CPR for a patient if the likely burdens of this intervention to the patient would seriously outweigh any expected benefits (e.g., mere continued existence until the next arrest). As with all medical decisions, a DNR order should be written by the physician only after a thorough consultation with the patient or surrogate and should be clearly documented in the medical record (Westphal & McKee, 2009). A DNR order may be folded into a more comprehensive POLST (discussed below).

The most vigorously disputed issue in the treatment limitation arena is still the status of artificial feeding and hydration (Wick & Zanny, 2009). The courts have been unanimous in holding that artificial feeding tubes (of all kinds) are merely another form of medical intervention that may be withheld or withdrawn under the same circumstances that would justify withholding or withdrawal of any other type of medical intervention such as a respirator, dialysis, or antibiotic use. Major medical professional groups endorse this position (Truog et al., 2008). The contrary position is that feeding and hydration, even when they can be achieved only through tubes surgically or forcibly inserted into the patient's body, are fundamentally different and more morally elemental than medical treatment, and therefore they should be maintained as long as they might physiologically keep the patient alive. A number of state legislatures reflect this argument in their living will or durable power of attorney (DPOA) statutes (discussed below) that are intended to severely constrain the rights of patients and surrogate decision makers to authorize the removal of feeding tubes (Tucker, 2009). Both the practical wisdom and the constitutionality of these purported restrictions are extremely questionable, but a fuller discussion of this matter is beyond the scope of the present chapter.

The federal Patient Self-Determination Act (PSDA), Pub. L. 101–508, Title IV, §§ 4206, 4751, went into effect in 1991. The PSDA mandates that hospitals, nursing homes, home health agencies, hospices, health maintenance organizations, and preferred provider organizations participating in the Medicare and Medicaid programs perform the following actions at the time a person is admitted or enrolled: (a) provide written information to individuals about their right to make their own medical decisions to the extent guaranteed by applicable state law, and make available to them the organizational policy for effectuating that right for the organization's patients; (b) ask patients whether they have completed an AD already and, if the response is yes, have a system for recording the patient's AD; (c) offer currently capable individuals a chance to execute an AD if they have not previously done so; (d) not discriminate in the provision of care based on the presence or absence of an AD; (e) create a system to assure compliance with relevant state laws on medical decision making; and (f) educate institutional/organizational staff and the community about patients' rights pertaining to medical decision making.

When the patient or surrogate refuses aggressive, technologically intensive medical interventions, the physician nonetheless has the legal obligation to offer basic palliative (comfort, pain control, and emotional support) and hygiene measures (Imhof & Kaskie, 2008). Failure to do so could constitute negligence or form the basis for professional discipline. Good palliative care may sometimes include the practice of palliative sedation (also called total, terminal, or controlled sedation) for distress or suffering during the dying process that cannot otherwise be treated satisfactorily (Mularski et al., 2009).

In every state, it is a criminal offense (as a form of homicide) for a physician to engage in positive or affirmative actions that are intended to speed up a patient's death (such as administering a lethal injection), even if a competent patient requested such action (Stern & Difonzo, 2009). Similarly, in every state except Oregon, Vermont, and Washington (Drum, White, Taitano, & Horner-Johnson, 2010) (and possibly Montana), it is criminal for a physician to go along with a patient's request that the physician supply the patient with the means to hurry up his or her own death (such as writing a prescription for a lethal dose of a medication, knowing fully well that the patient intends to commit suicide by taking that lethal dose) (Bollman, 2010). The U.S. Supreme Court has unanimously rejected the assertion that individuals have a federal constitutional right to physician-assisted death (PAD) (*Vacco v. Quill*, 1997; *Washington v. Glucksberg*, 1997).

Conversely, a patient, or more usually the patient's family, may insist on initiating or continuing medical treatment ("doing everything possible") that the clinician believes is futile in terms of patient benefit. Neither a patient nor a family possesses a legal right to demand, nor does a physician owe a duty to provide, nonbeneficial medical treatment (Cantor, 2010; Truog, 2008–2009; Whitmer, Hurst, Prins, Shepard, & McVey, 2009). On the rare occasions when courts have become involved prospectively with the futility issue, the judicial opinions generally have been confusing, inconsistent, and poorly reasoned. However, no court has ever held a provider liable after the fact for failure to begin or perpetuate futile interventions for a critically ill patient, even when the family was insisting on doing everything technologically possible. In practice, clinicians usually seem to take the path of least resistance in such circumstances and "treat the family," often out of misapprehension about potential liability exposure. In the vast majority of cases, better physician–family communication, in which the realistic (that is, negative) implications of "doing everything possible" are clearly delineated, can avoid serious disagreement over how to proceed.

INFLUENCE OF THE LEGAL ENVIRONMENT ON END-OF-LIFE CARE AND ADVANCE MEDICAL PLANNING

Overview of Advance Medical Planning

Over the past four decades, a lot of attention has been concentrated on advance or prospective health care planning as a mechanism for individuals to maintain a degree of control over their future medical treatment even if, at some point, they become physically and/or mentally incapable of making and expressing important decisions about their own care. Advocates of ACP also suggest that it may help people and their families avoid unwanted court involvement in medical treatment decisions, conserve limited health care resources in a manner consistent with patient autonomy or self-determination (Halpern & Emanuel, 2012; Nicholas, Langa, Iwashyna, & Weir, 2011), and diminish the emotional or psychological stress on family and friends that occurs in difficult crisis circumstances.

Two chief types of ADs are available for use in prospective (before-the-fact) health care planning. Statutes explicitly authorizing individuals to execute ADs have been enacted in every state; many of these state statutes (sometimes called "natural death acts") are modeled on the Uniform Health Care Decisions Act adopted by the National Conference of Commissioners on Uniform State Laws (1993). In some other countries (Great Britain, for instance), ADs have been recognized by the courts even though they have not been codified in statutory form.

One legal advance planning mechanism is the proxy directive, usu-ally a DPOA for health care. The proxy directive is an AD that enables an individual to voluntarily designate another person—called a health care agent, surrogate, proxy, or attorney-in-fact—to make health care decisions in the event that the principal (the individual who has delegated away decision-making authority) subsequently loses decision-making capacity through illness or accident. Many states have enacted statutes that des-ignate a legal hierarchy of family members and other persons who may make decisions on behalf of decisionally incapacitated patients when no guardian has been appointed or instruction directive (discussed below) has been written; in those jurisdictions, a DPOA may clarify which per-son has the authority to decide when two persons otherwise would have equal status (such as the patient's siblings) within the hierarchy. In addi-tion, a DPOA is valuable when a person prefers to name a nonrelative as the future decision maker. For instance, it is common in the gay commu-nity for individuals to appoint domestic partners or friends, rather than family members, as their health care agents.

Unlike the situation created with an ordinary power of attorney, the authority of an agent under a DPOA is not automatically ended when the principal subsequently becomes decisionally incapacitated. The agent's decision-making authority may become effective immediately (an immedi-ate DPOA) upon execution of the document, or it may "spring" into action when a specifically delineated event (such as "when my physician certifies that I am unable to make my own medical decisions") has taken place. The DPOA would then endure beyond that triggering event. The principal may terminate or revoke the arrangement at any time, so long as the principal remains mentally competent to do so.

One limitation of the DPOA device is the legal and practical require-ment that the person who would like to delegate certain decision-making authority to an agent actually have available a suitable, willing, and able person to whom to delegate that authority. The DPOA does not help people (the "unbefriended" population) who do not have someone else whom they can trust to make future personal decisions for them.

By contrast, an instruction (living will)–type AD documents an individual's desires about wanted, limited, or unwanted life-sustaining medical treatments (LSMTs) in case the person at some point becomes cognitively or emotionally incapacitated or is unable to communicate treatment wishes at all. These instructions may be detailed (in the sense of relating to specific medical treatments in particular clinical situations), general (such as "no extraordinary measures"), or phrased in terms of a patient's personal values (like "Life is sacred, so keep me alive forever regardless of pain or expense" or "Just don't let me suffer").

Proxy and instruction directives are not mutually exclusive. Some AD documents combine the instruction and proxy elements. Only a presently capable person may execute a valid AD. The AD becomes effective only when the person creating the AD subsequently lacks decisional capacity concerning a particular medical treatment issue; if the patient currently possesses sufficient decisional capacity and ability to communicate choices, there is no need for anyone to turn to an AD for advice.

Consistently, courts and state legislatures have made it clear that AD statutes are not intended to be the exclusive means by which patients may exercise the right to make future decisions about medical treatment. For example, a patient might convey concerns regarding future medical treatment orally to the physician during an office visit, with the physician documenting the patient's words in the medical chart. When that person subsequently becomes unable to make personal medical decisions, his/her oral instructions are just as legally valid as would be a written document executed in compliance with all the formalities contained in the state's AD statute. Nonetheless, even though a legally valid AD may be oral, it is much more likely to be followed by the health care system if it takes the form of a written document.

Problems With Advance Directives

Despite substantial positive public attention, unfortunately, psychological resistance to the contemplation of illness and death, coupled with inertia and legal complexities complicating the execution of an AD, keeps the rate of AD completion low among the general public (Bravo, Dubois, & Wagneur, 2008). Personal characteristics may influence AD completion rates among members of different population groups. Although nursing home residents are more likely to complete an AD than community-dwelling older persons, the PSDA expressly forbids any health care provider from requiring a patient/ resident to execute an AD as a condition of admission or receiving services.

Moreover, even when the law is clear and the patient has timely executed an instruction directive, health care providers often are unclear about when the living will applies and are uncomfortable about deciding when a patient is on a dying trajectory that warrants triggering the declaration's instructions. Also, health care providers sometimes find a living will's instructions either too broad or too narrow to provide useful guidance in a specific situation. Misunderstandings may be exacerbated by the reluctance of many physicians to engage patients in meaningful EOL discussions in a timely manner (Mack et al., 2012).

Thus, there is a significant body of evidence that, often, patients' previously stated wishes concerning LSMT are not respected and implemented by health care providers, and very often they are also not followed by families that are supposed to be acting as the patient's surrogate. Critically ill patients frequently receive more aggressive medical treatment than they had earlier said they would want (Fagerlin & Schneider, 2004).

State AD statutes specifically excuse a health care provider who decides, for reasons of personal conscience, not to carry out the explicitly stated treatment preferences of a patient or surrogate, so long as that provider does not impede efforts to have the patient transferred to the care of a different provider who is willing to respect the patient's AD. In the same vein, courts have declined to hold health care providers liable for failure to follow a patient's or surrogate's instructions to withdraw or withhold particular forms of treatment, on the grounds that providing life-prolonging intervention cannot cause the sort of injury or harm for which the tort system is designed to provide recognition and monetary compensation.

THE NEXT STEPS IN ADVANCE MEDICAL PLANNING

The POLST Paradigm Defined

"The evolution of advance directives has mirrored that of many new medical technologies: initial unbridled enthusiasm evolved into skepticism as empirical evidence raised questions about the current practice, followed by a wiser, more constrained application" (White & Arnold, 2011, p. 1485). Growing frustration with the inherent limitations of existing instruments for promoting the prospective autonomy of critically ill patients who may become decisionally incapacitated has led many attorneys, health care providers, and commentators to advocate the use of POLST forms as the next step in the evolution of health care advance planning law and policy. (The exact nomenclature varies among different jurisdictions; some states, New York for instance, use the acronym MOLST, or Medical Order for Life-Sustaining Treatment.) Unlike a traditional AD executed by a patient while still decisionally capable, POLST entails a medical order written by a physician (with the concurrence of the patient or surrogate) instructing other health care providers such as emergency medical squads about the treatment of a critically ill patient under specific factual situations.

POLST is intended for someone who has advanced, irreversible illness. "The POLST form is a more uniform, comprehensive, and portable method of documentation of patients' EOL treatment desires. Although the POLST form is not intended to replace advance directives executed by patients, it corrects many of the inadequacies of current AD forms and intends to lessen the discrepancy between a patient's end-of-life care preferences and the treatment(s) eventually provided by the patients' health care providers" (Spillers & Lamb, 2011, pp. 82–83). There is solid evidence that health care providers are much more likely to honor a patient's POLST across medical settings than they are to follow the patient's AD (Hickman et al., 2010).

At least 15 states have formally implemented the POLST Paradigm, with national coordination efforts being administered through the Center for Ethics in Health Care at the Oregon Health & Science University (www. ohsu.edu/polst). Many more states are in the process of developing or considering their own versions of POLST (Sabatino & Karp, 2011).

POLST Strategic Issues

There is an array of strategic issues with which states striving to successfully adopt and fulfill the POLST Paradigm must grapple (Hickman, Sabatino, Moss, & Nester, 2008).The initial set of strategic issues asks about what changes, if any, in current state law are necessary to authorize and/or encourage attending physicians to write POLSTs for appropriate patients and to authorize and/or encourage other health care professionals to respect and implement those POLSTs. One potential route (involving the most complex and controversial political ramifications) (Goodman, 2007) would be to propose legislative enactment of new, explicit statutory language.

Either as an alternative strategy to legislation or as a supplemental way of implementing the statutory change, explicit regulatory modifications could be sought to clarify the POLST-related rights and responsibilities of affected parties (Cerminara & Bogin, 2008). This approach would necessitate identifying which state agencies have relevant jurisdiction and ways to assure inter-agency coordination and cooperation in the administration of POLST oversight.

A third potential strategy would bypass, or at least delay, legislation and regulation in favor of action predicated on clinical consensus. Several states have already successfully pursued this approach. This approach entails obtaining explicit agreement from the relevant state agencies that current state statutes and regulations already permit physicians (and in some places other health care professionals) to write, patients and surrogates to agree to, and other health care providers to implement POLSTs. In this approach, the emphasis of change agents is placed on professional and public education rather than on trying to amend the law. The clinical consensus strategy relies mainly on common state legislative provisions such as the "Preservation of Existing Rights" clause found in Florida's AD statute:

The provisions of [Chapter 765] are cumulative to the existing law regarding an individual's right to consent, or refuse to consent, to medical treatment and do not impair any existing rights or responsibilities which a health care provider, a patient, including a minor, competent or incompetent person, or a patient's family may have under the common law, Federal Constitution, State Constitution, or statutes of this state. (Fla. Stat. § 765.106)

The argument would be that current common (that is, judge-made) law and constitutional law already protect the liberty rights of patients to make contemporaneous and prospective medical decisions and to secure the assistance of their physicians in effectuating those liberty rights by, for example, documenting a POLST instructing other health care providers on behalf of the patient.

Assuming that either a statutory or regulatory change strategy is pursued to promote the POLST Paradigm in a state, a myriad of policy questions need to be addressed in the legislative or rule-making drafting stage. There is a wide divergence among states with up-and-running POLST programs regarding how they have resolved these questions (Sabatino & Karp, 2011).

For instance, decisions need to be made about the specific content of the adopted POLST form and whether that content should be incorporated into statute or regulation or only described in broad terms. Typical POLST forms presently in use contain separate sections dealing with: CPR attempts; medical interventions (full treatment vs. comfort measures only); use of antibiotics; provision of artificially administered nutrition and hydration; reason for the orders (documenting the physician's conversations with the patient and/or surrogate); and signatures of the physician and (depending upon the particular jurisdiction) the patient or surrogate. States in which POLST is just emerging might comport with or deviate from this particular structure. When a statute or regulation does incorporate specific POLST form content, a question arises whether the explicitly approved form must be used by physicians in order for the POLST to be considered valid or, alternatively, whether a somewhat deviating but nonetheless comparable form would be legally acceptable.

A further legal and policy-drafting question is whether to require health care providers to offer the POLST option to patients. If so, which specific providers would be covered? Should the requirement encompass all patients or only certain categories of persons? What timing requirements (for instance, at the time of admission to a health care institution, as now specified in the PSDA), if any, should be delineated? What is the penalty for provider noncompliance? Another, likely very politically contentious, issue relates to who, beside physicians, should be granted the legal power to write POLSTs. Should this authority be extended, for example, to advance practice nurses or physicians' assistants, as has happened already in several jurisdictions?

A different strategic conundrum concerns the extent of the authority that a statute or regulation grants surrogates to consent to a POLST on behalf of a patient who lacks enough present cognitive and emotional capacity to decide and speak personally about medical treatment concerns. The desire to facilitate the writing of POLSTs, even when concurrence must come from a surrogate instead of the patient, must be balanced against the need to protect decisionally compromised patients from surrogates who, unfortunately (Rosenberg, 2010), may not be worthy of the trust bestowed upon them.

One of the largest impediments to successful POLST implementation has been health care providers' anxieties about the risk of possible lawsuits brought against them by disgruntled family members. Overcoming that vastly exaggerated but strongly and sincerely held apprehension is vital to achieving successful POLST implementation. Thus, the good faith legal immunity provisions necessarily built into POLST statutes and/or regulations must be drafted carefully, balancing encouragement of provider compliance with POLSTs against the need for some form of accountability for the actors involved. On a related note, there is a question about whether provider compliance with a valid POLST should be mandated. If so, what is the proper range of sanctions for a failure to comply with the mandate?

Other operational issues also need to be resolved in the legislative or regulatory drafting stage. May a provider rely, in withholding certain kinds of treatment, on copies or faxes of the POLST document? Must those copies or faxes be printed on paper of a particular color and/or size so as to be identifiable readily? Alternatively, must the original document always be available? If there is a material conflict between the physician's instructions in a patient's POLST and that patient's own earlier written AD, which document governs? What about POLST forms with some sections not completed? In the absence of a totally completed POLST form, should there be a presumption that maximum aggressive medical intervention must be rendered? Finally (although this enumeration of issues does not purport to be comprehensive), there is the matter of portability of the POLST as a patient travels between different jurisdictions. Should a state's legislation or regulations stipulate that providers in that state may (or must) recognize and implement POLSTs validly executed in other jurisdictions, in return for reciprocal respect for its own POLSTs by the other jurisdictions?

Storing and Retrieving POLST Forms

The goal of POLST proponents is to achieve legal recognition of the POLST Paradigm, educating physicians (and any other authorized health care providers) to discuss POLST possibilities with patients and their surrogates and to write a POLST when appropriate and agreed to, and convincing health care providers to implement their patients' valid POLSTs if and when the designated circumstances have materialized. Once that initial goal has been achieved, an additional set of legally tinged policy and practice issues would emerge concerning the storage and retrieval of POLST forms (or AD forms, for that matter [Grant, 2011]) so that they are readily available when needed.

One obvious, straightforward way to handle the storage and retrieval issue is the proverbial "form under the refrigerator magnet" method, with its equally obvious problem of inaccessibility of the document if an emergency situation involving the patient occurs outside of the patient's home. To avoid that frequent, foreseeable operational shortcoming, other options must be considered.

As physicians, hospitals, and other health care facilities move steadily in their documentation of all patient information from paper toward electronic medical records, it is desirable that a patient's electronic medical records include the POLST, if one exists. Making that happen, though, will implicate all of the potential legal issues that might apply to electronic medical records generally (Carter, 2011; Hall, 2010; Hoffman & Podgurski, 2009).

In addition to encouraging the incorporation of POLST forms into individual patients' electronic medical records, states eventually will need to consider establishing, through either legislative or regulatory recognition (and an accompanying appropriation of public funds) or through some type of voluntary arrangement, the creation of a central registry to facilitate both immediate form retrieval and quantitative research on the effectiveness of the POLST mechanism. Several states are at various stages of planning or implementing such central registries, and a taxonomy of associated legal issues has already begun to emerge.

Most fundamentally, should submission of every written POLST form to the central registry be required? Who (the physician, the patient, and/or others) would be mandated to submit? If submission were not required, then who (if anyone) would be permitted to electively submit a POLST to the registry? What immunity from criminal and civil liability or other legal protections for POLST submitters should be embedded in statute or regulation? What penalties, if any, should be imposed on mandated submitters who fail to comply with submission requirements? Who should be granted access to the data compiled within the POLST registry, and under what conditions? What specific procedures should be imposed to assure that the registry complies with the confidentiality and data security requirements of the Health Insurance Portability and Accountability Act (HIPAA), Pub. L. 104–191

(1996), codified at 42 U.S.C. § 1301 et seq. and 42 C.F.R. Part 160 and Part 164, and corresponding state laws regarding personal health information?

Additional challenges arising in the development and implementation of a POLST registry mechanism include quality control processes for maximizing the accuracy (in other words, the correct form for the correct patient) and timeliness of information entered into and stored within the registry. Potential questions pertaining to the civil liability of individuals and/or entities negligently entering data into, or negligently maintaining, a registry need to be anticipated and managed proactively; these questions involve, for instance, determining who would have standing to sue, defining the applicable standards of care to which the parties would be held accountable, and delineating the types and amount of damages for breach of duty.

Policy Issues for Health Care Institutions

Besides attention to the sort of public policy issues outlined above that may need to be addressed through the development of legislation and/or regulation, moving forward in promoting the POLST Paradigm to enhance patient autonomy and improve the quality of medical treatment for the critically ill will require individual health care providers (most notably, hospitals, nursing homes, rehabilitation facilities, and assisted living facilities) to confront several interrelated internal policy questions, ideally in a proactive stance. Specifically, despite a statutory or regulatory overlay, each institutional health care provider will likely retain substantial discretion about how POLSTs written by physicians for the patients they serve are to be reconciled and integrated with existing institutional bylaws and protocols regarding the treatment of critically ill persons.

For example, will the institutional provider presently caring for a particular patient recognize and act upon a POLST signed by a physician who earlier cared for that patient in the community or in another institutional provider, but who does not have active admitting and treating privileges within the current provider? Conversely, will the provider limit its recognition of POLSTs to those that are written by physicians who are members of that provider's medical staff? In a connected vein, even if state law permits non-physicians to write POLSTs in consultation with patients or their surrogates, would any particular institutional health care provider elect to recognize and implement a POLST written by a non-physician?

CONCLUSION

There is good evidence that, for a significant percentage of patients, medical treatment near the EOL substantially deviates from the patient's wishes, even when the patient has timely executed an AD that complies with state law. Improving this situation presents an opportunity for productive inter-professional collaboration in which the contributions of legal, ethical, clinical, and social expertise to the delivery of excellent medical care will be essential.

Case Study

Mrs. P is an 85-year-old, severely demented widow who was admitted to a nursing home from a hospital about 2 years ago. She had been hospitalized for treatment of a hip fracture incurred in an automobile accident when she was still driving. She now also suffers from chronic lymphocytic leukemia and hypertension. Before the hospitalization that led to her present nursing home admission, Mrs. P had lived in an apartment with a cousin with whom she has maintained close contact.

Mrs. P seemed to do well in the nursing home, even though her dementia became progressively more severe. She paces and talks to herself a lot. She periodically needs blood transfusions to control her leukemia. During these transfusions, Mrs. P cannot understand what is happening and sometimes vigorously resists the procedure despite the best efforts of facility staff, who are dismayed by her consternation, to calm her. Before administering the transfusion, it is necessary to give her a sedative and then physically hold her in bed while the procedure is begun. Otherwise, Mrs. P would remove the transfusion apparatus.

A year before the accident that began this chain of events, Mrs. P had gone to a legal aid office and executed advance medical directives. One document was a DPOA for health care naming the cousin as Mrs. P's decision-making agent if necessary. The other document was an instruction directive (living will) stating, among other things, "If I ever become unable to make and express my own treatment wishes, I do not want medical interventions that prolong my life if I have an incurable or irreversible terminal disease."

The nurses are upset when they have to restrain Mrs. P to transfuse her. Mrs. P's physician is apprehensive about potential negative legal consequences if the transfusions are discontinued at this point.

What should the physician and nursing staff do regarding Mrs. P? Are the physician's legal apprehensions well-founded?

- Do Mrs. P's ADs help or hinder the decision-making process?
- What could have been done differently in the drafting of Mrs. P's ADs?
- Would the writing of a POLST have helped with the decision-making process in this case? When, where, and by whom might a POLST have been written?

REFERENCES

Bollman, C. (2010). A dignified death? Don't forget about the physically disabled and those not terminally ill: An analysis of physician-assisted suicide laws. *Southern Illinois University Law Journal, 34*(2), 395–415.

Bravo, G., Dubois, M. F., & Wagneur, B. (2008). Assessing the effectiveness of interventions to promote advance directives among older adults: A systematic review and multi-level analysis. *Social Science and Medicine, 67*(7), 1122–1132.

Cantor, N. L. (2010). No ethical or legal imperative to provide life support to a permanently unaware patient. *American Journal of Bioethics, 10*(3), 58–59.

Carter, B. (2011). Electronic medical records: A prescription for increased medical malpractice liability? *Vanderbilt Journal of Entertainment & Technology Law, 13*(2), 385–406.

Cerminara, K. L., & Bogin, S. M. (2008). A paper about a piece of paper: Regulatory action as the most effective way to promote use of physician orders for life-sustaining treatment. *Journal of Legal Medicine, 29*(3), 479–503.

Cruzan v. Director, Missouri Department of Health, 497 U.S. 261 (1990).

Drum, C. E., White, G., Taitano, G., & Horner-Johnson, W. (2010). The Oregon Death with Dignity Act: Results of a literature review and naturalistic inquiry. *Disability and Health Journal, 3*(1), 3–15.

Fagerlin, A., & Schneider, C. E. (2004). Enough: The failure of the living will. *Hastings Center Report, 34*(2), 30–42.

Florida Statutes Section 765.106, available at http://www.leg.state.fl.us/Statutes/index.cfm?App_mode=Display_Statute&Search_String=&URL=0700-0799/0765/Sections/0765.106.html

Goodman, K. (2007). Ethics schmethics: The Schiavo case and the culture wars. *University of Miami Law Review, 61*(3), 863–870.

Grant, J. K. (2011). The advance directive registry or lockbox: A model proposal and call to legislative action. *Journal of Legislation, 37*(1), 81–107.

Hall, M. A. (2010). Property, privacy, and the pursuit of interconnected electronic medical records. *Iowa Law Review, 95*(2), 631–663.

Halpern, S. D., & Emanuel, E. J. (2012). Advance directives and cost savings: Greater clarity and perpetual confusion. *Archives of Internal Medicine, 172*(3), 266–267.

Hickman, S. E., Nelson, C. A, Perrin, N. A., Moss, A. H., Hammes, B. J., & Tolle, S. W. (2010). A comparison of methods to communicate treatment preferences in nursing facilities: Traditional practices versus the physician orders for life-sustaining treatment program. *Journal of the American Geriatrics Society, 58*(7), 1241–1248.

Hickman, S. E., Sabatino, C., Moss, A. H., & Nester, J. W. (2008). The POLST (Physician Orders for Life-Sustaining Treatment) Paradigm to improve end-of-life care: Potential state legal barriers to implementation. *Journal of Law, Medicine & Ethics, 36*(1), 119–40.

Hoffman, S., & Podgurski, A. (2009). E-Health hazards: Provider liability and electronic health record systems. *Berkeley Technology Law Journal, 24*(4), 1523–1581.

Imhof, S. L., & Kaskie, B. (2008). Promoting a "good death": Determinants of pain-management policies in the United States. *Journal of Health Politics, Policy & Law, 33*(5), 907–941.

Mack, J. W., Cronin, A., Taback, N., Huskamp, H. A., Keating, N. L., Malin, J. L.,… Weeks, J. C. (2012). End-of-life care discussions among patients with advanced cancer. *Annals of Internal Medicine, 156*(3), 204–210.

Matter of Quinlan (1976). 355 A. 2d 647.

Mularski, R. A., Puntillo, K., Varkey, B., Erstad, B. L., Grap, M. J., Gilbert, H. C., Sessler, C. S. (2009). Pain management within the palliative and end-of-life care experience in the ICU. *Chest, 135*(5), 1360–1369.

National Conference of Commissioners on Uniform State Laws. (1993). *Uniform health care decisions act*. Chicago, IL: Author.

Nicholas, L. H., Langa, K. M., Iwashyna, T. J., & Weir, D. R. (2011). Regional variation in the association between advance directives and end-of-life Medicare expenditures. *Journal of the American Medical Association, 306*(13), 1447–1453.

Rosenberg, J. A. (2010). Regrettably unfair: Brooke Aster and other elderly in New York. *Pace Law Review, 30*(3), 1004–1060.

Sabatino, C. P., & Karp, N. (2011). *Improving advanced illness care: The evolution of state POLST programs*. Washington, DC: AARP Public Policy Institute.

Spillers, S. C., & Lamb, B. (2011). Is the POLST model desirable for Florida? *Florida Public Health Review, 8*, 80–90.

Stern, R. C., & Difonzo, J. H. (2009). Stopping for death: Re-framing our perspective on the end of life. *University of Florida Journal of Law and Public Policy, 20*(2), 387–437.

Truog, R. D. (2008–2009). Medical futility. *Georgia State University Law Review, 25*(4), 985–1002.

Truog, R. D., Campbell, M. L., Curtis, J. R., Haas, C. E., Luce, J. M., Rubenfeld, G. D.,…American Academy of Critical Care Medicine (2008). Recommendations for end-of-life care in the intensive care unit: A consensus statement by the American Academy of Critical Care Medicine. *Critical Care Medicine, 36*(3), 953–963.

Tucker, K. L. (2009). The campaign to deny terminally ill patients information and choices at the end of life. *Journal of Legal Medicine, 30*(4), 495–514.

Vacco v. Quill, 521 U.S. 793 (1997).

Washington v. Glucksberg, 521 U.S. 702 (1997).

Westphal, D. M., & McKee, S. A. (2009). End-of-life decision making in the intensive care unit: Physician and nurse perspectives. *American Journal of Medical Quality, 24*(3), 222–228.

White, D. B., & Arnold, R. M. (2011). The evolution of advance directives. *Journal of the American Medical Association, 306*(13), 1485–1486.

Whitmer, M., Hurst, S., Prins, M., Shepard, K., & McVey, D. (2009). Medical futility: A paradigm as old as Hippocrates. *Dimensions of Critical Care Nursing, 28*(2), 67–71.

Wick, J. Y., & Zanny, G. R. (2009). Removing the feeding tube: A procedure with a contentious past. *Consultant Pharmacist, 24*(12), 874–883.

CHAPTER 6

Advance Care Planning and the Problem of Overtreatment

Nancy S. Jecker

Health professionals caring for critically ill and dying patients face daunting challenges. Deciding what treatments to recommend is complex for providers, and choosing among the available options can feel overwhelming for the patient and family. Even more challenging is the task of deciding with patients and families when treatments are no longer benefitting the patient and should be stopped. Shifting the focus of care from battling disease and prolonging life to providing palliative and comfort care often represents a pivotal moment in the trajectory of a patient's disease. Yet this pivotal moment is often poorly timed, coming later than it would ideally come. Providers often put off decisions to discuss withdrawing aggressive interventions, continuing to treat patients against their better judgment.

Overtreatment is a major concern among health professionals, and a source of moral distress. In the 1990s, Solomon et al. (1993) first found evidence that the majority of physicians and nurses were concerned about treatments that were overly burdensome, compared with only a small minority worried about undertreating patients. More recent findings show that overtreatment continues to be a major concern among providers (Sirovich, Woloshin, & Schwartz, 2011). Overtreatment often results in moral distress for health care professionals, especially in situations involving prolonging life in dying patients, inflicting harm, and dehumanizing patients (Wilkinson, 1987).

Overtreatment is driven by a variety of factors, including reimbursement incentives that encourage providers to perform more procedures,

75

while offering little or no remuneration for sitting down and talking with patients about advance care planning (ACP) and health care goals. Providers who reported inadequate time to spend with patients also reported increasing their ordering of tests and treatments, which is likely substituting for explanation and reassurance (Grady, 2011). Limited professional experience, especially the experience of supporting a dying patient, may provide an additional reason for overly aggressive treatment (O'Kane, 2011).

One result of failing to spend time discussing health care values and goals with patients is that when patients become incapacitated, ACP has usually not occurred. In such cases, treatment decisions are left by default to family members, who may have little or no clear direction from the patient about treatment preferences. Family members may feel obligated to "do everything possible," or may think this is the only or best way to demonstrate their love for and devotion to the patient (Schneiderman, Faber-Langendoen, & Jecker, 1994). Under such circumstances, it is easy to see how providers can end up giving patients more treatment than they believe is in the patient's best interest, and continuing with aggressive treatment well past the point of helping the patient. When a well-intentioned family member presses for aggressive interventions, providers often feel reluctant to go against that person's wishes. All of these factors together can conspire to make it more likely that providers find themselves doing more procedures, ordering more tests, and making more referrals than they ideally believe they should (Sirovich et al., 2011).

This chapter addresses the problem of overtreatment by focusing on the importance of ACP as one of many tools needed to improve the care of critically ill patients. I first clarify the definition of overtreatment and why it is a problem for patients, families, and the health care team. Next, I draw attention to two important values that underlie ACP. First, the value of honesty, which supports engaging in critical conversations with patients and families, and coming to terms with the reality of a patient's situation. Second, I consider the fragile thing called hope and explore the relationship between hope and honesty. I argue that, properly understood, hope aligns with honesty, offering the prospect of meaningful closure for patients and families.

THE PROBLEM OF OVERTREATMENT

Giving patients more treatment than is medically appropriate is bad for everyone. It is first and foremost bad for the patient. For example, futile attempts at CPR can result in cracked ribs, hasty intubation can damage the trachea, and iatrogenic effects are associated with many other medical procedures. When patients are heavily sedated or unconscious, overtreatment can be dehumanizing. It treats the patient not as a person we are trying to help, but as a body, or body part, where we are trying to produce an effect:

get the heart beating, make the lungs breath, hydrate and nourish the body. When the justification for treating the patient is to meet the demands of family members who insist on "doing everything," this exploits the patient. In the broadest sense, to exploit someone means to take unfair advantage of them (Wertheimer, 1996). On a Kantian analysis, the problem with exploitation is that it violates the dignity of the patient. Kant held that persons have an inherent worth and dignity, and therefore must always be treated as ends, and never as means only. If the patient is treated solely as a means to realize others' (e.g., a loved one's) ends, this violates the requirement to respect persons.

For family members, overtreating the patient does a different kind of damage. As long as a loved one is aggressively treated, it becomes psychologically more difficult to face and accept the reality of the patient's impending death or deterioration. As Martin (2008) notes, hope plays a framing role in relation to our uptake, interpretation, and deliberative use of information. In this manner, hope can lead families to ignore or downplay the fact that treatment is not producing a desired state of affairs. Health professionals unwittingly encourage such an approach when they continue treatment against all odds based on vague and unsubstantiated ideas, such as the idea that optimism or a "fighting spirit" benefits the patient's health, or is life-prolonging (Schneiderman, 2005). Overtreatment can also create an ethical force all its own, leading those who surround the patient to conclude that the right thing to do is "everything," or that fighting the disease is always the best, most honorable ideal. In the grips of such ideas, holding back and doing less can become exceedingly difficult. For family members, doing less may seem like a failure to love the patient enough, or to meet one's family obligation. Such an ethic ignores the fact that there are other, better ways to care for patients. Health professionals can model more appropriate caring by emphasizing palliative and comfort measures, and by assuring family members that their loved one will not be abandoned.

Finally, overtreatment is bad for providers because it undermines their integrity as health professionals, representing a breach of the duty to advocate on behalf of the patient's best interests. It is not surprising that overtreatment creates "moral distress" for providers, understood as the suffering that occurs when the right course of action is known but cannot be carried out because of institutional or other constraints (Jameton, 1984; Wilkinson, 1987). Moral distress in this situation arises because providers fail to uphold professional standards of care, which require doing what is in the patient's best interest and avoiding harm to the patient.

Moral distress is not just a "bad feeling." It has been demonstrated to be seriously detrimental to the provider's family relationships and professional performance, culminating in a loss of focus, reduced patience, and burnout (McClendon & Buckner, 2007; Meltzer & Huckabay, 2004). It affects physical well-being, self-image, spirituality, personal relationships, and job satisfaction (Elpern, Covert, & Kleinpell, 2005; Silen, Tang, Wadensten, & Ahlstrom, 2008; Wilkinson, 1987). Physical symptoms include heart palpitations, diarrhea, headaches, fatigue, and insomnia (Elpern et al., 2005; Silen et al., 2008; Wilkinson, 1987). A hallmark of moral distress is often an external and uncontrollable circumstance preventing an individual from doing the right thing (Russell, 2012; Webster & Baylis, 2000). One example of an external circumstance frustrating a provider's attempt to withhold or withdraw treatment might be a family member's demands to "do everything." Another might be fear of a legal challenge by family members if treatment is withdrawn or withheld. Situations involving the provision of heroic interventions to attempt to save terminal and dying patients are associated with some of the highest levels of moral distress (Elpern et al., 2005; McClendon & Buckner, 2007). Although nurses are particularly vulnerable, any provider can experience moral distress when overtreating a patient (Russell, 2012).

Understanding overtreatment requires not only specifying why it is a problem, but also how it relates to other problems that arise in the care of critically ill and dying patients. There is a close connection between the problem of overtreatment and the provision of futile interventions. The American Medical Association (1999) describes futile treatment as involving aggressive treatment to sustain life in individuals that are not likely to survive or achieve a successful outcome. So defined, using a futile intervention is a sufficient condition for overtreatment. Futility itself is closely linked to the psychological phenomenon of moral distress discussed above. While moral distress can arise in a variety of contexts, evidence suggests that it is most often preceded by incidents of futile treatment (Mobley, Rady, Verheijde, Patel, & Larson, 2007).

However, medical futility and overtreatment do not mean exactly the same thing. There are instances where overtreatment occurs without the use of futile interventions. For instance, an aggressive but beneficial surgery may qualify as overtreating the patient because a less aggressive and equally beneficial method of treatment, such as medical management, is available. Here, the surgery helps the patient and so it does not meet the definition of medical futility; however, the surgery does count as an instance of overtreatment.

There is a close connection between overtreatment and threats to the professional integrity of health care providers. This arises because physicians and other health care providers have a beneficence-based obligation to do what is best for their patient. When providers feel compelled to act in violation of this professional value, it undermines their professional integrity. "Integrity" in this sense refers to acting in accordance with one's most fundamental moral values and commitments. Williams (1981) describes a person of integrity as someone whose moral dispositions are so deeply ingrained and whose moral principles are so firmly held that the person nearly always acts in accordance with them. Not only is integrity undermined by continuing with inappropriate or futile medical interventions, such interventions can also distract the medical team from focusing on palliative care options that would truly benefit the patient. The failure to do the right thing is compounded when the provider not only uses treatments that are not helping the patient, but also refrains from the aggressive use of beneficial, palliative care options.

Of course, a provider may also overtreat a patient without any loss of integrity or feeling of moral distress. A self-assured provider, for example, may confidently pursue futile interventions because the provider sees the use of high-technology instruments is an end in itself, perhaps enhancing professional self-image and increasing self-esteem. Or, economic incentives may create a climate where it becomes normal for providers to perform procedures with the goal of gaining reimbursement, regardless of whether those procedures actually help the patient or are in the patient's best interests. When an economic model replaces traditional beneficence, providers come to regard fees as the goal of services and may be less likely to feel moral distress about overtreatment because it aligns with this goal. However, in both of these instances, providers are exploiting the patient. Exploitation in this instance builds on the Kantian idea noted above; it involves not only a purely instrumental utilization of a person for one's own advantage, or for the sake of one's own ends, but also a utilization that clearly harms the patient (Buchanan, 1985). In these instances, there is no ethical justification for overtreatment, and the goal of helping the sick should be reinstated.

History of the Problem

The interrelated problems of overtreatment, medical futility, and moral distress have become ubiquitous in health care. It is easy to forget that this was not always the case. For example, if we look back to the 1970s and 1980s, the legal and bioethical cases gaining attention were more likely to involve situations where patients or families asked to *withdraw treatment,* and the health care institution either felt it was improper to do so, or wanted legal immunity first. So, for example, in *In Re Quinlan* (1976), the family requested that treatment be stopped despite misgivings on the part of the institution. Likewise in *Saikewicz* (1977), *Brophy* (1986), *Conroy* (1985), *Cruzan* (1990), and other cases during this time, patients or family members requested that treatment be withheld or withdrawn.

During the decade of the 1990s we witnessed a reversal of this trend. Cases such as *Wanglie* (Angell, 1991; Miles, 1991), *Baby K* (1993), *Baby Ryan* (Kolata, 1994), *Hamilton* (Anonymous, 1994), and *Gilgunn* (1995) dealt with situations in which the patient, or more often the family, wished to *do everything possible* for a loved one. Thus, in Wanglie, the family wished to persist with treatment of an 86-year-old woman in a persistent vegetative state over the objections of doctors at Hennepin County Medical Center who wanted the patient removed from the respirator. Wanglie believed that life should be maintained as long as possible, no matter what the circumstances, and asserted that his wife, Helga Wanglie, shared his belief.

As noted already at the beginning of this chapter, there is ample evidence, beginning with Solomon's study in 1993, that health care professionals are concerned that the treatments they provide to patients at the end of life (EOL) are overly burdensome and that they are practicing more aggressively than they should. This is bad for patients and families, and creates moral distress among providers.

HONESTY AND HOPE

Falsehood is so easy, truth so difficult.

George Eliot, *Adam Bede*

How should we address the problem of overtreatment? One response to patient and family requests for treatment that is futile or falls outside the parameters of professional standards is to abide by such requests. We could simply accede to demands and give patients and families what they ask for. In support of this approach it could be said that patients and families, not health professionals, are on the receiving end of care; they must live through the experience of overly burdensome care and futile treatment. If there is meaning and value in this struggle, then why should it be denied to them? One way of understanding such a strategy might be that pursuing even unlikely and statistically small life extensions can have value for patients and families who place value on both current life and on hope, where "hope" is defined as the *current* consumption of the prospect of future survival (Menzel, 2011). Thus, one possible justification for overtreating patients is that it provides patients and families the benefit of hope.

Another argument in support of such an approach is that it is more humane and compassionate to let patients retain false beliefs if such beliefs offer comfort. According to this approach, fidelity to truth is misplaced at the EOL. The physician's highest duty is not to disclose the unvarnished truth, but rather to offer patients and families solace in a situation that is otherwise grim. Arguing along these lines, Lantos and Meadow (2011) urge physicians to resuscitate so-called slow codes. They argue that physicians should give the impression of aggressive resuscitative efforts when patients or families request this, even though no genuine effort need be made. In support of such an approach, they claim it is "kinder and gentler" because it signals caring, avoids confrontation, and nurtures hope. In this manner, patients can be spared the painful truth for as long as possible.

Yet this approach belies the true meaning of hope. "Hope" does not mean the same thing as refusing to give up. After all, consider the case where a person refuses to give up and insists on making her best effort, without having any hope that such efforts will bear fruit or be successful (Menzel, 2011). For example, a provider may attempt CPR, fully expecting that it will fail to resuscitate the patient. Here, the provider is refusing to give up, despite having no hope. Under these circumstances, "current consumption of the prospect of future survival" does not come into play as an added benefit of overtreating. Moreover, a hope that interferes with the hopeful person's engagement with and ability to pursue her own values is best thought of as "false hope" (Groopman, 2003). Like moral distress, false hope is at odds with a person's underlying thoughts and feelings. Like self-deception, it encourages a person to look away from reality and construct an alternative story.

A more promising response to patients' or families' requests for inappropriate treatment is to begin early on a process of encouraging honesty and frank communication about the goals of treatment and the range of medically appropriate treatment choices. The American Medical Association, Council on Ethical and Judicial Affairs recommends such an approach. The council instructs physicians to routinely engage patients in ACP regardless of their health status or diagnosis; assist patients with thinking about their values, perspectives on quality of life, and goals if faced with a life-threatening illness or injury; and encourage patients to make their views known to family members and intimates (American Medical Association, 2010). The council notes that outcomes in EOL care are strongly related to ACP, especially the quality of communication between clinicians and patients. While the primary value supporting ACP is respect for patient self-determination, the practical outcome of this approach is to ease burdens on family members and other surrogate decision makers by providing guidance for health care decisions. Another practical effect of ACP can be to uphold the value of honesty in facing medicine's limits, and the limits of life and quality of life. Thus, ACP done well helps to prevent patients from receiving care they do not desire, and helps to prevent denials of medically appropriate care they would want at the EOL. *Value of ACP*

Despite these advantages, it may feel easier in the short run to put off distressing moments for another day. After all, continuing to pursue aggressive treatments, however burdensome, often requires making no change. Thus, everyone may be tempted to think that no decision has been made. By contrast, being truthful about a patient's poor prognosis may require changing the course of treatment, and this in turn may create discomfort. For providers, honesty in the face of a patient's impending death or deterioration may feel like an admission of failure. For family members, being truthful about a patient's situation may require grappling with the loss of a loved one, and of a relationship central to one's life and identity. For patients, honesty may require confronting death and the dying process.

Yet, despite the difficulty of facing such choices, dealing honestly with patients is an ethical requirement. This requirement is based primarily on the more fundamental idea of respect for patient autonomy. The ethical principle of autonomy holds that patients should be allowed to be self-determining and self-governing when they are able. This means not only that health care providers should not stand in the way of what a competent patient wants to do, they should also work to facilitate patient autonomy by providing patients with the information required to make an informed health care decision. The American Medical Association, Council on Ethical and Judicial Affairs recognizes veracity, a commitment to truth and accuracy, as one of the fundamental elements of the patient–physician relationship, and acknowledges the patient's right both to receive information from physicians and to discuss the benefits, risks, and costs of appropriate treatment alternatives (American Medical Association Council on Ethical and Judicial Affairs, 1999). Upholding patient autonomy requires not only comprehensive, accurate, and objective transmission of information to the patient, it also demands a process of communication and ACP that fosters the patient's understanding and future goals (Beauchamp & Childress, 2008). An important part of ACP is encouraging patients to use advance directives (ADs) to formally convey their wishes about medical decisions in the event that they become incapacitated in the future and are unable to make their own health care decisions. Tools, such as the living will and durable power of attorney (DPOA) for health care, are important means for patients to ensure that their values are upheld. *Mom*

ADs have recently come under fire on a number of grounds. Critics argue that people cannot accurately predict what medical treatments they would want in the future, either because they do not have sufficient knowledge and experience to know, or because they have false preconceptions or misunderstandings about what is at stake. For example, the findings of the Study to Understand Prognoses and Preferences for Outcomes and Risks of Treatment (SUPPORT Principal Investigators, 1995) demonstrated that people who thought they would not want certain treatments change their minds when actually faced with a decision to decline treatment and die. Individuals have also been shown to overestimate the impact that having a specific disability will have on their lives, for example, discounting the many positive aspects of their lives that would remain and would be unaffected by the disability (Fried, Bradley, & O'Leary, 2006; Loewenstein, 2005; Loewenstein & Schkade, 1999; Ubel, 2006). Yet, proponents of ADs note that such concerns do not show that ADs should be dispensed with, but show instead the need for more education and support on the part of health care professionals. Some of the limitations of ADs arise because these tools may be narrowly constructed, static documents that leave little room for individuals to fully explore and express their wishes. Recent proposals provide promising avenues for addressing these and related concerns (Levi & Green, 2010). All things considered, it is better for patients to make the best decision they can make on behalf of their future selves, with as much support as possible, rather than not weighing in at all on future health care choices. As part of a larger process of ACP, ADs can help people grow in their understanding of what is important to them in their life, and in the process of their life's ending.

Despite acknowledging the value of ACP, it has been argued that tools such as ADs are of limited practical value because only a small percentage of people, even among those with life-threatening illness, ever avail themselves of these tools (Schneiderman, Pearlman, Kaplan, Anderson, & Rosenberg, 1992). In response, it can be said that the use of ADs, and the broader practice of ACP, are unlikely to become a routine part of health care without structural changes in the organization of health care and health care reimbursement. For example, until providers are reimbursed for offering assistance with ACP, rather than expected to do so without compensation, the practice is unlikely to become widespread. This was the idea behind a proposed section of the 2010 national health care reform legislation (the Patient Protection and Affordable Care Act [PPACA]), entitled "Advance Care Planning Consultation." This section called for reimbursement for a clinician visit in which the clinician explained ACP, living wills, the role of a health care proxy, and orders regarding life-sustaining treatments. Unfortunately, this section of PPACA was distorted by politicians and commentators into a mandate by which older and disabled individuals would be forced to forego life-sustaining treatment (Tinetti, 2012). Thus, despite the fact that seriously ill patients are at risk for receiving highly burdensome care with limited or no benefit, there was little public support for PPACA's ACP proposal. The fact that politicians and the media were able to mislead large segments of the public into equating ACP with "death panels" designed to deny patients necessary treatment is instructive. It suggests the public is fearful that they will receive too little, not too much, care (Fried & Drickamer, 2010).

In addition to patient fears about being denied medically needed treatments, substantial proportions of patients may not want to plan for their EOL care, believing that it is better to take things one day at a time, that it is impossible to plan the future, or simply finding it too difficult to contemplate serious illness and death (Fried & Drickamer, 2010). This suggests that even if reimbursement structures were amended to encourage ACP, providers will continue to encounter obstacles. Inevitably, some patients and families will face medical choices for which they have not prepared. To increase utilization of ACP requires health care facilities and communities to create a climate that encourages critical conversations among providers and patients so that patients feel empowered, rather than threatened by, the prospect of ACP. Providers need to educate patients about using ACP as a tool to strengthen their self-determination and support choices among a range of medically reasonable alternatives (Tulsky, 2005).

Realizing these values requires humility on the part of physicians, as well as heightened awareness of the hidden messages their statements can have for patients and families. Solomon (1993) conducted in-depth interviews with 20 physicians identified as caring for the highest proportion of critically and terminally ill patients at a university-affiliated teaching hospital, and described empirically how physicians think and talk about the concept of futility with their patients. The physicians reported feeling extreme distress, including anger, resentment, and uncertainty, when asked to provide what they considered to be futile treatments. Many felt that insistence by families on the provision of treatment was "both a burden on patients and an abrogation of the physician's responsibility to make professional judgments" (Solomon, 1993, p. 232). Solomon also found that "part of their angst comes not simply from the pressure to provide burdensome treatment, but also from an inability to find the right language and conceptual framework for talking about the problem with patients and families" (Solomon, 1993, p. 232). Physicians used the concept of futility in conversations with patients both to denote medical efficacy and to render evaluative quality-of-life judgments, but appeared unaware of the evaluative component. Thus, we generally distinguish between a physiological effect, on the one hand, and a *benefit* to the patient, on the other hand. A ventilator, for instance, may produce a physiological effect on the patient's body, such as keeping the lungs breathing, yet still be futile because it does not benefit the patient. When the focus is exclusively on producing effects, rather than benefits, providers can easily miss opportunities to engage in values discussions with patients and families. According to Solomon (1993), "All but one physician seemed unaware of the double meaning they ascribed to the word [futility]" (p. 233). Physicians must be prepared to be open and honest about their personal and professional values, even when these diverge from the patient's or family's. They also must be prepared to accept whatever reasonable option the patient or family decides upon. Physicians should refer patients to appropriate providers when requested treatments violate their personal values. Likewise, when a provider regards a treatment as clearly futile, but there is a lack of professional consensus or no clear standard of care, a referral should also be made to a provider willing to offer the treatment (Schneiderman & Jecker, 2011).

DEATH AND DYING

Death, the most awful of evils, is nothing to us, seeing that, when we are, death is not come, and, when death is come, we are not.

Epicurus, *The Enchiridion*

Another important reason that ACP is not widespread is our general reticence to talk about death. Too often, clinicians are reluctant to use the words "death" or "dying," even when caring for terminally and critically ill patients. This tacit omission may lead patients and families to assume that all is well or that things are at least stable for the time being. Stambovsky (2011) notes that "loath to hobble any momentum of hope, we intimate the possibility of recovery, which may compel families to insist upon continuing treatments" (p. 197). In this way, providers can unwittingly lead patients along corridors of hope and make their inevitable encounter with a loved one's deterioration and death all the more difficult. By contrast, when the requirements of honesty are fully met, patients and families have the opportunity to face their situation, show courage, and take comfort in being able to trust and rely on their providers. Becoming "master clinicians," able to facilitate critical conversations with patients and families, is especially challenging in a culture that shuns talking about death (Back, Arnold, & Tulsky, 2009).

Even while we intellectually recognize that death is the natural and inevitable outcome of every life, many of us at the same time assume that a patient's death is an evil, to be avoided at all costs. The idea that death is always something we should resist is in fact enshrined in statutes in a handful of states, which allow persons completing a "directive to physicians" to request that every possible treatment be employed in the event they become incapacitated, irrespective of whether the treatment is beneficial or futile. For example, in Nevada a patient can direct, "I desire that my life be prolonged to the greatest extent possible, without regard to my condition, the chances I have for recovery or long-term survival, or the costs of the procedures" (Nevada Revised Statue, 1993). The practical effect of such laws can be to discourage health professionals seeking to practice responsible medicine. As noted already, although physicians should accept whatever reasonable option the patient chooses and should refer to another provider when appropriate, there will be instances where a patient's preferences can be ethically overridden. Thus, when a treatment is clearly futile based on empirical evidence and widespread professional consensus, it is ethically permissible to withhold or withdraw treatment (Schneiderman & Jecker, 2011). In such cases, there may be no reasonable prospect of finding a willing alternate provider for the disputed treatment.

Is there any philosophical basis for our tendency to regard death as an evil, to be avoided at all costs? As Epicurus noted long ago: death cannot possibly harm the person who dies, because once we die, whatever happens no longer causes us to suffer. In other words, death leaves us immune to future harm. Likewise, philosophers, such as Lucretius, have pointed out that it is irrational to think of death as bad because we do not think that the nonexistence preceding our births was bad. When we compare the time before we existed to a future time when we are dead and no longer exist, we see that the two are mirror images, alike in all respects.

Although death itself is not an evil to the one who dies, contemplating our future nonexistence and preparing for the dying process is a formidable challenge to the living. Yet this challenge brings rewards, namely: the prospect of dying well and living more fully. Since we know that death, that closing of the circle, is our fate, we have every reason to treat it with the same foresight and planning that we treat the rest of our lives. Just as the unexamined life is not worth living, the unexamined death can feel empty and meaningless to the dying person. Understood as a distinctively human good, death contemplation and planning can be a counterpoise to hubris. Rather than feeling invincible and overconfident about our place in the universe, contemplating mortality reminds us that our human life is temporary and will end. Preparing for this ending can create perspective. It furnishes an opportunity to reflect on our life's value and on the goods and values that will outlast us.

REFERENCES

American Medical Association. (1999). Medical futility in end-of-life care: Report of the Council on Ethical and Judicial Affairs. *Journal of the American Medical Association, 281*(10), 937–941.

American Medical Association. (2010). *Advance care planning: Report of the Council on Ethical and Judicial Affairs.* Retrieved from http://www.ama-assn.org/resources/doc/ethics/ceja-4i10.pdf. Accessed April 4, 2012.

American Medical Association Council on Ethical and Judicial Affairs. (1990). Fundamental elements of the patient-physician relationship. *JAMA, 262,* 3/33.

Angell, M. (1991). The case of Helga Wanglie. *New England Journal of Medicine, 325,* 311–312.

Anonymous. (1994, February 12). Hospital fights parents' wish to keep life support for a "brain dead" child. *New York Times.*

In the Matter of Baby K (1994). 16 F.3d 590 (4th Cir.).

Back, A., Arnold, R., & Tulsky, J. (2009). *Mastering communication with seriously ill patients: Balancing honesty with empathy and hope.* New York, NY: Oxford University Press.

Beauchamp T., & Childress, J. (2008). *Principles of biomedical ethics* (6th ed.). New York, NY: Oxford University Press.

Brophy v. New England Sinai Hospital, Inc. (1986) 398 Mass. 417.

Buchanan, A. (1985). *Ethics, efficiency, and the market.* Totowa, NJ: Rowman and Allanheld.

Cruzan v. Director, Missouri Department of Health, 497 US 261, 110 S Ct. 2841 (1990).

Durable power of attorney for health care (1993). *Nev. Rev. Sta. Ann, 499,* 800.

Elpern, E. H., Covert, B., & Kleinpell, R. (2005). Moral distress of staff nurses in a medical intensive care unit. *American Journal of Critical Care, 14*(6), 523–530.

Fried, T. R., Bradley, E. H., & O'Leary, J. (2006). Changes in prognostic awareness among seriously ill older persons and their caregivers. *Journal of Palliative Medicine, 9*(1), 61–69.

Fried, T. R., & Drickamer, M. (2010). Garnering support for advance care planning. *Journal of the American Medical Association, 303*(3), 269–270.

Gilgunn v. Massachusetts General Hospital, (1995), No. 92–4820, Mass Super Ct Civ Action Suffolk Co. April 22, 1995.

Grady, D. (2011). Reasons for overtreatment. *Archives of Internal Medicine, 171*(17), 1586–1586.

Groopman, J. (2003). *The anatomy of hope*. New York, NY: Random House.

In Re Quinlan, 70 N. J. 10, 355 *A. 2d* 647 (1976).

Jameton, D. (1984). *Nursing practice: The ethical issues*. Englewood Cliffs, NJ: Prentice Hall.

Kolata, G. (1994, December 27). Battle over a baby's future raises hard ethical issues. *New York Times*, A1.

Lantos, J. D., & Meadow, W. L. (2011). Should the "slow code" be resuscitated? *American Journal of Bioethics, 11*(11), 8–12.

Levi, B. H., & Green, M. J. (2010). Too soon to give up: Re-examining the value of advance directives. *American Journal of Bioethics, 10*(4), 3–22.

Loewenstein, G. (2005). Projection bias in medical decision making. *Medical Decision Making, 25*(1), 96–105.

Loewenstein, G., & Schkade, D. (1999). Wouldn't it be nice? Predicting future feelings. In D. Kahneman, E. Diener, & N. Schwartz (Eds.), *Well-being: The foundations of hedonic psychology* (pp. 85–105). New York, NY: Russell Sage.

Martin, A. M. (2008). Hope and exploitation. *Hastings Center Report, 38*(5), 49–55.

Matter of Conroy (1983) 457 A.2d 1232 *N.J. Super. Ct*. Feb 02, 1983, revised, 486 *A. 2d* 1209 N.J. Jan 17, 1985.

McClendon, H., & Buckner, E. B. (2007). Distressing situations in the intensive care unit. *Dimensions of Critical Care Nursing, 26*(5), 199–206.

Meltzer, L. S., & Huckabay, L. M. (2004). Critical care nurses' perceptions of futile care and its effect on burnout. *American Journal of Critical Care, 13*(3), 202–208.

Menzel, P. T. (2011). The value of life at the end of life: a critical assessment of hope and other factors. *Journal of Law, Medicine, and Ethics, 39*(2), 215–223.

Miles, S. (1991). Informed demand for "Non-beneficial" medical treatment. *New England Journal of Medicine, 325*, 312–315.

Mobley, M. J., Rady, M. Y., Verheijde, J. L., Patel, B., & Larson, J. S. (2007). The relationship between moral distress and perception of futile care in the critical care unit. *Intensive and Critical Care Nursing, 23*, 256–263.

O'Kane, M. (2011). Peace at the end. *Archives of Internal Medicine, 171*(17), 1527–1527.

Russell, A. (2012). Moral distress in neuroscience nursing: An evolutionary concept analysis. *Journal of Neuroscience Nursing, 44*(1), 15–24.

Schneiderman, L. J. (2005). The perils of hope. *Cambridge Quarterly of Healthcare Ethics, 14*, 235–239.

Schneiderman, L. J., Faber-Langendoen, K., & Jecker, N. S. (1994). Beyond futility to an ethic of care. *American Journal of Medicine, 96*, 110–114.

Schneiderman, L. J., & Jecker, N. S. (2011). *Wrong medicine: doctors, patients, and futile treatment* (2nd ed.). Baltimore, MD: Johns Hopkins University Press.

Schneiderman, L. J., Pearlman, R. A., Kaplan, R. M., Anderson, J. P., & Rosenberg, E. M. (1992). Relationship of general advance directive instructions to specific life-sustaining treatment preferences in patients with serious illness. *Archives of Internal Medicine, 152*, 2114–2122.

Silen, M., Tang, P. F., Wadensten, B., & Ahlstrom, G. (2008). Workplace distress and ethical dilemmas in neuroscience nursing. *Journal of Neuroscience Nursing, 40*(4), 222–231.

Sirovich, B. E., Woloshin, S., & Schwartz, L. M. (2011). Too little? Too much? Primary care physicians views on U.S. health care: A brief report. *Archives of Internal Medicine, 171*(17), 1582–1585.

Solomon, M. Z., O'Donnell, L., Jennings, B., Guilfoy, V., Wolf, S. M., Nolan, K., ... Donnelley, S., (1993). Decisions near the end of life: Professional views on life-sustaining treatments. *American Journal of Public Health, 83*(1), 14–23.

Solomon, M. Z. (1993). How physicians talk about futility: Making words mean too many things. *Journal of Law, Medicine, and Ethics, 21*, 231–237.

Stambovsky, M. (2011). A personal reflection: The slippery slope of hope. *Dimensions of Critical Care Nursing, 30*(4), 196–197.

Superintendent of Belchertown State School & another v. Joseph Saikewicz (1977) 373 Mass. 728.

SUPPORT Principal Investigators. (1995). A Controlled Trial to Understand Prognoses and Preferences for Outcomes and Risks of Treatment (SUPPORT). *Journal of the American Medical Association, 274*, 1591–1598.

Tinetti, M. E. (2012). The retreat from advance care planning. *Journal of the American Medical Association, 307*(9), 915–916.

Tulsky, J. A. (2005). Beyond advance directives: Importance of communication skills at the end of life. *Journal of the American Medical Association, 294*(3), 359–366.

Ubel, P. A. (2006). *You're stronger than you think.* New York, NY: McGraw Hill.

Webster, G. C., & Baylis, F. (2000). Moral residue. In S. B. Rubin & L. Zoloth (Eds.), *Margin of error: The ethics of mistakes in the practice of medicine* (pp. 217–232). Hagerstown, MD: University Publishing Group.

Wertheimer, A. (1996). *Exploitation.* Princeton, NJ: Princeton University Press.

Wilkinson, J. M. (1987). Moral distress in nursing practice: Experience and effect. *Nursing Forum, 23*(1), 16–29.

William, B. (1981). Utilitarianism and moral self-indulgence. In B. Williams (Ed.), *Moral luck* (pp. 40–53). Cambridge, UK: Cambridge University Press.

CHAPTER 7

Religion, Spirituality, and Culture in Advance Care Planning

Beverly Lunsford

A STORY OF BELIEF AND END-OF-LIFE CARE DECISION MAKING

Henry and his wife, Virginia, had just moved into a retirement village in the same area as their son, Richard, and his family. Each of them had multiple health problems and Virginia was getting frail. Henry was hospitalized suddenly for a severe sinus infection and became unconscious within 48 hours. Virginia and Richard agreed for the doctors to intubate Henry just to help his breathing as the infection resolved. The other son, John, from Washington State, and their daughter, Vicki, from Vermont, came to visit their father, but when the doctors indicated it would be a while until their father's infection was controlled and he regained consciousness, they decided to go back home and return when he was better.

However, 10 days later, Henry was still unconscious and on a ventilator. The doctors wanted to insert a "peg tube" so he could get nutrition, as Henry had been unconscious and unable to eat during his hospital stay. At first, Virginia thought this was a good idea, again, to get Henry through this rough time. But the night before the surgery, she had the distinct sense that she should not sign the consent for surgery; she didn't think Henry would want this. It didn't seem to her that Henry was getting better. She wasn't even sure he had known her or responded to her presence during the past 5 days. She and Henry had never spoken about

(continued)

(continued)

what to do in this type of situation. While they knew they were getting older, they had not anticipated anything like this.

John and Vicki couldn't believe their mother would even consider not giving their father the nutrition that he needed to survive. They were sure their father would want to live. Besides, John was a devout Christian and was certain that not providing nutrition is contrary to the Church's teaching.

Virginia's pastor and Richard were with her that morning as she approached her husband's bed to try to discern what to do. The pastor had listened patiently to each of them as they expressed uncertainty as to the right thing to do. The pastor had also waited with them through the last 10 days that had been a roller coaster experience, with each doctor providing conflicting messages each day: "His blood gases are better today"; "His hemoglobin is dropping today"; "The infection seems to be improving today"; "He shows no signs of regaining consciousness." Richard knew his father had not shown any signs of life during the past week. His father had been a happy and active person all his life, and he would not want to lie here like this. The pastor helped them review the surgeon's report that stated Henry's condition was grave and he might not survive the surgery, and encouraged them that God is with them and hears their pain and uncertainty. The pastor arranged a conference call with Vicki and John, who were still upset that this would violate Church law, and told them their father couldn't survive without surgery. The palliative care team met with them to discuss the events of the past 10 days, reviewed the relevant medical information, and the continued deterioration in Henry's condition. There was considerable uncertainty that Henry would survive surgery.

After several hours of discussion and reflection, Virginia did not sign the consent for surgery, as she didn't want Henry to experience any additional pain or suffering. The palliative care team decided to give him what nutrition they could through IV feedings. They cared for Henry and he died peacefully 3 days later, never regaining consciousness.

This story illustrates some of the very difficult issues that families face when the medical prognosis is uncertain, family members disagree, religious teaching is interpreted differently by family members, and the very sick family member has not engaged in advance care planning (ACP). This chapter examines the importance of spirituality with serious, life-threatening illness and impending death, as well as how spirituality and religion may inform decision making around issues of medical treatment and intravenous feeding, ACP, and supportive care.

THE IMPORTANCE OF RELIGION AND SPIRITUALITY
IN ADVANCE CARE PLANNING

In considering how much religious and spiritual beliefs impact health care decision making and ACP, it is important to examine a recent Gallup Poll that indicates 92% of respondents ($N = 1,018$ adults nationwide) in the United States believe in God (Gallup Poll, 2011). In addition, 58% ($N = 2,973$ adults nationwide) consider religion to be very important in their lives, and more than 40% of adults in the United States attend religious services weekly (Pew Research Center, 2012). These high percentages indicate that there is good reason to consider how religious and spiritual needs impact ACP.

Research in health care practices provides evidence to indicate many people also believe there is value in health care professionals addressing spiritual issues. Surveys of people receiving health care have found that more than two-thirds of inpatients (e.g., King & Bushwick, 1994) and outpatients (e.g., Ehman Ott, Short, Ciampa, & Hansen-Flaschen, 1999; McCord et al., 2004) would like their physicians to ask about their spiritual beliefs and/or needs in at least some circumstances. However, even when people may be willing to discuss ACP and spirituality with health care professionals, research indicates the provider must initiate the conversation (Pautex, Herrmann, & Zulian, 2008). Moreover, the ability to talk with health care professionals about health care decisions becomes increasingly important as illnesses progress and become more complex. Thus, it is imperative that medical, nursing, social work, chaplain and other healthcare professionals are able to help patients and their families explore the religious and spiritual dimensions that guide their health care decision making and ACP.

As medical, nursing, social work, and chaplaincy professionals have worked to improve palliative and end-of-life (EOL) care, there has been increasing attention to the importance of spiritual and religious dimensions of individuals. In more recent medical literature, Sulmasy (2002) described the biopsychosocial-spiritual model for comprehensive medical care of individuals and families, which recognizes that people experience health and illness in many dimensions, including religious and spiritual domains (also see Katerndahl, 2008).

DISCUSSING RELIGIOUS AND SPIRITUAL ASPECTS OF
ADVANCE CARE PLANNING

While many health care professionals may recognize religion and spirituality as important, several reasons have been identified to explain why health care professionals may not provide spiritual care to patients and their loved ones. First, professional caregivers do not feel they have the training, knowledge, or skills to be able to talk with patients and their families about these topics (Balboni et al., 2010; Brush & Daly, 2000; Draper & McSherry, 2002).

Another reason is that professional caregivers anticipate that patients and their loved ones may interpret conversations about spiritual matters as proselytizing, or conversely, that the patient or members of the patient's support network may try to proselytize them.

Many health care professionals do not talk with those for whom they provide care about spiritual matters because they, like many people (including patients and their loved ones), view spiritual care as the realm of clergy, pastors, and other spiritual leaders. Indeed, the topics of religion and spirituality are widely discussed among theologians. However, being a theologian or member of the clergy is not a requirement for supporting patients and their loved ones as they integrate religion and spirituality into health care decision making and ACP. It is important for all professional caregivers to see their role as members of a team providing care that includes spiritual care. This may be likened to the management of pain for a person with cancer. All members of the health care team and family play a role in relieving pain, for example, recognition and reporting, ordering medication, providing medications and comfort care, or addressing spiritual concerns that may cause or exacerbate physical symptoms and pain.

Spiritual concerns are part of the series of health concerns to be addressed.

DEFINING RELIGION AND SPIRITUALITY

Many people use the concepts of religion and spirituality interchangeably, but while they are related, they are not the same. Some people find a spiritual home in religion, either organized (as part of a faith community) or on a very private, personal level as a set of beliefs that may or may not draw from one or more religious traditions. Other people do not consider themselves religious; instead, they may experience a sense of awe and reverence when they experience nature, immerse themselves in solitude, be transported by music or other creative arts, or come face to face with the edges of life as we know it, perhaps by encountering birth or death.

Two broad working definitions can help distinguish religion and spirituality. Religion provides a specific set of beliefs, values, and traditions. Religion also gives specific meaning to events and experiences in life, such as the origins of life or the existence of an afterlife. Religion is also understood as a concept that gives expression to the sense of the extraordinary, describes the concept of transcendence, and provides a language in which to speak of spiritual things.

Spirituality is a broader concept that has to do with the need of all people to find ultimate meaning in life and to confront the mysteries of life and death. A definition of spirituality from an interprofessional consensus conference (Puchalski et al., 2009) is that spirituality is the aspect of humanity that refers to the way individuals seek and express meaning and purpose

Religion vs. Spirituality

and the way they experience their connectedness to the moment as well as self, others, nature, and the significant or sacred.

This for the explanation, meaning, and purpose takes a unique form that is integral to each individual (though not always conscious). It may be expressed in many different ways including religious practices, philosophical commitment or scientific ideal, art, music, literature, a connection to nature, and relationships with family and/or community. The search for meaning and purpose has also been described as a universal characteristic that is part of what makes us human. *Sanders' 5 Dimensions*

Sanders (2002) identified five dimensions of spirituality that lend a *of* greater understanding to the multiple facets of this concept. The first dimension of spirituality is meaning, which can include that which provides sig- *Spirit-* nificance in one's life, those aspects that offer purpose, and/or the way one *uality* makes sense of the world. The second dimension is value, which includes one's beliefs and standards; one's sense of truth; and beauty and worth of thought, object, or behavior. Transcendence is the third common aspect across various definitions of spirituality and it is one's sense of awareness of dimensions beyond one's self. The next dimension is that of connectedness, for example, the feeling of relationship with self, others, God/higher power, and even the environment (or nature). The final dimension is that of always becoming. This involves the sense of continued unfolding of life, which demands reflection and experience. It includes a sense of who one is and how one knows. These five dimensions help to illustrate the broad nature of spirituality, which can include religious expression, relationships, music, art and nature, and/or other belief systems.

Peters (2010) identifies five tasks of religion and spirituality that underscore the importance of spirituality in the well-being of human beings. The tasks include: (a) confronting one's finitude and vulnerability; (b) uncovering meaning, value, and dignity in illness and death; (c) developing meaning, purpose, and connectedness to others; (d) seeking faith, hope, love, and forgiveness in the midst of fear and despair; and (e) engendering serenity and transcendence, which can buffer stress. These tasks also illustrate the importance of the spiritual for health care decision making and ACP. The tasks of confronting one's finitude and vulnerability, as well as seeking hope in the midst of fear and despair, can be catalysts for expressing one's wishes in ACP. Conversely, if one is not able to consider the possibility of dying, it precludes the desire to express one's wishes and plan for EOL.

One must consider her own mortality in order to plan for her end of life.

SPIRITUAL ASSESSMENT AND ADVANCE CARE PLANNING

One way to approach ACP is within the context of a holistic health assessment that includes a spiritual assessment (Chrash, Mulich, & Patton, 2011). As part of the spiritual assessment, the health care professional can explore specific concerns about the distinction between prolonging life versus prolonging death, and sanctity versus quality of life. In addition, a spiritual assessment would address specific religious concerns about initiating and terminating life-support technologies and appropriate medication to relieve suffering, while maintaining awareness of hastening, or not hastening, death.

In many respects, ACP provides the space and time to address spiritual and existential aspects experienced during serious, life-threatening illness and death. When encouraged to talk about what the illness means to them, the sick individual and/or their loved ones may wonder why this is happening to them. These questions can lead to existential exploration of what gives the individual meaning and purpose in spite of the presence of disease. Providing space for existential discussions can help the health care professional support the patient and loved ones in discovering sources of hope, as well as identifying more supportive ways to journey with the patient and their significant persons during worsening illness and eventual death. The process of ACP can provide opportunities for the sick person to discuss more intimate matters with family and friends. It can be very helpful for professional caregivers to help patients and their loved ones to explore the value of their shared lives, feelings of love, exchanges of forgiveness for real or imagined events, and disclosing previously unspoken truths.

One aspect of the spiritual dimension is that of "always becoming," and ACP can provide the opportunity to express desires for completing unfinished business or goals, doing or seeing particular events or places before dying, as well as desires for presence and rituals around dying. These discussions can provide the individual and his or her family a much-needed sense of control and possibility for continued growth and hope.

The ability to contemplate the reality of eventual death can also enable people to live life more fully in the present. Religious, spiritual, and philosophical teachings remind us that we cannot live life to its fullest unless we have confronted the possibility of our dying. Watson (2011) expresses this concept in observing, "The end (conclusion) of life leads us to think about the end (purpose) of life" (p. 45). This opportunity for growth can enhance the person's coping and resilience for facing the unknown as the illness worsens.

THE MEETING OF SPIRITUALITY, RELIGION, AND CULTURE

The dimensions of spirituality, religion, and culture may overlap within the individual, making culture, religion, and spiritual beliefs difficult to distinguish or separate. Culture may be described as the various ways of living and thinking that are developed and shared by a particular group of people

(Leininger, 1980). Spirituality can be shaped entirely by culture, determined by life experiences unrelated to culture, or influenced by both culture and personal experience (Martsolf, 1997). Indeed religion, spirituality, and culture can be deeply intertwined concepts.

The concept of cultural humility can be helpful in knowing how to approach other people about their beliefs, values, and personal preferences (Tervalon & Murray-Garcia, 1998). Cultural humility is in contrast to cultural competence, which suggests one can learn the patient's culture (or fully understand someone else's spirituality), as opposed to considering the effect of the health care provider's worldview and focusing on the particular beliefs and behaviors of certain groups of people. Rather, one can develop a greater self-awareness of one's own assumptions and beliefs that impact understanding and goal setting in working with individuals in health care encounters. Greater self-awareness on behalf of professional care providers facilitates the ability to develop a respectful partnership for person-centered interviewing, and exploring the patient's and their loved one's priorities, goals, and capacities, which are unique to each individual. Further, cultural humility enables the health care professional to negotiate each person's perspective to arrive at a consensus for goals of care and an agreeable plan of action, including developing an advance care plan.

CROSS-CULTURAL INFLUENCES AND ADVANCE CARE PLANNING

Spiritual values and beliefs are deeply intertwined with cultural influences. Thus, they impact health care decision making and ACP in several ways, including:

1. Historical cross-cultural abuses and prejudices of disadvantaged minority groups' health care;
2. Cultural biases about "Western" values and medicine by both health care professionals and the individuals served;
3. Requests for nondisclosure of health care information to the person who is ill;
4. Different cultural and spiritual values regarding what constitutes life, treatment withdrawal, place of death, and manner of death; and
5. Misunderstanding about rituals at EOL, as well as misunderstandings that may arise from cultural and language differences.

The above five elements may help to explain the lower rates for completing advance directives among individuals from several ethnic backgrounds, including Asians, Hispanics, and African Americans (Searight & Gafford, 2005). The first element listed above indicates there may be a general distrust

[handwritten: common — advance directives - more in whites]

of the U.S. health care system due to historical prejudices and discrimination, along with perceived and real disparities in access to care.

CONFLICTS WITH "WESTERN" MEDICAL SYSTEM VALUES

The second element refers to the locus of health care decision making in the United States that is widely influenced by Western medical values placing an emphasis on autonomy and individualism. Emphasis on the highly valued principle of autonomy and the Western value of physician beneficence, which may still be valued by older Americans, can potentially clash with values that are highly regarded in indigenous, interdependent, and community-based cultures and religions.

Three critical cultural and religious perspectives may differ from the widely regarded medical value of autonomy, thereby influencing EOL treatment and ACP—communicating bad news, locus of decision making, and the value of ACP. These differing perspectives can influence the course of discussions about goals of care and implementation of a previously documented ACP or, if a current ACP does not exist, developing an ACP for the first time. *Cultural roadblocks in EOL plan—*

Communicating bad news is when the health care professional informs the individual about a health care condition that indicates it is a life-threatening illness, or the exacerbation of a pre-existing condition that indicates more imminent death. In such cases, Western cultural values may infer that autonomy and the person's inherent "right to know" are important to uphold for the patient to weigh treatment options. Therefore, health care professionals may feel they have a "duty" to give the patient full disclosure about their illness, and the patient's loved ones may be seen as having a secondary or supportive role, rather than a role as primary decision maker.

However, in indigenous and interdependent cultures, family and loved ones and even religious leaders may be viewed as part of a communal decision-making body. These differences in values may be especially difficult to sort out when there are religious, spiritual, cultural, and language differences that may involve interpreters, different conversation styles, differing customs regarding personal space, eye contact, touch, and learning styles that differ from those of health care professionals. *Orthodox Jews*

Nondisclosure

It is not unusual for a patient's family or friends who are aware of the impending "bad news" to request nondisclosure—to ask that the sick individual not be told the "bad news." There are many reasons for families or loved ones to request nondisclosure.

Some cultures maintain high reverence for the physician as expert and authority and defer to the physician to make EOL decisions. In some cultures, the special status of the elderly includes the value of not burdening older adults unnecessarily when they are ill (Candib, 2002; Holland, Geary, Marchini, & Tross, 1987; Yeo & Hikuyeda, 2000). Another reason can be the belief that open discussion of serious illness may provoke unnecessary depression or anxiety for the sick person. Others may view discussion about serious illness and death with the sick individual as disrespectful or impolite; direct disclosure may even be perceived as inhumane (Searight & Gafford, 2005).

Some people hold the belief that speaking aloud or thinking consciously about a condition may cause the illness or death to become real. In other words, one's thoughts and one's words are very powerful and may be self-fulfilling.

Families may feel that direct disclosure of diagnosis and/or prognosis may eliminate hope for the person who is seriously ill. If hope is shattered, people may not continue to enjoy or engage in life. Patients may feel like they are already dead, even though they are still living (Candib, 2002).

Others may request nondisclosure because they may feel that it is in "God's" hands and they shouldn't try to influence the outcome. It is important to trust God, and believe in "God's will be done."

Such requests may also be based on real past experiences, such as major depression or even a previous suicide attempt. The family may be concerned about depression that may either be a pre-existing condition, or that the anxiety of illness and imminent dying may create depression that may influence the individual's willingness to live and to engage in ACP (Liu et al., 1999; Matsumura et al., 2002).

When nondisclosure is requested, health care professionals can be obligated to not reveal that the diagnosis is actually terminal and help the sick individual to maintain optimism and hope (Searight & Gafford, 2005). Thus, nondisclosure can be a professional dilemma for health care professionals who value individual autonomy and the individual's "right to know" to make decisions about health care treatments and decisions about what is important as death draws near. What does a health care professional do?

When family or friends request nondisclosure it is important to determine the cause and whether the reasons and fears are proportional to reality, based on real previous experiences, or differences in perception of family role in decision making. When the reason for nondisclosure is based on cultural and/or religiously defined roles, then it can be important to explore who makes decisions, who is included in the discussions about the major illness, and whether full disclosure is acceptable. It may be helpful to negotiate nondisclosure with families, offering a statement of respect for their position and concern, and asking why the request of nondisclosure is being *re: informing ill person of their condition.*

Best option

made. It can be helpful to determine if loved ones have discussed desires for disclosure or nondisclosure with the patient and, if not, to explore what the patient's decision might possibly be if he or she could choose for themselves. Another approach is to discuss with members of the patient's support network the possibility of confirming with the sick person how much information about their disease and prognosis he or she wants to receive. If the sick individual requests full disclosure, then let the family know that you will comply. If the person asks that you talk only to the family, then affirm that you will respect the sick individual's wishes and talk with the family.

Health care professionals can explore the family's concerns to provide additional education and support, and to establish who they would like to make decisions. If reasons for requesting nondisclosure are based on previous experience with mental health concerns, then it might be helpful to obtain psychological assistance to determine how much information to deliver, and provide referrals for ongoing psychological support.

BELIEF, PAIN, AND ADVANCE CARE PLANNING

Another dimension that leads to disparities in how people approach illness and ACP is in relation to the different ways that people view pain and suffering based on religious and spiritual beliefs. Deriving deep religious significance in the experience of pain has implications for addressing pain and suffering that may accompany the dying process. The individual facing the potential for death, or the family facing the potential death of a loved one, may not only seek to treat the cause of the impending death, but they may search for meaning in these experiences, including experiences of pain.

Some may view pain as a form of divine punishment, either for one's own sins, the sins of other people, and/or the sins of one's previous lives. Eastern belief systems, such as Hinduism, believe that pain and suffering are from misdeeds in previous lives. The attempt to avoid pain may be seen as avoiding the natural consequences of being human.

Despite more contemporary religious teachings to the contrary, Christianity, Judaism, and traditional Islam relate pain and suffering to punishment. Pain may be viewed as a means of atonement for one's own sins or the sins of humanity. This is illustrated in the Christian tradition of Jesus's crucifixion for atonement of sin and the Hindu belief that there is virtue in the endurance of pain.

Cusick (2003) notes that punishment is not always seen as a negative experience, but rather as a time for potential growth. Some people believe that pain and suffering provide greater insight into the soul and the possibility of spiritual transformation. Pain and suffering can force the individual to dig deep within himself/herself for strength to endure and experience mystical transformation. Transcendence may be seen as an opportunity arising from the pain experience.

Another perspective of the importance of pain in relation to spirituality is that of a test or competition. There may be a sense of virtue in seeing how much pain and suffering one can handle or endure. Voluntary endurance of pain and suffering may offer the opportunity to discover one's own limits and/or strengths, the opportunity to connect with one's self at an intimate level. This is especially possible when the individual and/or family views pain or suffering while dying as something that is intended to draw them closer to God.

What one believes about the origin and purpose of pain may impact the desire to engage in ACP, as it may be viewed as action intended to shorten time or lessen the degree of suffering. Viewing illness and pain as punishment, individuals may be disinclined to do anything to anticipate or plan for reducing or relieving the suffering through ACP. Consequently, interpretations of pain and suffering can influence the willingness of individuals and their support networks to utilize advanced directives (ADs) as a way of directing their EOL and/or dying experiences, especially to relieve potential suffering (Cusick, 2003). *Pain & the perception that suffering is some sort of atonement for sins...*

RELIGIOUS PERSPECTIVES ON ADVANCE CARE PLANNING AND ADVANCE DIRECTIVES

While ADs are intended for individuals to record their wishes for health care should they be unable to communicate them when they are extremely sick or unconscious, that is, to indicate when to discontinue (or not initiate) life-support technologies, ADs have also emerged to ensure that religiously sanctioned care is given. Several religious groups have developed their own religious ADs out of concern there may be undertreatment via life-support technologies, that is, treatment might be prematurely discontinued, denied, or withheld at times when such actions may violate religious principles.

Religious concerns arise when there is a greater obligation to preserve life than there is concern for the "right to die." In addition, there may be concerns about limits set on health care and health care expenditures that threaten the very value of life.

An example of guidance regarding health care decision making within a religious context is a Catholic Health Association of the United States (CHAUSA, 2009) publication that provides guidance to help people express their wishes regarding health care treatments. It states, "There is no ready made answer that applies to all situations" (p. 17), but goes on to provide discussion of various considerations for assessing burdens and benefits of treatment decisions. It describes Catholic moral teaching and what the teaching may mean in various medical situations.

Another approach for ensuring religious principles and doctrine are followed is for individuals to name a specific religious health care proxy to act in the event the individual lacks capacity or is unable to communicate his or her own wishes and preferences (Massachusetts Catholic Conference, 2010). In this case, the religious direction is stated as follows:

> I direct my Health Care Agent to make decisions based on my Health Care Agent's assessment of my personal wishes, moral values and religious beliefs as stated below or as he/she otherwise knows: (here state your personal wishes or moral religious beliefs.) An example of such moral and religious beliefs is the following: I am a Roman Catholic. It is my wish that my Health Care Agent make health care decisions for me, which are consistent with the authentic teaching of the Catholic Church and based upon my profound respect for life and my belief in eternal life (p. 12).

Then the document goes on to stipulate several specific instructions for appropriate pain medication that will not cause or hasten death, food and water when capable of sustaining life, standard comfort care, and special instructions if pregnant.

A religious organization representing Orthodox Jews has developed the Jewish Health Care Proxy (Agudath Israel of America, 2008). This document appoints and directs an agent to make health care decisions in accord with Jewish law and custom, specifically in accordance with strict Orthodox interpretation and tradition. In addition, a specific Orthodox rabbi is named for consultation if there are any questions as to requirements of Jewish law and custom. This document includes directions for organ and tissue donation and disposition of the dead body.

Certainly these specific documents can provide the context for critical discussions among the health care professionals, the patient, and their loved ones to identify values and preferences that arise from their religious beliefs. However, Grodin (1993) argues that because of the complexity of EOL events and the interpretational dimensions of health care decision making at EOL, there are both strengths and weaknesses to specific religious ADs that can actually serve to undermine the goals of the individual for achieving religious and health care goals (Grodin, 1993). The specific documents and requirements to seek religious consultation may be too rigid to accommodate the range of choices and decisions that may need to be considered. For instance, given the complexity of illnesses and medical options, can written instructions cover all conditions and possibilities that may arise for a given person? Could the specificity of instructions actually lead to controversy and confusion?

Controversy and confusion can arise due to numerous factors. ACP can be focused on issues of autonomy, empowerment, and the individual's rights—principles, which may be in contrast to religious doctrine that may be more concerned with duty, obligation, community, and beneficence (Steinberg, 1989).

Families and friends may be unable to see the specific reality of the individual's condition when they are still hoping for a cure or another treatment. The judgment of families and friends can also be obscured by their own anticipatory grief of the loss, or by previous experiences they have encountered. In addition, the family and friends may receive even different interpretations from chaplains, clergy, and other people they turn to for spiritual support.

CONCLUSION

A holistic assessment of the religious and spiritual dimensions of an individual's life can facilitate existential exploration as a part of ACP. A critical aspect of integrating religion and spirituality in ACP is recognizing the individuals' ability to choose wisely based on their own faith journey and acknowledging that each person has unique attributes and conscience to discern what is right for them.

Similarly, health care professionals may have their own meaning in life challenged by their experiences of their patient's struggles and suffering, and by the stresses they encounter while providing health care. The health care professional that accompanies patients and their loved ones on their journey of discerning what is right for them within the given circumstances must recognize that his or her own decisions may have been different. Yet, the health care professional must be willing to be nonjudgmental and remain supportive—to provide compassionate care for people facing very difficult situations.

Health care professionals must be able to help patients and their families explore the religious and spiritual dimensions that guide their decision making, not to be able to convince them of a "right" way, but to be able to guide them in reviewing possible options and resources, and expressing their preferences and values to guide others who may be advocating or speaking on their behalf. Journeying with the individual in the quest to connect more deeply with what is meaningful can enable the patient to engage more fully in ACP. Knowledge of the differences in values, beliefs, and preferences, in addition to the need to partner with the individuals and families to negotiate care within the patient's religion, spirituality, and culture are critical for good health care decision making.

REFERENCES

Agudath Israel of America. (2008). *Halachic health care proxy*. New York, NY: Author.

Balboni, T., Paulk, M., Balboni, M., Phelps, A., Loggers, E., Wright, A., . . . Prigerson, H. (2010). Provision of spiritual care to patients with advanced cancer: associations with medical care and quality of life near death. *Journal of Clinical Oncology, 28*(3), 445–452.

Brush, B., & Daly, P. (2000). Assessing spirituality in primary care practice: Is there time? *Clinical Excellence for Nurse Practitioners, 4*, 67–71.

Candib, L. (2002). Truth telling and advance planning at the end of life: Problems with autonomy in a multicultural world. *Families, Systems & Health, 20*(2), 13–28.

Catholic Health Association of the United States. (CHAUSA). (2009). *Advance directives: A guide to help you express your health care wishes.* Washington, DC: Author. Retrieved from www.chausa.org/searchresults.aspx?searchtext=advance+dire ctives

Chrash, M., Mulich, B., & Patton, C. (2011). The APN role in holistic assessment and integration of spiritual assessment for advance care planning. *Journal of the American Academy of Nurse Practitioners, 23*(10), 530–536.

Cusick, J. (2003). Spirituality and voluntary pain. *American Pain Society Bulletin, 13*(5). Retrieved from http://www.ampainsoc.org/pub/bulletin/sep03/path1. htm

Draper, P., & McSherry, W. (2002). A critical view of spirituality and spiritual assessment. *Journal of Advanced Nursing, 39*(1), 1–2.

Ehman, J., Ott, B., Short, T., Ciampa, R., & Hansen-Flaschen, J. (1999). Do patients want physicians to inquire about their spiritual or religious beliefs if they become gravely ill? *Archives of Internal Medicine, 159*(15), 1803–1806.

Gallup Poll. (2011). More than 9 in 10 Americans continue to believe in God. Retrieved from http://www.gallup.com/poll/147887/americans-continue-believe-god.aspx

Grodin, M. A. (1993). Religious advance directives: The convergence of law, religion, medicine, and public health. *American Journal of Public Health, 83*, 899–904.

Holland, J., Geary, N., Marchini, A., & Tross, S. (1987). An international survey of physician attitudes and practice in regard to revealing the diagnosis of cancer. *Cancer Investigation, 5*, 151–154.

Katerndahl, D. A. (2008). Impact of spiritual symptoms and their interactions on health services and life satisfaction. *Annals of Family Medicine, 6*(5), 412–420.

King, D. E., & Bushwick, R. (1994). Beliefs and attitudes of hospital inpatients about faith healing and prayer. *Journal of Family Practice, 39*(4), 349–352.

Leininger, M. (1980). Caring: A central focus for nursing and health care services. *Nursing and Health Care, 1*(10), 135–143, 176.

Liu, J., Lin, W., Chen, Y., Wu, H., Yao, N., Chen, L., et al. (1999). The status of the do-not-resuscitate order in Chinese clinical trial patients in a cancer centre. *Journal Medical Ethics, 25*, 309–314.

McCord, G., Gilchrist, V., Grossman, S., King, B., McCormick, K., Oprandi, A., Srivastava, M. (2004). Discussing spirituality with patients: A rational and ethical approach. *Annals of Family Medicine, 2*(4), 356–361.

Martsolf, D. (1997). Cultural aspects of spirituality in cancer care. *Seminars in Oncology Nursing, 13*(4), 231–236.

Massachusetts Catholic Conference (2012). Appointing a healthcare agent in Massachusetts a Catholic guide. Massachusetts Catholic Conference, West End Place 150 Staniford Street First Floor, Boston, Massachusetts 02114-2511. Retrieved from http://stjohnswampscott.org/Parish_Events_files/Health%20 Care%20Proxy.pdf

Matsumura, S., Bito, S., Liu, H., Kahn, K., Fukuhara, S., Kagawa-Singer, M., et al. (2002). Acculturation of attitudes toward end-of-life care: A cross-cultural survey of Japanese Americans and Japanese. *Journal of General Internal Medicine, 17,* 531–539.

Pautex, S., Herrmann, F., & Zulian, G. (2008). Role of advance directives in palliative care units: A prospective study. *Palliative Medicine, 22,* 835–841.

Peters, J. (2010). *Module # 10: Introduction to palliative & hospice care.* VISN 3 Geriatric Research, Education & Clinical Center (GRECC). Retrieved from http://www.nynj.va.gov/docs/Module10.pdf

Pew Research Center. (2012). *Religion.* Retrieved from http://www.pollingreport.com/religion.htm

Puchalski, C., Ferrell, B., Virani, R., Otis-Green, S., Baird, P., Bull, J.,...Sulmasy, D. (2009). Improving the quality of spiritual care as a dimension of palliative care: The report of the consensus conference. *Journal of Palliative Medicine, 12*(10), 885–904.

Sanders, C. (2002). *Challenges for spiritual care-giving in the millennium.* Retrieved from http://contemporarynurse.com/12.2/12–2p107.html

Searight, H., & Gafford, J. (2005). It's like playing with your destiny: Bosnian immigrants' views of advance directives and end-of-life decision-making. *Journal of Immigrant Health, 7*(3), 195–203.

Steinberg, A. (1989). Bioethics: secular philosophy, Jewish law and modern medicine. *Israel Journal of Medical Sciences, 25*(7), 404.

Sulmasy, D. P. (2002). A biopsychosocial-spiritual model for the care of patients at the end of life. *The Gerontologist, 42,* 24–33.

Tervalon, M., & Murray-Garcia, J. (1998). Cultural humility versus cultural competence: A critical distinction in defining physician training outcomes in multicultural education. *Journal of Healthcare for the Poor and Underserved, 9*(2), 117–125.

Watson, M. (2011). Spiritual aspects of advance care planning in advance care planning in end of life care. In K. Thomas & B. Lobo (Eds.), *Advance care planning in end of life care* (pp. 45–54). New York, NY: Oxford University Press.

Yeo, G., & Hikuyeda, N. (2000). Cultural issues in end-of-life decision making among Asians and Pacific Islanders in the United States. In K. Braun, J. Pietsch, & P. Blanchette (Eds.), *Cultural issues in end-of-life decision making* (pp. 101–125). Thousand Oaks, CA: Sage.

Best Practices for Communicating About End-of-Life Care

Introduction

Susana Lauraine McCune

When advance care planning (ACP) and advance directives (ADs) are successful, they can help ensure patients receive the health care they desire—no more and no less—during life and through death. Research has shown that ongoing communication is the key to successful ACP. Yet due to lack of effective communication among health care providers, patients, and their loved ones, ADs and ACP have been underutilized by professional care providers and members of the general public.

In Part II the authors present successful models and best practices to help professional care providers foster ongoing communication with patients and their loved ones about ADs and ACPs. The conceptual models and clinical best practices presented in this part help accomplish what has previously been difficult to achieve—developing and documenting effective ADs and ACPs and providing for quality of life at end of life (EOL).

In Chapter 8, physician Stu Farber and his wife, Annalu Farber, offer compelling examples of the ways in which uncertainty and competing autonomies can influence ACP and delivery of EOL care. They ask straightforward questions that ignite the process of ACP. In clear, concise, and honest language, they discuss complex reasons that patients and families resist discussing EOL care and formulating an AD, as well as look at challenges to honoring ADs when they are activated. The Farbers pose helpful questions to encourage employing values and the meaning of life as guiding lights to facilitate communication about ACP. They conceptualize a network of relationships in which communication about EOL care is provided in a vital community.

In Chapter 9, social work and gerontology professor Kathy Black points out how three prevalent trajectories of decline will influence EOL in the 21st century. She discusses the need for planning for EOL care in advance using a long-range, holistic perspective of care needs by key domains, including psychological, social, cultural, spiritual, medical, physical, and financial considerations. Black informs us about behavioral change models that have been applied to ACP and discusses ways in which health care providers' understanding of personality styles can help in doing effective ACP.

In Chapter 10, Susana Lauraine McCune outlines what she calls an "Interdisciplinary Relational Model of Care©" (IRMOC) that invites practitioners, whether they are physicians, psychologists, nurses, social workers, or other professionals working with persons dealing with life-threatening illness, to move from a position of authority and objectivity to a position of partnership and vulnerability. Drawing on relational psychological theory, the IRMOC sees patient and clinician as partners, or companions, in relation to dying and death with both parties profoundly affected by the interactional encounter. McCune argues against a traditional "hands-off" stance in which clinicians aspire for objectivity and dispassion, calling instead for compassion—the condition of suffering together—as well as the use of specific therapeutic communication skills to transform practice in dealing with EOL concerns and ACP.

In Chapter 11, social worker and former president of the Association for Death Education and Counseling Ben Wolfe discusses how ADs are used to facilitate communication among patients, family members, and health care providers. He uses a dramatic personal story to illustrate the twists and turns and complexities of ACP, emphasizing the need for an individualized approach that reflects the uniqueness of each person and his/her family system and the changing dynamics of dealing with dying and death in real life. Wolfe draws on his many years as a grief counselor to give professionals ideas and strategies for encouraging individuals and their families to engage in "conversations that matter" far in advance of a life-threatening crisis.

In Chapter 12, Mercedes Bern-Klug, Jane Dohrmann, and Patrick A. Dolan, Jr., describe contemporary nursing homes, the multiple roles long-term care facilities play in the community, and the variety of care needs residents of these nursing homes may have. They discuss challenges and opportunities related to ACP in nursing homes from the perspective of the nursing home residents and their health care agents, highlighting the enormous responsibility of proxy decision makers and pointing out the need to consider the emotional, psychological, and spiritual concerns they face. Finally, the authors demonstrate common ACP challenges and opportunities through the lens of three popular television game shows, *Jeopardy*, *Wheel of Fortune*, and *Let's Make a Deal*.

In Chapter 13, palliative care physician Cory Ingram outlines an innovative model for guiding families to understand dementia as a terminal illness and to plan for the inevitable decline and death of their loved one. Dr. Ingram presents a compassionate, sensitive approach that delivers the person with dementia from anonymity, affirms caregivers' feelings of guilt, identifies the healing power of hope, and gently educates the caregiver about the futility of aggressive treatment and, in particular CPR, for persons in late stages of the disease. Through the effective communication fostered through Dr. Ingram's communications model Watch Over Me©, family members can do ACP that takes into consideration the expected course of the disease and helps the patient and family live well until the patient's death.

Finally, in Chapter 14, Joe Jack Davis, a general surgeon whose career has spanned four decades, helps us make friends with death by candidly discussing the consequences, sometimes intended, sometimes unintended, of medical treatment, compared and contrasted with an unmitigated disease process, showing ways in which natural death, resulting from natural disease processes can be less painful, involve less suffering, and engender death with dignity. Contrasting longevity with quality of life, Davis clearly delineates the quality of life consequences of "heroic measures" and "do everything possible" requests. Dramatically, Dr. Davis shares his personal AD that is based on a medically specific and values-based rationale and written in terms that provide clinicians and his family clear guidance about the care leading to the "good death" and "dying well" that he desires at the end of his life. Based on his years of practical experience, he stresses the importance of talking with one's loved ones and naming someone to act on one's behalf if one is no longer able to speak for oneself.

CHAPTER 8

It Ain't Easy: Making Life and Death Decisions Before the Crisis

Stu Farber
Annalu Farber

If there is a condition that everyone in this wide, contentious, diverse world shares, it is this one: mortality. We can say with 100% certainty that all of us are going to die. We all know this, and yet we have been immeasurably slow in recognizing that many of the people we love are not dying the way they would choose.

Goodman, 2012

Working within the reality of mortality, coming to death is then an inevitable part of life, an event to be lived rather than a problem to be solved. Ideally, we would live the end of our life from the same values that have given meaning to the story of our life up to that time. But in a medical crisis there is little time, language, or ritual to guide patients and families in conceptualizing or expressing their values and goals (Farber & Farber, 2006). Completing an advance directive (AD) opens up the opportunity to communicate to our community the quality of life that we would find acceptable and how we would want to live the end of our life, should a time come when we cannot act on our own behalf.

In the AD we can state our preferences for care and choose an agent to advocate for us. Even so, there are many challenges to the completion and actual application of ADs. For example, some people aren't yet convinced that death is inevitable. Others worry that talking about death will bring the event to pass. Still others, seeing themselves as wholly independent, refuse to talk about serious illness and end of life (EOL) as a way of protecting themselves and their family from the emotional burden of such discussions. For those who do decide to create an AD, there is the more basic challenge of making decisions today about some unknown event in an unforeseeable future.

In this chapter we discuss two of these major challenges:

- *Uncertainty*: It is difficult and usually impossible to know the circumstances in which an AD will be used.
- *Autonomy and interdependence*: By its very nature living with serious illness diminishes a person's autonomy and increases interdependence within his/her community and the care team that is serving him or her.

UNCERTAINTY

A person completing an AD is being asked to make life and death decisions for a medical event that will happen at an unknown time in the future under unknown circumstances. In this context, logically completing such a form is difficult, and it may be a primary reason why very few people, whether healthy or seriously ill, ever complete an AD. Once the AD is completed, it then lies dormant until a medical crisis activates it.

Challenges arise when the specific circumstances of the medical crisis may not have been anticipated in the AD, which is all too common. And more importantly, at the time of crisis the choices in the AD are often not honored for a variety of reasons, two of them particularly common.

First, the surrogate decision maker chooses to ignore the AD believing that the current circumstances indicate a different course of action. During a medical crisis, emergency care may be rendered, resulting in intubation, mechanical ventilation, and admission to the intensive care unit (ICU) before the AD has the opportunity to be considered. The surrogate decision makers are left with a "living" family member who may or may not get better. The surrogate (variously called agent, proxy, or durable power of attorney for health care matters) is then asked to make the daunting decision of whether or not to withdraw life-supporting treatments.

Second, we see that uncertainty exists on multiple levels: The AD often does not anticipate the actual medical crisis that activates it, or how the surrogate decision maker may interpret events, or how medical providers will interpret treatment needs, or even the role of the AD when decisions need to be made. Such uncertainty has prompted several experts to recommend that ADs focusing primarily on treatment choices should be abandoned altogether because they are of little value when implemented (Tonnelli, 1996).

This brings us to what are called third-generation ADs. These focus less on specific medical procedures and more on the person's values as a way of guiding decision making. What are most certain in anticipating an unknown future health crisis are the values that define meaning and quality of life for the ill person. What makes life worth living? What constitutes quality of life for that person? Answers to these questions provide a firmer foundation to answer the question of which medical treatments are appropriate in unanticipated circumstances.

Equally important is that this document can be used to facilitate a conversation with family and community members, those who will support the patient and speak for that person if he/she is unable to do so for himself/herself. Each of us has a robust "lived story" that is filled with values, choices, and relationships that have provided meaning in our lives. Our family and community have access to this "lived story" even if we have not discussed the specifics of a particular medical situation. Talking with our agents about quality of life and how that is congruent with the life that we have lived will assist in assuring that medical treatments support the "lived story" of our life within our community. It is a vital way to help decrease uncertainty and increase the precision of medical decision making.

AUTONOMY AND INTERDEPENDENCE

Autonomy, the right of individuals to make decisions about how they want to live their life, is deeply ingrained in our culture. It is embedded in our laws and is a basic ethical tenet in medical decision making. The rise of ADs is based on the goal of extending patient autonomy (the right to make medical decisions based on personal choice) when the patient has lost capacity to speak for him/herself. It is anticipated that the choices expressed in the AD will be used to make medical decisions in an unknown future. Current ADs tend to focus on specific medical procedures, including cardiopulmonary resuscitation (CPR), mechanical ventilation, feeding tube, antibiotics, and designating a proxy or agent.

It is important to emphasize that the AD is giving instruction to the community that is caring for the patient. The instructions are directing a dynamic group of caregivers (family, friends, and health care professionals) who will be expected to both interpret and act on those instructions. However, this is not a one-way communication. The community will also be deeply affected by the responsibility given in these instructions. Thus, an AD depends heavily on the community that is receiving it.

Conflicting Autonomies

As previously mentioned, the belief in autonomy—the right of a patient to make medical decisions based on personal choice—is a basic tenet of both general and medical culture in the United States. The problem with the belief in autonomy is that, while it inspires all of us in living our lives, it just isn't true. By its very nature, serious illness diminishes personal autonomy and increases interdependence within our community. We live in a web of reciprocal relationships. Decisions that a patient makes will have an impact on the entire community, the family, and the medical providers.

Each individual in this web of relationships also possesses autonomy that may or may not agree with the decision made by the patient. If a seriously ill patient wants to go home for further care, do we consider the autonomy of the spouse who is already exhausted from past care giving and is now being asked to do even more? What about the medical team whose extensive clinical experience and wisdom may support a different story? What should clinicians do when they witness patients and families making decisions that they deeply grieve because they are certain that these choices will only add to the combined suffering of the patient and the family? (Farber, Egnew, & Farber, 2004).

The competing autonomies of the patient and all members of his/her community need to be acknowledged. However, when these multiple points of view are acknowledged, decision making becomes much more complicated and the utility of a fixed AD written before the medical crisis may well be of limited value. Ideally, medical decisions will integrate the viewpoints of the patient, the patient's community, and the medical community, acknowledging interdependence. The patient who has lost the capacity to make decisions is dependent on his or her community, and the community is both dependent on and is a guide to the medical team to make medical decisions that are respectful of the lived history of the patient. This complex process is rarely reduced to a single document that focuses primarily on medical procedures.

VALUES AND GOALS

What makes a life worth living? Isn't this really what we are trying to determine? How does any one person define living? For some it may be the physiological process of continuing to breathe, to stay physically here on this earth for as long as possible. For another, it is something more. If you were no longer able to feed yourself, bathe yourself, or manage any of your personal care needs, would that be intolerable? Or, could you accept that level of living as long as you were still able to recognize and communicate with your loved ones?

When someone clearly states what constitutes quality of life, especially identifying his or her bottom line, it is much more helpful to the community of caregivers (both personal and professional) than any of the boxes about medical treatments checked on the AD form. Values and goals, openly communicated, will give substance and guidance to a patient's agents should the time come for them to act on a loved one's behalf.

When we facilitate workshops to assist people in the completion of ADs, this is where we begin. Our workshops often use Five Wishes (available online at www.5wishes.com) as our working document. There are other good tools including My Directives (found at theconversation-project.org/), a website created by Ellen Goodman and Len Fishman to promote EOL planning and the use of ADs. Before we distribute the document, we begin with a guided experience that helps participants get in touch with what they value most in life. One such exercise, created by Steven Levine in his book *One Year to Live*, asks a series of questions about what the participants would do if they knew they only had 1 year left to live. The categories of questions include such things as, "What unfinished business would you complete?," "What things would you want to do with family and friends?," "Where would you travel?," "What would you want to say to loved ones?," and so on. At the end of the exercise most people notice themes that flow through their answers reflecting their values as well as goals. In our action-oriented lives taking time to think about values is often a new experience, even though it is these values that have created meaning in our lives.

Next, the Five Wishes AD document is handed out and participants are requested to turn to the last page. We instruct participants to complete the form backwards. Why do we start this way? Most AD documents place questions about how we want to live the EOL at the end of the document. This assumes that the questions of medical intervention, which are asked first, are primary to the quality of life we would choose to live. However, if we begin by contemplating our values to define a quality of life that is consistent with our lived history, questions about medical procedures become secondary, supporting our goals and values. In other words, the use of various medical procedures should be determined on the basis of their ability to help us achieve our quality-of-life goals. In the same vein, when we talk to our family and community about our ADs, the most important information that we can communicate is not whether or not we want CPR or other aggressive treatments. It is the story that describes when quality of life is present and when it is not. It is a tool to guide the agent in knowing when the patient is no longer living a life with meaning.

We are beings who inherently create meaning in story form. So, thinking of future possibilities in terms of the story of a life, given some unforeseen diminishment, helps to identify both what is worth living for and what would be intolerable. That will be as unique for each person as the life story that he/she has created. One certainty is that values are more stable and constant than the medical facts of an unknown future. Encouraging conversations about values and goals between individuals and their agent is one of the best ways to reduce uncertainty when the unknown future arrives.

What we cannot know is what the future has in store. What we can be certain of today is what we value. Values do not tend to shift with changing circumstances.

CASE STUDIES

The following three clinical cases offer an illustration of both the challenges and potential value of using completed ADs as a basis for medical decision making. In each case, the extent to which the family or community had a conversation about values and goals is critical to the outcome.

Case 1: Alan

Alan was a 50-year-old palliative care physician who understood the importance of planning ahead for a health care crisis. Alan had a large community of friends and a loving relationship with his wife. He completed an AD clearly stating his wish not to be resuscitated or intubated under any circumstances. Alan's appointed agent was a long-time friend who knew him and his values well. He discussed his definition of quality of life with her and made clear that anything short of his current quality of life would not be acceptable to him. He purposefully chose not to have his wife of 20 years be his agent because he knew it would be emotionally difficult for her to carry out his wishes. He was concerned that she would likely provide more medical care than he would want.

Alan was on vacation when he leaned against a railing that gave way, and he fell 15 feet to the hard ground. Alan knew immediately that he had a serious injury because he couldn't feel anything below his shoulders and couldn't move his arms or legs. As his wife rushed to his side, he looked at her and said goodbye, expecting that he would die from what would be determined to be cervical 5–6 spinal cord trauma that would leave him a functional cervical level-4 tetraplegic (totally paralyzed from the shoulders down). Alan was air ambulanced to the regional trauma center, where emergency surgery was performed to stabilize his spine. He regained consciousness and initially regained some function in his arms allowing for full extension of his elbows and limited use of his fingers. The doctors told him he could likely become "independent in transfers" and mobile in a power wheelchair. He discussed these issues with his wife and his agent friend, and he said that he was willing to see what life would be like "scooting around" in a motorized wheelchair, though he never formally changed his AD.

(continued)

Case 1: Alan   *(continued)*

After a second spine stabilizing surgery, Alan's mental status markedly declined. He lost all motor function from his neck down, and post surgery he was unable to be weaned off the ventilator, so he became ventilator dependent. He was unable to reliably speak to communicate his wishes. Exhaustive evaluation suggested his mental and motor changes were due to a rare demyelinating process that might resolve over several months. His agent decided to maintain all medical care but at the same time to honor his instruction not to accept resuscitation. She hoped to give Alan time to "awaken," so that he could decide for himself whether he wanted to continue his current level of care focusing on recovery or to transition to comfort care. His wife and many of his friends felt that Alan would not find his current quality of life acceptable and wanted to shift him to comfort care. The agent, supported by several other close friends of Alan's, was adamant that she couldn't make an irreversible decision that would certainly lead to Alan's death. She reasoned that he still had the chance to regain capacity to make his own decision and found it especially difficult after Alan had said he was willing to see what life would be like when scooting around in a motorized wheelchair.

Six weeks after his initial surgery, Alan was still hospitalized, he had a tracheostomy placed to maintain long-term, ventilatory support, and discharge plans were being made for him to be transferred to a long-term acute care facility. Alan's palliative care colleagues were distressed that he was receiving care totally at odds with his "lived story" despite all of his advance planning.

Alan's case illustrates several common challenges of even the most well thought out AD.

- His AD could not anticipate the actual medical events that occurred in his medical crisis, or the way in which he became ventilator dependent (uncertainty; competing autonomy of patient's wishes and surgical team).
- His agent believed Alan "changed his mind" during discussions after the accident (agent uncertainty about the appropriateness of the AD instructions due to changed circumstances).
- Later, Alan's agent was unwilling to make a life-and-death decision with the possibility of his cognitive recovery, however unlikely, even knowing that Alan's wife disagreed with this choice (competing autonomies among AD, agent, and Alan's wife).

At this point in Alan's story, he is living a life that is inconsistent with his "lived history" and his well-documented AD without any likelihood of a change in the care plan in the near future. Alan's AD has not influenced the medical care he has received or the outcomes of care.

Case 2: Florence

Florence was a lively 91-year-old woman who had been blessed with an active mind and a body healthy enough to allow her to live independently and pursue her love of music. She was the leader of two weekly flute groups; she had season subscriptions to the symphony and ballet, a large circle of friends, and a granddaughter who visited her regularly. She also had a son in California who was her legal next of kin. Florence had verbally designated him as her surrogate decision maker.

Florence was resistant to filling out an AD or to discussing what she wanted in case of a medical crisis because she thought it was depressing, and she wanted to focus on the joy of living. She did eventually share with her son that she didn't want to live on machines, be in an ICU, or live in a nursing home. At her son's insistence, Florence finally signed an AD documenting these wishes.

Then it happened that Florence had a large left-middle cerebral artery stroke that initially left her unconscious, though not needing ICU care. Her son specified that she should be designated as do not resuscitate (DNR) and do not intubate (DNI) patient, consistent with her AD. As the stroke evolved, Florence awoke with total expressive aphasia, dense hemiplegia, and severe dysphagia with secondary aspiration pneumonia on antibiotics. She was able to nod or blink in response to simple questions but otherwise needed total care and had a feeding tube placed due to her high aspiration risk. The level of care that Florence needed could only be provided in an institutional setting. There she received a gastrostomy tube for nutrition. Given her resistance to talking about "death," her son asked that all medical discussions be with him and his daughter excluding his mother. Florence's son readily acknowledged that she would find her new quality of life a "purgatory," but as her son, he was also unable to "let her starve or die from an infection that could easily be treated with antibiotics." The neurology team told the son that Florence might improve over time, though it could take 6 to 12 weeks before they would know her new baseline.

Florence's case also illustrates common challenges in implementing an AD; particularly, the often unclear and distressing decisions that the

(continued)

Case 2: Florence *(continued)*

agent is asked to make in murky circumstances when a loved one has not been willing to talk about his/her wishes.

- Florence's AD did not anticipate the actual medical events that occurred in her medical crisis (uncertainty).
- Her son and granddaughter's interpretation of what was in her best interest ignored Florence's documented wishes and, therefore, precluded her from being involved in her own medical decisions (dependence on community; competing autonomies).
- The culture of a skilled nursing facility is to extend life within the limits of the DNR, so it will likely prolong her "living in purgatory." Florence will be living a life inconsistent with her "lived history" (interdependence in community; competing autonomies).
- Florence's AD did not influence the care she received.

Case 3: Betty

Betty was an 84-year-old woman who several years before had experienced a blood clot to her brain causing an embolic stroke from atrial fibrillation resulting in mild executive function diminishment. At that time, she and her mildly demented husband of 60 years decided to accept an offer to live in an apartment in the home of their daughter and son-in-law. Betty and her husband felt they had done a good job of financial and health care planning, including creating ADs, through a reputable estate planning attorney in Arizona while they were still living actively in that community. Betty's daughter, a retired trust executive, and her son-in-law, a palliative care physician, were designated agents for both parents. In addition, over the years that they lived together, Betty's son-in-law had initiated conversations about what would constitute quality of life for Betty and her husband, attempting to clarify their values and goals of care.

In the fall of her 84th year, Betty was found by her husband on the floor of their bathroom unresponsive. He called his son-in-law at work and was instructed to call 911. Betty's daughter was out of town on business and was expected to return late that evening. Upon evaluation in the emergency room (ER), Betty was found to have a dissecting, ascending aortic aneurism including her left carotid artery. In consultation with her son-in-law, the surgeon said that given the extent of the aneurism,

(continued)

Case 3: Betty *(continued)*

the fact that she was unconscious when found, her prior stroke history, her age, and the preferences she had documented in her signed Physicians Orders for Life-Sustaining Treatment or POLST (a one-page document used in Washington State by people with advanced illness to inform all care providers of the person's care goals), surgery was not recommended. Betty woke up and was transferred to the ICU for close observation, with medical treatment including IV infusion to reduce her blood pressure and pain medication. Betty's daughter returned home at midnight and decided to get a few hours sleep before going to the hospital to see her mother. At 2:30 a.m., the daughter received a call from her very distraught mother wanting to know when she could come home.

The next morning Betty's daughter and husband arrived at the ICU early and requested a meeting with a palliative care physician. Because Betty's prognosis was poor, the daughter contacted her brothers and the grandchildren to advise them that they should come soon. The palliative care doctor talked to Betty, her daughter, and husband compassionately and honestly about the certainty of her prognosis: Betty's life was at an end; she had minutes to perhaps 2 weeks left to live. Betty responded with a mix of terror and acceptance. Her daughter asked the doctor about planning to bring her mother home on hospice care. The doctor explained that they wanted to keep Betty for a few days to see if she could be stabilized a bit more before sending her home.

The daughter and her brothers were fully on board with Betty's wishes, spelled out clearly in her ADs, that when her time came she did not want to be in the hospital, and furthermore that she wanted to be cared for at home. Even in light of the eminently terminal prognosis, the doctor's eyes reflected her fear of taking Betty off the intravenous medications. She recommended that Betty stay in the ICU through the weekend. It was Friday and Betty's daughter knew that it would be challenging to arrange a hospice intake over the weekend. Besides, she had clearly heard the doctor say that her mother could die in 10 minutes or at most 2 weeks.

The daughter turned to her mother and asked, "Do you understand what the doctor is telling you?" Betty replied fearfully, "I think she's saying I'm going to die." Her daughter said gently, "Yes, and she is saying that they would like you to stay in the hospital a few more days to become more stable before going home. That also means that there is a possibility that you may not leave the hospital." Betty's shocked reply was, "You mean I might die here? I want to go home!" Even so, the doctor

(continued)

Case 3: Betty   *(continued)*

was reluctant to agree that going home was a good choice. Finally, in emotional distress, the daughter asked her own husband to intervene in communicating the family's desire to bring her mother home. Hospice was contacted and Betty was transferred to her daughter's home on hospice care late that afternoon. She died peacefully, holding her husband's hand and attended by her daughter and son-in-law 48 hours later.

Betty's case illustrates that even a well-planned and well-communicated AD is not without its challenges. It also helps us to see that Betty's willingness to have the conversation about what constituted quality of life for her allowed her agent to feel certainty in being a strong advocate for Betty's goals.

- Betty's goals were communicated consistently over time and they were wholly congruent with her "lived history" (desired outcome was achieved; individual and family autonomy issues were addressed in ongoing conversations before the crisis).
- Betty's AD was clear to her and made clear to her family. She had stated that she did not want to be in the hospital for any reason. Given the crisis that landed her in the ER and then the ICU, it was less clear to the medical team because it was at odds with the immediacy of her medical condition (medical team uncertainty; competing autonomies and goals).
- Betty trusted her appointed agents, her daughter and son-in-law, to carry out her wishes and was willing to have ongoing, meaningful discussions with them about what constituted quality of life. This allowed her agents to advocate clearly and assertively on her behalf when the crisis occurred (interdependence in community; reduced uncertainty; clarity of goals).

In contrast to Florence's story, Betty's AD was effective because it was illuminated by ongoing family discussions that focused on understanding Betty's quality-of-life goals. These conversations laid the foundation for medical decision making.

SUMMARY

ADs are a good beginning to EOL care planning, especially those that address one's quality of life before asking about medical treatments. However, if we are to transform the lived experience of the last days of life in this culture, we must find a way to facilitate the conversations that will breathe life into ADs, bringing clarity to the decision-making process for the family and agent and ultimately the professional care team.

Perhaps as an example we should look to the radical shift in birthing in the 1970s that transformed childbirth from a medical event to a life-cycle family event. Birthing plans became the norm and are actively in use today. A birth plan spells out the detailed personal values that define a quality birth—who will be present, where the birth will ideally take place, what procedures will or will not add to the quality of the experience, and what is the bottom-line quality-of-life experience if a less-than-optimal situation should occur. Birthing plans are also created in community and in conversation with the provider, the family, and the doula.

There are two great bookend mysteries in life—birth and death. Doesn't it make sense to plan for, and talk about, how we want to live the last days of our life as robustly as we plan for birthing life into this world? This would allow all affected parties to be prepared for and be respectful of the individual's values and goals. When we have these conversations with a loved one, we don't focus on death and dying. We focus instead on how the person wants to live, because that is really what is being decided. We offer here some questions that we have found help facilitate this conversation:

- In your life, have you had experience being with people at the EOL?
  - What was that like for you?
  - What was your role in that circumstance?
- How would you describe what makes your life worth living?
  - What if you were no longer able to do _____?
  - What would be a quality of life that would be acceptable?
- Who and what are the people, places, things, and activities that are important to you?
- Where do you imagine yourself being in the last days of your life?
  - What would that look like?
  - Who would be with you?
  - What would you be doing?

In our family, these conversations are approached casually; they are interspersed with other conversation. Often the topic comes up naturally in asking about someone's life experiences, or when a friend or family member is ill or has died, or when we have seen something in a movie that stirs the conversation. The trick is to examine our own discomfort in having the conversation and begin to accept that mortality, birth and death, is indeed the common denominator for us all. Perhaps it is a subject that should be moved from taboo topic to table talk.

REFERENCES

Farber, S., Egnew, T., & Farber, A. (2004). What is a respectful death? In J. Berzoff & P. Silverman (Eds.), *Living with dying: A comprehensive resource for healthcare practitioners* (pp. 102–127). New York, NY: Columbia University Press.

Farber, A., & Farber, S. (2006). A respectful death model: Difficult conversations at the end of life. In R. Katz & T. Johnson (Eds.), *When professionals weep: Emotional and countertransference responses in end-of-life care* (pp. 221–236). New York, NY: Routledge.

Goodman, E. (2012). Die the way you want to. *Harvard Business Review, 90*(1–2), 58–59.

Tonnelli, M. R. (1996). Pulling the plug on living wills. A critical analysis of advance directives. *Chest, 110*, 116–122.

CHAPTER 9

Advance Care Planning: Considerations for Practice With Older Adults

Kathy Black

The end of life must be understood as a period that typically spans ☆☆ *years, not just weeks or months.*

Lynn, 2005

As the average life expectancy continues to increase in the United States, an unprecedented number of people are living longer (Murphy, Xu, & Kochanek, 2012). Today, many Americans will live well into their eighth, ninth, and even tenth decades of life. According to the U.S. Census, older adults aged 85, and specifically those aged 90 and older, constitute the fastest-growing age group (Werner, 2011). However, the vast majority of the nation's older population will experience declining health and functional incapacity as they age. More than 9 out of 10 older adults have at least one chronic condition, and nearly three quarters have at least two or more (Centers for Disease Control and Prevention, 2011).   *stats on health cards. of oldest old*

TRAJECTORIES OF DECLINE AT THE END OF LIFE

The demographic aging trend coupled with the advances of U.S. medical care has shaped the end of life for most Americans (Lynn, 2005). Although the bulk of interest in EOL care appropriately focuses on the last days and weeks of those imminently dying, research suggests that the majority of Americans follow fairly typical courses or trajectories of care needs over the last months, and even years of life (Lynn, 2005). Figure 9.1 denotes the three general trajectories of decline leading to death.

The three trajectories of decline represent the EOL course for more than 9 out of 10 Americans (Lynn, 2005). In the first trajectory, people will experience long periods of good functioning, with a few weeks or months of rapid decline in which a fatal illness becomes overwhelming, leading to death. Cancer represents the most common cause of this type of trajectory,

FIGURE 9.1 Trajectories of Decline at the EOL.

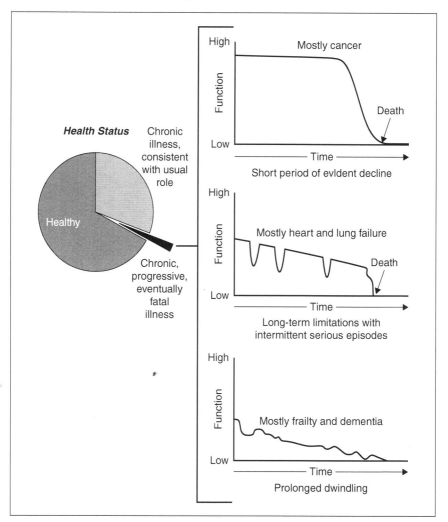

SOURCE: Lynn, J., & Adamson, D. M. (2003). *Living well at the end of life. Adapting health care to serious chronic illness in old age.* Washington, DC: Rand Health.

with approximately 20% of Americans following this course, peaking around age 65.

The second trajectory, faced by approximately 25% of Americans, is exemplified by a slow decline in functional status, with sporadic exacerbations of two primary chronic conditions; chronic heart failure and emphysema (Lynn, 2005). After years of living with increasingly poorer health, people following this course will experience death rather suddenly and ultimately die from chronic organ system failure mostly in their eighth decade of life.

The final trajectory, representing about 40% of all people, is typified by a long-term dwindling of function, requiring years of personal care. About half of this population will have serious cognitive failure during the course of decline. Death will follow after a minor physiological challenge such as influenza, urinary tract infection, pneumonia, or a broken bone in which the body will be unable to recover. Many in this group suffer from frailty and/or dementia and will generally live into their 80s.

Combined, the latter two trajectories represent the EOL course for the majority of Americans. According to Lynn (2005), about two thirds of all Americans will succumb to one of four primary conditions: chronic heart failure, emphysema, frailty, or dementia. These EOL trajectories span a period of years, providing ample time to plan in advance.

RECONCEPTUALIZING PLANNING IN ADVANCE FOR CARE

Advance care planning (ACP) is an increasingly important issue for older Americans, their families, and their network of health care providers. Growing interest regarding ACP has been fueled by the nation's palliative and EOL care movement, which aims to better prepare people for their experiences throughout the latter years. The prominence of planning for health-related care in advance has been recognized by such key organizations as Institute of Medicine (Field & Cassel, 1997), National Institutes of Health (NIH, 2005), American Geriatrics Society (Lynn, 1997), and the National Consensus Project for Quality Palliative Care (2009). Philanthropic endeavors in improving EOL care include the Soros Foundation *Project on Death in America* (2012; www.soros.org) and the Robert Wood Johnson Foundation (2012) *Last Acts* campaign (www.rwjf.org). Public-based movements include *Americans for Better Care for the Dying* (2012; www.abcd-caring.org) and *National Healthcare Decisions Day* (2012; www.nhdd.org).

The concept of ACP has both traditional and evolving applications. Historically, ACP has referred primarily to advance directives (ADs), such as the living will and durable power of attorney for health care, which prepare adults for future medical decision making. In 1991, the Federal Patient Self-Determination Act mandated health care organizations and providers to address ADs with their adult patients (United States Public

The spiritual + emotional aspect of EoL Planning

Law 101–508, 1990). However, the focus on the documents has failed to address the broader elements of ACP (Gillick, 2004; Lorenz et al., 2004). Increasingly, ACP is viewed as a process and not a task (Hawkins, Ditto, Danks, & Smucker, 2005; Ludwick & Baughman, 2011), and as a social and not legal or autonomous activity (Romer & Hammes, 2004; Van Leuven, 2011). Today, there is widespread acknowledgment that ACP requires clarification of underlying values and goals to guide future health care decisions (Gessert, Forbes, & Bern-Klug, 2001), and applies to broader domains in life and health than mere medical decision making (Friedemann, Newman, Seff, & Dunlop, 2004; Zweig, Popejoy, Parker-Oliver, & Meadows, 2010).

Research suggests that older people require care in a variety of life domains, including social, financial, environmental, and health (Friedemann et al., 2004), and that future care needs can be anticipated as a result of common disease trajectories (Lynn, 2005). Yet much of the focus on planning for EOL care has centered on the needs of those imminently dying (Beckstrand, Callister, & Kirchhoff, 2006). Although there has been increasing attention on the holistic needs of dying people and their families (Heyland et al., 2006; Steinhauser et al., 2000; Teno, Casey, Welch, & Edgman-Levitan, 2001), relatively little attention has focused on the comprehensive needs of those whose EOL trajectories are extended prior to the final months of life. Therefore, ACP requires a long-range, holistic approach that addresses multiple considerations for practice. *RIGHT → the experiences of*

ACP throughout the EOL is a distinct area of professional practice between people and their providers. *the older Betty Asks anxiety* ACP has been defined as "a means of communication and negotiation about the patient's life goals and the care that will be received in the final years of life" (Teno & Lynn, 2005, p. 205). This view is consistent with both patient- and family-centered care that addresses an individual's needs, goals, preferences, cultural traditions, family situation, and values (Feinberg, 2012). In a special *Hastings Center Report on Improving Care at the End of Life*, Asch (2005) suggests that ACP should help people imagine not only what physical changes may occur, but also what social, technological, and financial resources they might require to maintain themselves after the onset of serious illness and disability. Therefore, future care considerations involve attention to social supports, home and safety needs, financial concerns, and health-related issues (Friedemann et al., 2004).

MULTIPLE CARE CONSIDERATIONS BY DOMAIN

Planning for care throughout the EOL is multifaceted and wide-ranging. The broad scope of EOL practice includes the following life domains: psychological, social, cultural, spiritual, medical, physical, and financial (Bern-Klug, Kramer, & Linder, 2005). As noted in Table 9.1, ACP addresses a variety of key questions by domain in order to prepare for future care needs that are either foreseeable or likely to occur. ACPs can include arrangements for services and supports that are to be provided at home or in a community setting through informal or formal care providers including family, friends, or paid staff. Family and friends are the predominant providers of both long-term and EOL care, particularly in the last year of life (Wolff, Dy, Frick, & Kasper, 2007), and about 10 million Americans with chronic illness or disabilities use formal long-term care services for personal needs (Rodgers & Komaisr, 2003). The goals of care for people essentially require melding medical- and community-based services. Therefore, professional practice in this area requires a multifaceted approach. The section below reviews select ACP aspects for consideration by domain.

TABLE 9.1
Key Questions by Domains of Care Needs Throughout the EOL

Psychological	Is the person cognitively able to recognize progressive disease manifestations and understand future care options? How is the person coping with the prospect of declining health and future needs?
Social	What social supports (formal and informal) are available to assist the person in the future? Is the caregiver capable of providing care for the extent and duration of anticipated needs?
Cultural	How does the person's ethnicity affect perceived and expected needs? What cultural traditions exist regarding health and end-of-life care?
Spiritual	Is the person aware of future care desires and values? How does the person view needs in the broader context of his/her life?
Medical	How will the person maintain and meet chronic health needs? How will the person manage future medical care and decision making?
Physical	What will be needed to ensure that the person can manage safely at home in the days ahead? What arrangements need to be considered in anticipation of the person's likely needs?
Financial	What financial resources are available to the client for meeting future care needs? What will be needed to help manage the client's resources to provide future care?

SOURCE: Black (2007). Reprinted with permission.

Psychological Considerations

Key psychological considerations include foremost the cognitive capacity to engage in planning. Although all adults are presumed to have the capacity to participate in health care and other life decisions, older adults in particular are known to possess low levels of health literacy; that is, the capacity to obtain, process, and understand basic health information and services needed to make appropriate health decisions (Centers for Disease Control and Prevention, 2009). At later stages of life, a number of factors can impact cognitive status. For example, dementia afflicts an estimated 5.2 million persons in the United States, suggesting that one in seven older adults in their 70s have dementia (Plassman et al., 2007). The percentage of older adults with dementia increases with advancing age, with estimates of prevalence at more than 4 out of 10 (44.5%) by later adulthood (Kukull & Bowen, 2002). Research suggests that persons with dementia have limited understanding of the natural progression of dementing conditions, are uncomfortable setting goals for EOL care, and have had little substantive communication with professionals regarding EOL planning (Gessert et al., 2001). Despite cognitive impairment that may eventually preclude communication, research suggests that people in the early to middle stages of the disease course are able to express preferences for care (Whitlatch & Feinberg, 2003) and should be included in clarifying values for ACP to the extent that they desire and are able (Karel, Moye, Bank, & Azar, 2007).

Social Considerations

Social considerations are quite prominent in ACP. This includes key informal networks and significant others in the person's life, such as family and friends. Such persons may be helpful in serving as surrogate decision makers or providing care in the future. As previously stated, ACP is not entirely an autonomous undertaking, as decisions made often necessitate consideration of impact on others. However, it is also important to note that older people do not need to involve others, and, without their expressed approval to engage others, in many cases, practitioner communication with others may be prohibited under the *Health Insurance and Privacy Protection Act* (HIPPA). For a variety of reasons, many older adults may have dwindling networks of others in their lives. For example, a study conducted by systematic random sampling of older adults and ACP in Florida revealed that the majority of persons anticipating the need for future care in their lives relied more so on friends (81%) than relatives (42%) (Black, Reynolds, & Osman, 2008).

It is important to ascertain whether informal supports are willing, able, and available to serve as surrogate decision makers or caregivers. For example, a systematic review on surrogate decision makers found that at least one third experienced a negative emotional burden such as stress, guilt, and doubt over their decisions, and the negative effects were often substantial and typically lasted months or, in some cases, years (Wendler & Rid, 2011). Conversely, research also suggests that increased communication with surrogates is effective in facilitating ACP decisions by increasing understanding about personal goals and preferences (Kirchhoff, Hammes, Kehl, Briggs, & Brown, 2010).

People vary greatly in their reliance on family in planning for future care needs as a result of family structure as well as current and past familial relationships (Roberto, Allen, & Blieszner, 2001), with some people preferring to receive formal care through providers such as home care agencies over family members. Moreover, there are serious concerns about caregiver burden. Research indicates that caregivers have competing responsibilities and roles and high levels of stress in EOL issues related to caregiving (Haley, 2003). In addition, the costs of future care for access to ongoing treatment, transportation, medications, and supplies can impose serious financial burdens on caregivers as well as older adults (Haley, 2003). In their pioneering work and recommendations, the Family Caregiver Alliance has called for the comprehensive assessment of caregiver capacity to provide care as an important practice and policy standard in consideration of all care plans (Family Caregiver Alliance, 2006).

Cultural Considerations

Culture has become increasingly identified as an important aspect of ACP. Culture may have an important impact on how people's specific ethnic views impact their attitudes regarding treatment wishes, ADs, and decision making about terminal care (Perkins, Geppert, Gonzales, Coretez, & Hazuda, 2002). Cultural issues that impact decision making include language, locus of decision making, fatalistic beliefs, gender and power issues in relationships, and sociopolitical and historical factors that might influence beliefs regarding illness, health care, and death (Ersek, Kagawa-Singer, Barnes, Blackhall, & Koenig, 1998). For example, not wanting to talk about future care needs was a key finding in focus group interviews with both Hispanic elders and their adult children, despite the importance of family relationships (Gutheil & Heyman, 2006) and other research showing clear preferences for less aggressive and comfort-focused care (Kelley, Wenger, & Sarkisian, 2010). Other research investigating preferences for aggressive care at the EOL revealed that, compared to Caucasians, African Americans and Hispanics preferred dying in the hospital, wanted life-prolonging drugs, and were significantly less than Caucasians to want potentially life-shortening palliative drugs (Barnato, Anthony, Skinner, Gallagher, & Fisher, 2009). Therefore, ACP should be tailored to address the specific cultural influences (Ersek et al., 1998; Perkins et al., 2002) and sociodemographic characteristics of age, gender, ethnicity, and education (Hopp, 2000; Kelley et al., 2010).

Spiritual Considerations

Spiritual factors associated with ACP broadly involve existential issues regarding the purpose and meaning in life as well as other highly valued concerns. For example, a meta-study on qualitative literature across international populations identified a spectrum of spirituality encompassing: spiritual despair (alienation, loss of self, dissonance), spiritual work (forgiveness, self-exploration, search for balance), and spiritual well-being (connection, self-actualization, consonance) (Williams, 2006). However, in a review on preferences for care at the EOL, the Agency for Healthcare Research and Quality has found that many persons are unaware of their desires, that desires change in the course of illness, and that discussions with providers and others can facilitate a better understanding of personal values and goals for future care (Kass-Bartelmes, Hughes, & Rutherford, 2003). Helpful approaches to discern spirituality can be found in the prolific work of David Hodge (2001, 2005).

Medical Considerations

Medical circumstances represent perhaps one of the most important considerations in ACP. For example, ACP preferences have been found to change over time due to health (Hawkins et al., 2005) and are related to declining health manifestations (Fried et al., 2006). Research on patients in the latter stages of a terminal disease course identified several coping concerns dealing with physical changes and managing financial demands (Farber, Egnew, Herman-Bertsch, Taylor, & Guldin, 2003). Therefore, ACP is typically conducted at several times during a person's illness so that needs can be continually reassessed (Byock, 2001). *Importance of re-thinking ACP as a person's condition progresses*

Physical Considerations

To best meet comprehensive ACP needs, it is critically important to consider physical aspects of the person's life, such as the match between their current degree of functioning and projected needs. This involves assessing the physical environment of the home as well as the *fit* between the older person and his or her residential setting (Pynoos, 1990). That is, it is important to ensure the right balance between the demands of the person's ability to deal with their environment (Lawton & Nahemow, 1977). Moreover, physical needs, as well as one's physical environment, are further compounded by psychological, social, medical, and financial circumstances that affect future and end-of-life care plans. That is, the physical environment is the result of the dynamic interaction between people, social processes, and relationships (Yen & Syme, 1999). Therefore, though identified as a distinct domain here, physical needs must be viewed within a comprehensive context.

Financial Considerations

Financial considerations represent a critical, yet often under-considered, aspect of planning. Understanding one's finances is important to best plan for the costs of future care needs. In most cases, a variety of factors converge with financial issues to impact ACP. For example, factors influencing plans for future nursing home care included affordability and insurance availability, as well as health and functional status and the availability of formal and informal support (Mitsuko, Chapin, Macmillan, & Zimmerman, 2004). Helpful resources to assess future care costs can be found at the National Clearinghouse for Long-Term Care Information at www.longtermcare.gov, which provides detailed costs throughout the continuum of care by geographical location (U.S. Department of Health and Human Services, 2012).

BEHAVIORAL CHANGE MODEL FOR PLANNING

Increasingly, ACP is viewed as a health behavior and applied to various behavioral change models including the Transtheoretical Model (TTM) of behavior change (Fried, Bullock, Iannone, & O'Leary, 2009; Fried et al., 2010; Pearlman, Cole, Patrick, Starks, & Cain, 1995). Initially identified by Prochaska and DiClemente (1983) and applied to smoking behavior, the model has since been applied to other behaviors. For example, in application to ACP, behavior change is viewed along a continuum ranging from: (a) precontemplation (e.g., not thinking about ACP); (b) contemplation (e.g., actively thinking about ACP); (c) preparation (e.g., commitment to engage in ACP); (d) action (e.g., undertaking ACP); and (e) maintenance (e.g., ongoing changes to ACP). Research has found that older adults are in different stages of readiness, as identified by different components of the model, as a result of many perceived benefits and barriers to planning, and that ACP does not represent the totality of one's planning for the EOL (Fried et al., 2009). Furthermore, past experiences with health care decision making for others represented a strong influence on their own perceptions of susceptibility and engagement in ACP. Additional research on the model suggests that a majority of older patients were found to be stuck in the precontemplation stage due to lack of communication with their providers (Fried et al., 2010). Recommendations from the study suggest tailoring discussions based on personal readiness to change and recommend that such discussions occur through non-medical settings, with other providers and paraprofessionals.

Personality Styles Associated With Decision Making

Distinct personality styles have been associated with ACP. In one grouping, personalities were identified in five subtypes, including: (a) Scramblers: forced to act in response to a serious health crisis; (b) Reluctant Consenters: pushed to make a change in care arrangements by relatives and professionals who notice a decline in health and functional independence; (c) Wake-up Caller: change care arrangements in response to a near crisis while health continues to deteriorate, thereby requiring greater levels of care; and (d) Advance Planners: research long-term care options and plan ahead while still healthy (Maloney, Finn, Bloom, & Andresen, 1996). Other research has identified (a) Avoiders: who try not to think about future care issues; (b) Thinkers: who are aware of future care needs, but make no plans; (c) Planners: who think about and make concrete plans regarding their future care needs; and (d) Consenters: who adopt the plans devised by family members and others (Steele, Pinquart, & Sorenson, 2003). Accordingly, people differ in their willingness to plan ahead (Bailly & DePoy, 1995). Although research suggests that many people want to know what to expect in the course of their illness (Beisecker, 1988; Steinhauser et al., 2000) and services available to provide long-term care (Kane & Kane, 2001), others may be cognitively limited or unable to be involved in ACP.

CONCLUSION

This chapter has discussed considerations for ACP practice with older adults using a reconceptualization of traditional planning based solely on future health care decision making to a longer range, holistic view that incorporates multiple life domains. The importance of ACP with older people was discussed and trajectories of decline leading to the EOL were presented. Multiple care needs were addressed along with key domains for consideration in ACP practice with older adults. A behavioral change model (TTM) for ACP practice was presented along with research on personality styles associated with planning in advance for care.

REFERENCES

Americans for Better Care for the Dying. (2012). Retrieved from http://www.abcd-caring.org

Asch, A. (2005). Recognizing death while affirming life. In *Improving end-of-life care: Why has it been so difficult? Hastings Center Report Special, 35*, S31–S36.

Bailly, D. J., & DePoy, E. (1995). Older people's responses to education about advance Directives. *Health & Social Work, 20*, 223–228.

Barnato, A. E., Anthony, D. L., Skinner, J., Gallagher, P. M., & Fisher, E. S. (2009). Racial and ethnic differences in preferences for end-of-life treatment. *Journal of General Internal Medicine, 24*(6), 695–701.

Beckstrand, R. L., Callister, L. C., & Kirchhoff, K. T. (2006). Providing a "good death": Critical care nurses' suggestions for improving end-of-life care. *American Journal of Critical Care, 15,* 38–45.

Beisecker, A. E. (1988). Aging and the desire for information and input in medical decisions: Patient consumerism in medical encounters. *The Gerontologist, 28,* 330–335.

Bern-Klug, M., Kramer, B. J., & Linder, J. F. (2005). All aboard: Advancing the social work research agenda in end of life and palliative care. *Journal of Social Work in End of life and Palliative Care, 1,* 71–86.

Black, K. (2007). Advance care planning throughout the end of life: Focusing the Lens for Social Work. *Journal of Social Work in Palliative and End-of-Life Care, 3*(2), 39–58.

Black, K., Reynolds, S., & Osman, H. (2008). Factors associated with advance care planning among older adults in southwest Florida. *Journal of Applied Gerontology, 27*(1), 93–109.

Byock, I. R. (2001). End-of-life care: A public health crisis and an opportunity for managed care. *The American Journal of Managed Care, 7,* 1123–1132.

Centers for Disease Control and Prevention. (2009). *Improving health literacy for older Adults: Expert panel report 2009.* Atlanta, GA: U.S. Department of Health and Human Services.

Centers for Disease Control and Prevention. (2011). *Healthy aging: Helping people live long and productive lives and enjoy a good quality of life.* Atlanta, GA: National Center for Chronic Disease Prevention and Health Promotion.

Ersek, M., Kagawa-Singer, M., Barnes, D., Blackhall, L., & Koenig, B.A. (1998). Multicultural considerations in the use of advance directives. *Oncology Nursing Forum, 10,* 1683–1690.

Family Caregiver Alliance. (2006). *Caregiver assessment: Principles, guidelines and strategies for change.* Report from a National Consensus Development Conference (Vol. I). San Francisco, CA: Author.

Farber, S. J., Egnew, T. R., Herman-Bertsch, J. L., Taylor, T. R., & Goldin, G. E. (2003). Issues in end-of-life care: Patient, caregiver, and clinician perceptions. *Journal of Palliative Medicine, 6,* 19–31.

Field, M. J., & Cassel, C. K. (1997). *Approaching death: Improving care at the end of life.* Washington, DC: Institute of Medicine, National Academies Press.

Feinberg, L. (2012). *Moving toward person- and family-centered care.* Washington, DC: AARP Public Policy Institute.

Fried, T. R., Bullock, K., Iannone, L., & O'Leary, J. R. (2009). Understanding advance care planning as a process of health behavior change. *Journal of the American Geriatrics Society, 57,* 1547–1555.

Fried, T. R., Redding, C. A., Robbins, M. L., Paiva, A., O'Leary, J. R., & Iannone, L. (2010). Stages of change for the component behaviors of advance care planning. *Journal of the American Geriatrics Society, 58,* 2329–2336.

Fried, T. R., Byers, A. L., Gallo., W. T., Van Ness, P. H., Towle, V. R., O'Leary, J. R., & Dublin, J. A. (2006). Prospective study of health status preferences and changes in preferences over time in older adults. *Archives of Internal Medicine, 166*, 890–895.

Friedemann, M. L., Newman, F. L., Seff, L. R., & Dunlop, B. D. (2004). Planning for long-term care: Concept, definition, and measurement. *The Gerontologist, 44*, 520–530.

Gessert, C. E., Forbes, S., & Bern-Klug, M. (2001). Planning end-of-life care for patients with dementia: Roles of families and health professionals. *OMEGA, 42*, 173–291.

Gillick, M. (2004). Advance care planning. *New England Journal of Medicine, 350*, 7–8.

Gutheil, I. A., & Heyman, J. C. (2006). "They don't want to hear us": Hispanic elders and adult children speak about end-of-life planning. *Journal of Social Work in Palliative and End-of-life Care, 2*, 55–70.

Haley, W. E. (2003). Family caregivers of elderly patients with cancer: Understanding and minimizing the burden of care. *Journal of Supportive Oncology, 1*, 25–29.

Hawkins, N. A., Ditto, P. H., Danks, J. H., & Smucker, W. D. (2005). Micromanaging death: Process preferences, values, and goals in end-of-life medical decision making. *The Gerontologist, 5*, 107–117.

Heyland, D. K., Dodek, P., Rocker, G., Groll, D., Gafni, A., Pichora, D., et al. (2006). What matters most in end-of-life care: perceptions of seriously ill patients and their family members. *Canadian Medical Association Journal, 174*, 627–633.

Hodge, D. R. (2001). Spiritual assessment: A review of major qualitative methods and a new framework for assessing spirituality. *Social Work, 46*, 203–214.

Hodge, D. R. (2005). Spiritual life maps: A client-centered pictorial instrument for spiritual assessment, planning, and intervention. *Social Work, 50*, 77–87.

Hopp, F. P. (2000). Preferences for surrogate decision makers, informal communication, and advance directives among community-dwelling elders: Results from a national study. *Gerontologist, 40*(4), 449–457.

Kane, R. L., & Kane, R.A. (2001). What older people want from long-term care, and how they can get it. *Health Affairs, 20*, 114–127.

Karel, M. J., Moye, J., Bank, A., & Azar, A. R. (2007). Three models of assessing values for advance care planning: Comparing persons with and without dementia. *Journal of Aging and Health, 19*, 123–151.

Kass-Bartelmes, B. L., Hughes, R., & Rutherford, M. K. (2003). *Advance care planning: Preferences for care at the end of life.* Rockville, MD: Agency for Healthcare Research and Quality. Research in Action Issue #12. AHRQ Pub No. 03–0018.

Kelley, A., Wenger, N., & Sarkisian, C. (2010). Opinions: End-of-life care preferences and planning of older Latinos. *Journal of the American Geriatrics Society, 58*(6), 1109.

Kirchhoff, K. T., Hammes, B. J., Kehl, K. A., Briggs, R. A., & Brown, A. L. (2010). Effect of a disease-specific planning intervention on surrogate understanding of patient goals for future medical treatment. *Journal of the American Geriatrics Society, 58*(7), 1233.

Kukull, W. A., & Bowen, J. D. (2002). Dementia epidemiology. *Medical Clinics of North America, 86*, 573–590.

Lawton, M. P., & Nahemow, L. (1977). Ecology and aging process. In C. Eisendorfer & M. P. Lawton (Eds.), *The psychology of adult development and aging* (pp. 619–674). Washington, DC: American Psychological Association.

Lynn, J (1997). Measuring quality at the end-of-life: A statement of principles. *Journal of the American Geriatrics Society, 45*, 526–527.

Lynn, J. (2005). Living long in fragile health: The new demographics shape end-of-life care. In *Improving end-of-life care: Why has it been so difficult? Hastings Center Report Special, 35*, S14–S18.

Lynn, J., & Adamson, D. M. (2003). *Living well at the end of life. Adapting health care to serious chronic illness in old age.* Washington, DC: Rand Health.

Lorenz, K., Lynn, J., Morton, S. C., Dy, S., Mularski, R., Shugarman, L., et al. (2004). *End-of-life care and outcomes summary.* Evidence Report/Technology Assessment: Number 110. AHRQ Publication Number 05-E004–1, December 2004. Rockville, MD: Agency for Healthcare Research and Quality. Retrieved from http://www.ahrq.gov/clinic/epcsums/eolsum.htm. Last accessed January 24, 2006.

Ludwick, R., & Baughman, K. (2011). Advancing the advance care planning process. *International Journal of Older People Nursing, 6*(3), 163–164.

Maloney, S. K., Finn, F., Bloom, D. L., & Andresen, J. (1996). Personal decision-making styles and long-term care choices. *Health Care Financing Review, 18*, 141–156.

Mitsuko, N., Chapin, R. K., Macmillian, K., & Zimmerman, M. (2004). Decision making in long term care: Approaches used by older adults and implications for social work practice. *Journal of Gerontological Social Work, 43*, 79–102.

Murphy, S. L., Xu, J. Q., & Kochanek, K. D. (2012). Deaths: Preliminary data for 2010. *National Vital Statistics Reports, 60*(4). Hyattsville, MD: National Center for Health Statistics.

National Consensus Project for Quality Palliative Care. (2009). *Clinical practice guidelines for quality palliative care* (2nd ed.). Retrieved from http://www.national-consensusproject.org.

National Institutes of Health (NIH). (2005). *State-of-the-science conference statement on improving end- of-life care.* Bethesda, MD: National Institutes of Health.

National Healthcare Decisions Day. (2012). Retrieved from http://www.nhdd.org.

Pearlman, R. A., Cole, W. G., Patrick, D. L., Starks, H. E., & Cain, K. C. (1995). Advance care planning: Eliciting patient preferences for life-sustaining treatment. *Patient Education Counseling, 26*, 353–361.

Perkins, H. S., Geppert, C. M. A., Gonzales, A., Cortez, J. D., & Hazuda, H. P. (2002). Cross-cultural similarities and differences in attitudes about advance care planning. *Journal of General Internal Medicine, 17*(1), 48–57.

Plassman, B. L., Langa, K. M., Fisher, G. G., Heering, S. G., Weir, D. R., Ofstedal, M. B.,…Wallace, R. B. (2007). Prevalence of dementia in the United States: The aging, demographics, and memory study. *Neuroepidemiology, 29*, 125–133.

Prochaska, J. O., & DiClemente, C. C. (1983). Stages and processes of self-change of smoking: Toward an integrative model of change. *Journal of Consulting and Clinical Psychology, 51*(3), 390–395.

Pynoos, J. (1990). Public policy and aging-in-place: Identifying the problems and potential solutions. In Tilson (Ed.), *Aging-in-place: Supporting the frail elderly in residential environments* (pp. 167–208). Glenview, IL: Scott, Foreman.

Robert Wood Johnson Foundation. (2012). *Means to a better end: A report on dying in America today*. Retrieved from http://www.rwjf.org.

Roberto, K. A., Allen, K. R., & Blieszner, R. (2001). Older adults' preferences for future care: Formal plans and familial support. *Applied Developmental Science, 5*, 112–120.

Rodgers, S., & Komaisr, H. (2003). *Who needs long term care?* Washington, DC: Georgetown University Long Term Care Financing Project.

Romer, A. L., & Hammes, B. J. (2004). Communication, trust, and making choices: Advance care planning four years on. *Journal of Palliative Medicine, 7*, 335–340.

Steele, M., Pinquart, M., & Sorenson, S. (2003). Preparation dimensions and styles in long-term care. *Clinical Gerontologist, 26*, 105–122.

Steinhauser, K. E., Christakis, N. A., Clipp, E. C., McNeilly, M., McIntyre, L., & Tulsky, J. A. (2000). Factors considered important at the end of life by patients, family, physicians, and other care providers. *Journal of the American Medical Association, 284*, 2476–2482.

Soros Foundation. (2012). *Transforming the culture of dying: The project on death in America*. Retrieved from http://www.soros.org/initiative/pdia

Teno, J. M., & Lynn, J. (2005). Putting advance care planning into action. *The Journal of Clinical Ethics, 7*, 205–214.

Teno, J. M., Casey, V. A., Welch, L. C., & Edgman-Levitan, S. (2001). Patient-focused, family-centered end-of-life medical care views of the guidelines and bereaved family members. *Journal of Pain and Symptom Management, 22*, 738–751.

U.S. Department of Health and Human Services. (2012). *National clearinghouse for long-term care information*. Retrieved from www.longtermcare.gov

United States Public Law 101–508. (1990). *Patient self determination act*. Washington, DC: US Code.

Van Leuven, K. (2011). Advance care planning in healthy older adult. *Californian Journal of Health Promotion, 9*(2), 6–14.

Wendler, D., & Rid, A. (2011). Systematic review: The effect on surrogates of making treatment decisions for others. *Annals of Internal Medicine, 154*, 336–346.

Werner, C. A. (2011). *The older population: 2010 census briefs* (Report # C2010BR-09). Washinton, DC: U.S. Census Bureau.

Whitlatch, C. J., & Feinberg, L. F. (2003). Planning for the future together in culturally diverse families: Making everyday care decisions. *Alzheimer's Care Quarterly, 4*, 50–62.

Williams, A. L. (2006). Perspectives on spirituality at the end of life: A meta-summary. *Palliative & Supportive Care, 4*, 407–417.

Wolff, J. L., Dy, S. M., Frick, K. D., & Kasper, J. D. (2007). End-of-life care: Findings from a national survey of informal caregivers. *Archives of Internal Medicine, 167*, 40–46.

Yen, I. H., & Syme, S. L. (1999). The social environment and health: A discussion of the epidemiologic literature. *Annual Review of Public Health, 20*, 287–308.

Zweig, S. C., Popejoy, L. L., Parker-Oliver, D., & Meadows, S. E. (2010). The physician's role in patients' nursing home care: "She's a very courageous and lovely woman. I enjoy caring for her." *The Journal of the American Medical Association, 306*(13), 1468–1478.

CHAPTER 10

Worlds of Connection: Applying an Interdisciplinary Relational Model of Care© to Communicating About End of Life

Susana Lauraine McCune

DEATH IS NOT THE ENEMY

Death is a human universal. Death is inclusive. Death is multicultural and multiracial. Death is not ageist or sexist. Death is the great equalizer. Death impacts everyone who is living, and does so during all phases of the life span. Why then is modern American society so resistant to discussing death and the truths of aging and medical care that bring us to death? Our current medical culture and health care system appear driven to use all available medical care to prevent, or at least postpone, all deaths in all situations and at all costs.

Advanced medical technologies can extend life almost indefinitely. Sulmasy (2002) commented that "today's health professions seem to have become superb at addressing the physical finitude of the human body. Previously lethal diseases have either become curable or have been transformed into the chronic" (p. 24). Sulmasy notes here that while medicine has advanced to the point of being able to cure many lethal diseases, one effect of such advances is the current high prevalence of chronic diseases. This means that while more people are living longer, experiences of disease and frailty that lead to physical and mental incapacity over an extended duration of the life span are now common patient experiences that require long-term planning. Even though advanced medical technology has been able to cure deadly diseases and postpone death, the prominence of chronic diseases and new choices about which technologies to use and when to use them requires longer-term attention. This requires all of us, including clinicians, to give more attention to the prospect of extended medical care over a longer period of life. This in turn requires that clinicians be able to address the needs of whole human persons, and not just give attention to producing physiological effects on parts of the finite body that are most visibly affected by disease. However, contemporary medicine, as Sulmasy stated, "still stands justly accused of having failed to address itself to the needs of whole human persons and of preferring to limit its attention to the finitude of human bodies" (p. 24).

Holistic treatment of patients can help counteract the body-bound, or strictly physiological, understanding of the patient that technology has encouraged. Sulmasy (2002) observed that "genuinely holistic health care must address the totality of the patient's relational existence" (p. 24). Total care of the patient must also account for the ways in which the patient exists in relation not only to his/her disease, but also to the myriad factors—not solely the physical, but also the psychosocial dynamics that structure the patient's life. Sulmasy goes on to say that "the fundamental task of medicine, nursing, and the other health care professions is to minister to the suffering occasioned by the necessary physical finitude of human persons, in their living and in their dying" (p. 24). Toward this end, Sulmasy advocates a more comprehensive model of care that accounts for patients in the "fullest possible understanding of their wholeness—as persons grappling with their ultimate finitude" (p. 24).

A person's quest for psychological and existential meaning in the face of finitude continues across the life span (Reker & Chamberlain, 2000). The challenge for clinicians then is to recognize that companioning—accompanying—a patient as he or she conceptualizes and develops an advance care plan—a plan for dying and death—is as important as companioning a patient in developing a plan of care for curing disease—a plan for living.

Toward these ends, this chapter presents the Interdisciplinary Relational Model of Care© (IRMOC) as a theoretical framework that aspires to support clinicians' ability to engage with patients and their loved ones about advance care planning (ACP) for end-of-life (EOL) care and, in so doing, improve the quality and increase the frequency of communication about ACP. The tasks of this chapter are to bring together theoretical concepts and clinical skills that have until now been regarded and employed disparately. It will demonstrate how, when applied together, these concepts and skills can help clinicians feel more comfortable and confident conducting, and thus better facilitate, more frequent communication about ACP.

The chapter begins with a discussion of the historical impact that the presuppositions of objectivity, paternalism, and autonomy have had on patient–clinician models of care in which ACP takes place. Next, the chapter considers the ways in which these presuppositions perpetuate dynamics that relational psychology understands as counter- and cotransference (Orange, 1995, 2006). It will present emergent understanding from contemporary relational psychological theory that emphasizes compassion as a fundamental element in the patient–clinician relationship (Orange, 2006). This is followed by overviews of reflective practice and therapeutic communication skills that can help clinicians facilitate communication about ACP. The chapter concludes with a summary and a case study demonstrating the need for the IRMOC and ACP.

BEYOND OBJECTIVITY, PATERNALISM, AND AUTONOMY

The "objectification myth," which requires psychological distance in professional relationships, is detrimental to the patient and impairs clinical empathy.

Smith and Newton, 1984, p. 57

The birth of modern science began with the scientific and philosophical revolution of the 17th century, catalyzed by the work of philosopher Renee Decartes. Bordo (1987) observed that Decartes' "seventeenth-century rationalist project" has brought forward the "objectivist, mechanist presuppositions of modern science" (p. 1). Objectivity holds that each person exists independently of each other, and that people are able to view things and interact with others independent of—detached from—their emotions, thoughts, and biases. Bordo notes that since the 17th century, "The Cartesian epistemological ideals of clarity, detachment, and objectivity" have remained "largely unquestioned" (p. 4). As such, the presuppositions of clarity, detachment, and objectivity have become the underlying assumptions that have shaped the modern era. These ideals have also informed theoretical conceptualizations of the patient–clinician relationship, and influenced formulation of models of care. These models of care have been predominately based on what Bordo labels "absolute epistemic objectivity" (p. 2).

History demonstrates how over time, along with objectivity, the moral principles of paternalism and autonomy have also informed conceptual frameworks for models of care and paradigms for the patient–clinician relationship (Roter, 2000; Schermer, 2003; Smith & Newton, 1984). At the beginning of the 20th century, the patient–clinician model included a "paternalistic" ethic and physician privilege, which were based on the Hippocratic Oath. According to the paternalistic ethic, in this paradigm the professional care provider was held as an objective "authority" that delivered information, and power relations (Emanuel & Emanuel, 1992; Roter, 2000) inherent in the clinical relationship were not acknowledged.

Developed in parallel with, and in response to, paternalism, models for the patient–clinician relationship evolved that emphasized the role of patient autonomy. The principle of autonomy underscores the patient's right to make her or his own decisions about care (Schermer, 2003; Smith & Newton, 1984).

Models of care based on patient autonomy also emphasize the clinician's nondirectiveness and value-neutrality (Wachbroit & Wasserman, 1995). The clinician's value-neutrality is based on the underlying assumption that the clinician can be "objective" and, in so doing, the clinician's objectivity facilitates upholding a clinical distance to ensure that the clinician does not interfere with the patient's autonomy.

These three paradigms have thus at times intertwined and reinforced each other. In the objectivist, paternalist, and autonomous models, the clinician's and the patient's lived experiences are partitioned off from each other. The "autonomous patient" remains independent of the "objective clinician," and thus, the illusion of separateness is perpetuated. However, Smith (an internist) and Newton (a philosopher) recognized that "the old 'objective' medical tradition, which aims to separate me from my patient, is invoked as a mechanism—a very ineffective mechanism—to prevent such entanglement of our lives" (1984, p. 53). Smith and Newton concluded: "The myth of clinical distance between the patient and the physician is, after all, only a myth" (p. 53).

In contrast to objectivity, subjectivity describes the presence of one's personal thoughts and emotions, and one's unique personal reality. Smith and Newton (1984) captured the subtle, yet important, aspect of subjectivity in the clinical relationship: "To understand the patient, the physician must *see* the patient, which requires personal contact with the sphere of the subjective, a difficult skill to learn or teach" (p. 57).

Intersubjectivity extends subjectivity by recognizing the interactive features of human relatedness. Intersubjectivity, as Stolorow, Atwood, and Brandchaft stated, underscores the importance of the "reciprocal mutual influence" (1994/2004, p. 37) between the patient and the clinician. The paradigm of intersubjectivity acknowledges that relational interactions between people take place within an intersubjective sphere that is comprised of each person's subjectivity.

A new model for the patient–clinician relationship, the IRMOC aims to account for the importance of intersubjectivity. The IRMOC conceptualization stresses the importance of understanding the unique intersubjective experiences of the patient and the clinician and the mutual influence they have on each other. This paradigm also values and calls attention to the meaning of relationship. In this way, instead of emphasizing paternalism, objectivity, autonomy, and clinical distance, this new model recognizes the mutually reciprocal intersubjective spheres of engagement—the worlds of connection—between the patient and the clinician, and in so doing encourages mutual trust, suffering, and compassion.

A SHIFT TO RELATIONALITY: APPLYING THE INTERDISCIPLINARY MODEL OF CARE

In this new concept, the clinician is no longer the distant and objective authority in charge of making a patient well, and delivering information unidirectionally, as in the paternalistic model. Neither is the clinician the authority who listens unidirectionally, leaving the patient to make his/her "autonomous" choices in a vacuum, as in the autonomy model. Rather, in the IRMOC, the clinician is encouraged to shift his/her self-conceptualization to begin to see himself/herself as a professional who compassionately companions—or accompanies—the patient and does so with awareness of the ways in which the clinician is affected by the patient, and the patient is affected by the clinician. Such a shift can underscore the importance of relationality that is conditioned by—but certainly not limited to—medical professionals' concern with improving the body's condition. In so doing, the IRMOC suggests that a focus on relational psychological theories that incorporate counter- and cotransference, compassion, and therapeutic communication skills might help establish the intersubjective relationship as the basis of ACP situations.

The IRMOC is a model for conceptualizing the patient–clinician relationship that is based in relational psychological theory (e.g., Aron & Harris, 2005, 2011; Mitchell & Aron, 1999). This body of theory recognizes the importance of the patient–clinician relationship and acknowledges the importance of reciprocal mutual influence in the clinical relationship. Relational psychological theory is grounded in "respect for the personal realities of both participants" (Stolorow et al., 1994/2004, p. xii) and the understanding that contexts of relatedness and interaction between people are crucial. This relational conceptualization allows for the recognition and integration of both the patient's and the clinician's unique and mutually reciprocal intersubjective experiences. The IRMOC aims to undo the illusion of separateness and, instead, re-centers the focus on the relationship between patient and clinician.

In addition to a focus on relationship, the IRMOC encourages compassion and conversation in the spirit of discovery as a means of reaching mutual understanding about the patient's desired medical care, which is then documented through the process of ACP. The IRMOC also calls for reflective practice to help reveal clinicians' transference and countertransference. The aim of the IRMOC is not to require all care providers to become psychologists, but to recognize that clinicians can provide better care for the whole person with the aid of some understanding of vital psychological concepts.

Some might see the highly specific goals of care in psychotherapy as not always fitting the needs of clinicians facilitating communication about ACP in medical settings—settings in which at times a flurry of activity is occurring and quick life-and-death decisions may need to be made. However, psychological concepts are valuable in ACP. Psychological services are useful for individuals who wish to make thoughtful plans about their own future care (Haley, Larson, Kasl-Godley, Neimeyer, & Kwilosz, 2003). In addition, Haley et al. (2003) argue that psychology is not usually recognized as a part of the current paradigm for medical care. The omission of psychology in medical care and ACP situations may result in a gap in finding solutions that meet the psychological needs of patients.

UNSPOKEN CLINICAL REALITIES: TRANSFERENCE, COUNTERTRANSFERENCE, AND COTRANSFERENCE

Everyone is much more simply human than otherwise.

Sullivan, 1953, p. 32

Transference and *countertransference* are psychoanalytic concepts first identified by Sigmund Freud (1905/1955). *Transference* refers to the phenomenon in which patients transfer to the clinician feelings about persons who were important early in the patient's life. The American Psychological Association *Dictionary of Psychology* defines *countertransference* as the clinician's "unconscious reactions to the patient and to the patient's transference" (VandenBos, 2007, p. 239). Psychoanalytic theories, along with definitions of transference and countertransference, have evolved during the past century since Freud coined the terms. Today, relational psychological theory acknowledges that, as Stolorow and Lachmann (1995/2000) observed, "Transference and countertransference together form an intersubjective system of reciprocal mutual influence" (p. 42). This mutual influence can manifest as the clinician's countertransference. In relational psychological theory, countertransference is not seen as taboo in the patient–clinician relationship, but is seen instead as an instrument that is necessary to the relationship, as a means to inform the clinician's understanding.

Countertransference can arise for clinicians due to the nonreciprocal professional duty to care that is intrinsic to caring professions. Silver (1999) observed that while transference and countertransference exist in all human relationships, transference and countertransference are "most notable and potentially problematic in those relationships involving the 'imbalance of power' (p. 265) inherent in the 'power relationship of caring professions'"

(p. 267). These professional relationships—relationships in which the obligations and duty of caring are one-sided—can invite misplaced emotional responses and countertransference. Nonreciprocal professional relationships include nurse–patient relationships (O'Kelly, 1998), doctor–patient relationships (Stein, 1985), and relationships between social workers and patients (Berzoff & Kita, 2010), among others.

According to Silver (1999) countertransference emanates from both professional training and personal experience. It is therefore important for clinicians to recognize that their history, including personal experiences and professional training, "filters, informs, and organizes" their perceptions and responsiveness to patients (Orange, 1995, p. 63). Orange parses further the clinician's responses to the patient and the clinical setting and proposes that we reserve the term "countertransference" for the clinician's "reactive emotional memories that interfere with empathetic understanding" and "optimal responsiveness" to the patient (1995, p. 74). In contrast to countertransference, Orange introduced the term *cotransference* to describe influences of the clinician's history and personality that help to empathetically understand the patient's experience "through our [the clinician's] own equally subjective experience" (1995, p. 66). Orange (1995) concludes: "We must know and acknowledge our cotransference, our point of view or perspective, if we are to become capable of empathy" (p. 71).

Another source of counter- and cotransference can emerge from projection bias (Loewenstein, 2005). Projection bias occurs when one attempts to predict how another will behave, yet errs in the prediction as a result of underestimating or overestimating "differences between oneself and others" (Loewenstein, 2005, p. 99). In the case of ACP, the clinician may project his/her own projective biases into the ACP process.

One last yet important point about counter- and cotransference as conceptualized by Orange (2006) is that the clinician's "self-expectations" are vital. The author reminds us, as she reminds herself that, at times, "there is no way to fix the situation or 'cure' the patient, so I must accept my own powerlessness to help" (p. 16).

Counter- and cotransference are important in discussions about ACP because contemplating EOL care and facing mortality, whether one's own or that of another, can evoke existential anxiety, fear, and uncertainty in both the patient and the clinician. Attempting to maintain assumptions of objectivity, paternalism, and autonomy can camouflage the clinician's self-expectations, projection biases, feelings of powerlessness, and unconscious death anxieties. If these hidden assumptions remain unidentified and unacknowledged, they can lead the clinician to, perhaps unwittingly, project his/her own values into the patient's ACP process. The clinician may also defend against his/her own anxieties and fears about death. As a result, rather than helping the patient develop and document advance care plans, the clinician may unknowingly influence the patient's ACP formulation or avoid discussions about ACP, planning for EOL care, and death altogether.

Consequently, the IRMOC challenges clinicians to recognize the ways in which their self-expectations and personal views accompany, or are perhaps hidden by, assumptions from medical training and previous experiences. Relatedly, the IRMOC asks clinicians to reflect on the ways in which countertransference and projection bias can inadvertently influence the ability to facilitate communication about ACP with patients and their loved ones.

Reflective Practice: Discovering Countertransference and Cotransference

Counter- and cotransference involve personal matters, which can have public implications. These dynamics may at times either hinder or help a clinician's ability to facilitate communication about ACP. Only when counter- and cotransference are identified and understood can professionals ensure that they have made every effort to provide the best professional care assisting patients in developing their advance care plans. Therefore, clinicians must be able to identify the ways in which their personal experiences and professional training are impacting their clinical practice. At the same time, clinicians must both respect these experiences and advocate for the patient's advance care plans. To do this—specifically, to identify and address counter- and cotransference—requires reflective practice.

Reflective practice is the act of reflecting on the clinical encounter with the intent to evaluate and continually improve the clinician's proficiency. Reflection has the intent to assess and search for meaning, and to understand how the clinician has been affected by, and has responded to, the patient (Johns & Freshwater, 2005; Ruth-Sahd, 2003). In the process, clinicians ask themselves questions along the lines of: How have I been affected by this encounter with this patient? How has my personal past and professional training influenced my clinical receptivity and my responsiveness to this patient? How have these affected my ability to engage in communication about ACP? In prompting these questions the IRMOC promotes moments of quiet introspection and encourages compassion for both the patient and for the clinician.

COMPASSION IN THE CLINICAL RELATIONSHIP

Orange (2006) advocates for clinicians to restore compassion to a central role in the patient–clinician relationship (p. 7). She goes on to observe that in everyday English, "compassion" often connotes "pity or sympathy" and thus compassion could also imply the act of "being-nice-to-patients" (p. 14).

However, the IMROC's conceptualization of compassion goes beyond this everyday understanding. In keeping with Orange's interpretation, the IRMOC draws on the etymology of the word. The Latin origin of *compassion,* as Orange reminds us, is *suffering with.*

Orange (2006) notes that, complementarily, the Latin origin of the word *patient* is *patior*: *to suffer, or undergo.* Thus, "a patient is one who suffers, who bears what feels unbearable" (p. 15). In relationship to the patient, who is bearing what feels unbearable, the clinician's compassion is thus "a suffering-with, a bearing together" (p. 15). The author concludes that compassion is "a way of being-with" and is "both process and attitude" (p. 15). Orange advises, if "we are not too intent on naming pathologies and defenses or being right, but instead relentlessly seek to understand and accompany the sufferer, an implicitly interpretive system emerges" (p. 15). By seeking to understand and accompany—to *suffer with*—the patient (*the sufferer*), the clinician can help mitigate remaining echoes of paternalism and objectivity, and attenuate clinicians' tendency to "name pathologies," focus exclusively on physiology, and maintain the illusion of clinical distance. In this way, compassion can guide clinicians as they facilitate communication about ACP and EOL care.

Compassionate Communication

In the foreword to his book, Knapp (2007) notes that therapeutic communication skills are "universal principles among health and human service providers" (p. xi). They are effective ways of listening and responding in clinical relationships (Hammond, Hepworth, & Smith, 2002). These skills have been posited for inclusion in training curricula for nurses (Kluge & Glick, 2006), doctors (Back, Arnold, & Tulsky, 2009), social workers, and other helping professionals (Wolvin & Coakley, 1985). From a psychotherapeutic view, Orange (2011) has advocated a "readiness to listen and learn from the voice of the other [the patient] —as a clinical philosophy" (p. 15). However, there has been historically a lack of clinical training in these skills.

Many clinicians provide exquisitely compassionate care and sensitively engage in communication with patients. Yet the literature demonstrates that this is not the experience of many patients or their loved ones (Tulsky, 2004). At the same time, therapeutic communication skills have been widely identified as crucial to building clinician confidence in that such skills can enhance ACP by augmenting clinicians' interpersonal competence and increasing patient trust (Rodriguez et al., 2011; Skirbekk, Middelthon, Hjortdahl, & Finset, 2011). Improved therapeutic communication skills have also been shown to reduce professional health care providers' anxiety (Back et al., 2009; Fried, Bradley, O'Leary, & Byers, 2005). Moreover, Levinson (1994) and Roter (2000) propose that clinicians improve their communication skills as a way to reduce malpractice suits.

Schaffer and Norlander (2009) offer eight principles that underlie therapeutic communication in the health care setting. Together, these principles provide a supportive framework for clinicians to draw upon when communicating with patients and their advocates and loved ones. These principles can help clinicians skillfully facilitate communication about ACP. Schaffer and Norlander's principles have been adapted here, in conjunction with other authors' recommendations, to the particular imperatives of ACP:

- Ensure privacy and adequate time for ACP discussions.
- Assess patients' and their loved ones' and advocates' understanding of disease processes, treatment options, and effects of treatment. Respond by providing accurate information about diagnosis, prognosis, and effects of treatment simply and honestly while avoiding euphemisms and medical jargon. Give broad, realistic (not overly optimistic) time frames for possible effects of diseases and treatments in order to help the patient and his or her advocates take full advantage of "relevant and accurate information about the medical details of various clinical conditions and treatments" (Ditto, Hawkins, & Pizarro, 2005, p. 494) as they formulate and complete ADs.
- Encourage expression of feelings and elicit patients' values, beliefs, and care goals as guides for formulating ACP (Doukas & McCollough, 1991).
- Be empathetic and embody both a process and attitude of compassion (Orange, 2006).
- Arrange for follow-up. This final point is particularly noteworthy in ACP situations.

Follow-up in ACP is crucial because ACP is not a one-time event. Advance care plans should be revisited whenever patient's care needs, desires, and circumstances change.

An important additional component to the principles offered by Schaffer and Norlander is found in the SPIKES Protocol (Baile et al., 2000), which encourages clinicians to ask open-ended questions to reach increased understanding. Clinicians often mistakenly believe that asking open-ended questions and cultivating deeper understanding requires more time than is available. However, Stewart, Brown, and Weston (1989) found that this is not the case if clinicians follow basic communication principles, including paying attention to the patient's emotional schema, listening actively rather than controlling the discussion, and communicating empathetically.

It is also important for clinicians to recognize nonverbal communication cues—what Stolorow, Atwood, and Orange (2002) have identified as "unconscious nonverbal affective communication" (p. 85), such as a glance away, a change of focus or facial expression, a shift in posture such as leaning forward, or a subtle turn away. It is vital for clinicians to explore with the patient what these nonverbal signals might mean—that is, engaging with the patient in dialogue, with the aim of discovering the meaning of the unspoken. No less in importance, Orange (2006) advocates for "close and compassionate listening" (p. 15). An attitude of compassion affirms the "human worth of the patient" and conveys to the patient, "You are worth hearing and understanding" (p. 16). These skills, individually and collectively, can help clinicians participate relationally and engage compassionately in dialogue with patients to help formulate their ACPs. In so doing the clinician can engender and convey, as Orange advocates, both a process and an attitude of compassion.

HOPE, DEATH, AND COMMUNICATION: REFLECTIONS THAT INFORM THE IRMOC

The presence of death in life can evoke existential dilemmas and afford possibilities for completion, transformation, and transcendence (McCune, 2012). Understanding contained in the IRMOC, coupled with training in the areas of relational theory, counter- and cotransference, and therapeutic communication skills, can allow the existential dilemmas that can be evoked by advance planning for EOL care to emerge. Reflective practice can reveal and help clinicians attend to their own death anxiety and sense of personal loss—the cotransference—that can engender empathy and compassion. Moreover, reflective practice can help clinicians attend to projection biases as well as to unconscious and problematic defenses—the countertransference—that can emerge when facing mortality and engaging in communication with patients about EOL care, dying, and death. In so doing the clinician can more ethically advocate for the patient's ACP. The IRMOC can help clinicians engage in ACP with patients and their families by attaining deeper understanding of their role in the patients' final journey. This chapter is designed not to be a final answer or a nostrum, but rather as a starting point for compassionate inquiry that acknowledges the worlds of connection in the patient–clinician relationship, and as a source of support for clinicians as they engage with patients in facilitating communication about, and developing advance care plans for, the journey to EOL—a journey that each of us will inevitably take and a destination at which each of us will ultimately arrive.

YOUR WISH, MY COMMAND: FINDING SOLACE IN ADVANCE DIRECTIVES

Portions of the following section have been adapted from a previously published article (McCune, 2012).

In 2003, we had celebrated my mother's 80th birthday. She had lived for over 25 years with a rare degenerative nerve disease. Her health was declining even further due to congestive heart failure. Her health care power of attorney designated me as her health care advocate, with responsibility to enact her advance directives.

My mother was in and out of the emergency room and intensive care repeatedly over the course of three months. During one of these episodes, I stood in the hospital hallway with the doctor. He said to me, "Your mother needs a feeding tube."

I dug down deep within myself and found the strength to say: "No feeding tube." He looked puzzled. I explained: "My mother has advance directives. No feeding tube."

"You're murdering your mother!" He shouted at me. His face and his words are emblazoned in my memory.

Companioning a loved one through illness is difficult. Serving as a health care advocate for the patient is also difficult. Finding oneself in both roles simultaneously—companioning a loved one who is ill, and being called to serve that loved one by advocating for his or her medical care—is a doubly difficult set of experiences. I experienced the burden of advocating for the medical care the patient, my mother, desired when these choices were not those typically condoned by the medical establishment, as embodied by the doctor at the helm of my mother's case. In both capacities, I suffered from the clinician's failure to engage relationally through compassionate communication. The clinician failed to compassionately companion the patient, my mother, and her advocate, me, which would have helped ensure that the patient received no more, and no less, than her desired care.

Although years have passed since that day, I remain distressed by being accused of "murdering my mother." At the same time, I benefited at that moment from, and continue to find solace today in, the confidence my mother gave me to make decisions on her behalf through her advance care planning. I remain grateful for the gift of my mother's clear advance declaration of her choices for medical care and for her choices about how she wanted to die. She gave me the gift of a clearly thought-through and well-articulated position statement accompanied by clear communication about her values, EOL care goals, and choices for her death. As an advocate, I can't imagine making these difficult end-of-life care decisions on behalf of another without the gifts of certainty that my mother gave me by completing her advance directives, and communicating with me about her values, beliefs, and care goals.

I knew that advocating for my mother's choices meant she would die sooner. Yet, as the advocate my duty was to ensure her wishes were executed, rather than taking care of myself—delaying my grief about her death by postponing her death—by keeping her alive with a feeding tube she did not want. What my mother's specific EOL care choices were is secondary to the fact that she made her choices, communicated with me, her chosen advocate, about her choices, and signed papers to document her choices before they were needed. She did so while she was still able to make, articulate, and document them.

Subsequently, in my professional work providing psychological services with hospice I have sought to understand, through reflective practice, the ways in which my counter- and cotransference might influence my duty to advocate for patient's care choices. I continually seek to remind myself that regardless of the specifics of those choices, it is my duty to advocate for the patient's choices. In doing so, I have attempted to not impose my personal values or beliefs, while striving to embody compassion and use therapeutic communication skills. I have attempted to recognize and understand the ways in which I have been affected by my personal past and psychological training and by my patients and their loved ones—my counter- and cotransference. These personal and professional experiences have contributed to development of the IRMOC, which I hope will offer a practical theoretical model that recognizes the influences of clinicians' personal and professional experiences, encourages reflective practice and careful listening, and inspires compassionate companioning in the clinical setting and ACP situations.

REFERENCES

Aron, L., & Harris, A. (2005). *Relational psychoanalysis. Volume 2: Innovation and expansion*. Hillsdale, NJ: The Analytic Press.

Aron, L., & Harris, A. (2011). Relational psychoanalysis. In G. O. Gabbard, B. E. Litowitz & P. Williams (Eds.), *Textbook of Psychoanalysis* (2 ed., pp. 211–224): American Psychiatric Publishing.

Back, A., Arnold, R., & Tulsky, J. (2009). *Mastering communication with seriously ill patients: Balancing honesty with empathy and hope*. New York, NY: Cambridge University Press.

Baile, W. F., Buckman, R., Lenzi, R., Golber, G., Beale, E. A., & Kudelka, A. P. (2000). SPIKES—A six-step protocol for delivering bad news: Application to the patient with cancer. *The Oncologist, 5*, 302–311.

Berzoff, J., & Kita, E. (2010). Compassion fatigue and countertransference: Two different concepts. *Clinical Social Work Journal, 38*(3), 341–349. doi: 10.1007/s10615-010-0271-8

Bordo, S. R. (1987). *The flight to objectivity: Essays on cartesianism and culture.* New York, NY: State University of New York Press.

Ditto, P. H., Hawkins, N. A., & Pizarro, D. A. (2005). Imagining the end of life: On the psychology of advance medical decision making. *Motivation and Emotion, 29*(4), 475–496.

Doukas, D. J., & McCollough, L. B. (1991). The values history: The evaluation of the patient's values and advance directives. *Journal of Family Practice, 32,* 145–152.

Emanuel, E. J., & Emanuel, L. L. (1992). Four models of the physician patient relationship. *Journal of the American Medical Association, 267,* 2221–2226.

Freud, S. (1955). Fragment of an analysis of a case of hysteria (J. Strachey, Trans.). In J. Strachey (Ed.), *The standard edition of the complete psychological works of Sigmund Freud* (Vol. 7, pp. 1–122). London, UK: Hogarth Press. (Original work published in 1905).

Fried, T. R., Bradley, E. H., O'Leary, J. R., & Byers, A. L. (2005). Unmet desire for caregiver-patient communication and increased caregiver burden. *Journal of the American Geriatrics Society, 53*(1), 59–65. doi: 10.1111/j.1532–5415.2005.53011.x

Haley, W. E., Larson, D. G., Kasl-Godley, J., Neimeyer, R. A., & Kwilosz, D. M. (2003). Roles for psychologists in end-of-life care: Emerging models of practice. *Professional Psychology: Research and Practice, 34*(6), 626–633.

Hammond, D. C., Hepworth, D. H., & Smith, V. (2002). *Improving therapeutic communication: A guide for developing effective techniques.* San Francisco, CA: Jossey-Bass.

Johns, C., & Freshwater, D. (2005). Transforming nursing through reflective practice. *Recherche, 67,* 2.

Kluge, M. A., & Glick, L. (2006). Teaching therapeutic communication VIA camera cues and clues: the video inter-active (VIA) method. *The Journal of Nursing Education, 45*(11), 463.

Knapp, H. (2007). *Therapeutic communication: Developing professional skills.* Thousand Oaks, CA: Sage.

Kroft, S. (2009). *The cost of dying.* Retrieved from http://www.cbsnews.com/stories/2009/11/19/60minutes/main5711689.shtml?ta

Levinson, W. (1994). Physician-patient communication. *The Journal of the American Medical Association, 272*(20), 1619–1620.

Loewenstein, G. (2005). Projection bias in medical decision making. *Medical Decision Making, 25*(1), 96–104.

McCune, S. L. (2012). Living beyond the Other. *Pastoral Psychology.* Retrieved from http://link.springer.com/article/10.1007%2Fs11089-012-0466-8?LI=true#page-1 doi:10.1007/s11089-012-0466-8

McCune, S. L. (in press). Engaging a/r/tography to reveal countertransference: Enhancing self-awareness in caregiving professionals. *UNESCO Observatory E-Journal Multi-disciplinary Research in the Arts, 3*(1).

Mitchell, S. A., & Aron, L. (1999). *Relational psychoanalysis: The emergence of a tradition*. New York, NY: The Analytic Press.

O'Kelly, G. (1998). Countertransference in the nurse-patient relationship: A review of the literature. *Journal of Advanced Nursing, 28*(2), 391–397. doi: 10.1046/j.1365–2648.1998.00638.x

Orange, D. M. (1995). *Emotional understanding: Studies in psychoanalytic epistemology*. New York, NY: Guilford.

Orange, D. M. (2006). For whom the bell tolls: Context, complexity and compassion in psychoanalysis. *International Journal of Psychoanalytic Self Psychology, 1*(1), 5–21.

Orange, D. M. (2011). *The suffering stranger: Hermeneutics for everyday clinical practice*. New York, NY: Routledge.

Reker, G. T., & Chamberlain, K. (Eds.). (2000). *Exploring existential meaning: Optimizing human development across the lifespan*. Thousand Oaks, CA: Sage.

Rodriguez, K. L., Bayliss, N. K., Alexander, S. C., Jeffreys, A. S., Olsen, M. K., Pollak, K. I.,...Garrigues, S. K. (2011). Effect of patient and patient-oncologist relationship characteristics on communication about health-related quality of life. *Psycho-Oncology, 20*(9), 935–942. doi: 10.1002/pon.1829

Roter, D. (2000). The enduring and evolving nature of the patient-physician relationship. *Patient Education and Counseling, 39*(1), 5–15.

Ruth-Sahd, L. A. (2003). Reflective practice: A critical analysis of data-based studies and implications for nursing education. *Journal of Nursing Education, 42*(11), 488–497.

Schaffer, M., & Norlander, L. (2009). *Being present: A nurse's resource for end-of-life communication*. Indianapolis, IN: Sigma Theta Tau International Honor Society of Nursing.

Schermer, M. (2003). *The different faces of autonomy: patient autonomy in ethical theory and hospital practice* (Vol. 13). New York, NY: Springer.

Silver, M. (1999). Love, hate and other emotional interference in the lawyer/client relationship. *Clinical Law Review, 6*, 259–260.

Skirbekk, H., Middelthon, A.-L., Hjortdahl, P., & Finset, A. (2011). Mandates of trust in the doctor-patient relationship. *Qualitative Health Research, 21*(9), 1182–1190. doi: 10.1177/1049732311405685.

Smith, D. G., & Newton, L. H. (1984). Physician and patient: Respect for mutuality. *Theoretical Medicine and Bioethics, 5*(1), 43–60. doi: 10.1007/bf00489245

Stein, H. F. (1985). *The psycho-dynamics of medical practice: Unconscious factors in patient care*. Berkley, CA: University of California Press.

Stewart, M., Brown, J. B., & Weston, W. W. (1989). Patient-centered interviewing, III: Five provocative questions. *Canadian Family Physician, 35*, 159–161.

Stolorow, R. D., Atwood, G. E., & Brandchaft, B. (Eds.). (2004). *The intersubjective perspective*. Northvale, NJ: Jason Aronson (Orig. pub. 1994.)

Stolorow, R. D., Atwood, G. E., & Orange, D. (2002). *Worlds of experience: Interweaving philosophical and clinical dimensions in psychoanalysis.* New York, NY: Basic Books.

Stolorow, R., & Lachmann, F. (1995/2000). Transference—the organization of experience. In R. Stolorow, G. Atwood, & B. Brandchaft (Eds.), *Psychoanalytic treatment: An intersubjective approach* (pp. 28–46). Hillsdale, NJ: The Analytic Press.

Sullivan, H. (1953). *The interpersonal theory of psychiatry.* New York, NY: W. W. Norton.

Sulmasy, D. P. (2002). A biopsychosocial-spiritual model for the care of patients at the end of life. *Gerontologist, 42*(Spec No. 3), 24–33.

Tulsky, J. A. (2004). *NIH state-of-the-science conference on improving end-of-life care* (pp. 73–75). Bethesda, MD: National Institute of Health.

VandenBos, G. R. (2007). *Countertransference.* In *APA dictionary of psychology* (p. 239). Washington, DC: Author.

Wachbroit, R., & Wasserman, D. (1995). Patient autonomy and value-neutrality in nondirective genetic counseling. *Stanford Law & Policy Review, 6*(2), 103–111. Retrieved from: http://heinonline.org/HOL/LandingPage?collection=journa ls&handle=hein.journals/stanlp6&div=27&id=&page=

Wolvin, A. D., & Coakley, C. G. (1985). *Listening.* Dubuque, IA: William C. Brown.

CHAPTER 11

Conversations That Matter: Stories and Mobiles

Ben Wolfe

"Conversations that matter" are really about stories. So, let me start by telling you a story. A true story. My story.

It was during the fall of 1985. A typical day for me at the medical center seeing inpatients and outpatients dealing with grief issues ranging from just being diagnosed with cancer, to accidents, to grief after a death. I had planned on driving down the next day to a conference in St. Paul, Minnesota, a 2½ hour drive from Duluth where I was living and working. Life was good. My mother had died over thirteen years earlier from cancer and my father was, thank goodness, healthy. He had turned 75 years old the previous December and was living alone in an apartment. I also had a sister and a brother and their children living in the Twin Cities, and again, life was good.

Then the call arrived at the hospital. "Ben, dad's had a major stroke and the doctors don't think he will survive. How soon can you drive down?" Life was, in an instant, no longer "good." Life had changed. I had changed. My family had changed. In an instant, life became different. Now what? Will my dad survive the stroke over the next few hours, or the next couple of days, and if he does, if he does survive the stroke, what will his quality of life be like? I kept thinking, "He has to survive!" Working in a medical center myself, I knew outcomes after a stroke did not always turn out well and how in an instant life changes for not only the person who had the stroke, but also for his or her entire family and support system. I kept saying to myself in that short time between getting the phone call and getting my car keys, "He will come out of this without any problems...maybe."

I called my wife, shared with her the news, and then proceeded to meet her at our home so we could drive to the Twin Cities immediately. There were no cell phones then, so we made the 2½ hour drive wondering if we would even make it in time before he might die. I had the opportunity to be with my mother in December of 1971 when she was dying. She had a good death with family around, each of us having the opportunity to say what we needed before she died. But this was different. This was unexpected. This really was far from the radar screen.

We arrived at the hospital in St. Paul and immediately went to the ICU. There he was, lying in an ICU bed like all the patients I've worked with in our medical center. Machines and technology all working, or "waiting and ready" to work. But I did notice, at that moment, he was not on a ventilator. ICUs are places full of high-tech machines and, supposedly, of miracles, but people in ICUs die at a much higher rate than patients on regular hospital floors.

My father at that moment was able to say he loved me when I told him I was there. I was the lucky one I thought: he was alive at that moment and I had made it before he died. After a few moments in the ICU room with my father, I walked into the waiting room where the rest of my family had been waiting for the past couple of hours hoping he would live, but waiting for him to die.

The waiting room. In my professional work, I'd spent hours and hours in ICU waiting rooms, in pediatric intensive care units, in emergency rooms supporting patients and their loved ones... but this time, in this waiting room, it was different. This was not any family and this was not any ICU. This was my family and our waiting room. This was our father, our grandfather, our father-in-law. This was Mr. Independent. This was a man, the youngest of five children raised on a farm, who emigrated to the United States from Canada when he was a teenager, only to have his eldest brother who was caring for him die in a car accident. This was a man who worked hard, very hard: who married, had three children and six grandchildren; who cared for his wife through her cancer and who lived alone, and independently, for the past 14 years.

Today, I can still see that waiting room. All of our family there. All of our family at that moment looking at me—looking at me to help them figure out what to do next. Why me? I knew why me. I was the "grief guy." I was the one who worked with "these types of families during these types of scenarios." I was the guy they were now expecting to help them during this difficult time. We talked, and talked, and talked.

But it did not take us very long to make one major decision: because there was no health care directive in those days, we knew we would be the ones to make the decision about what type of care would be provided for him as the minutes and hours rolled by. We, his family who, thank goodness, knew what he always requested from us, needed to tell his physician and health care providers that we did not want any artificial ventilation used, and we wanted him to be allowed to die with dignity. No CPR.

Each of us in that room knew what he wanted regarding end-of-life (EOL) issues. Each of us had heard him tell us his wishes for years after our mother died.

"Whatever happens to me do not let them use advanced life support on me…I do not want anything that will diminish my quality of life. You have to promise me you will not let them ventilate me or do anything that will not allow me to die with dignity." Over and over again he would share these sentiments with each of us. With his children, his grandchildren, and all those close to him. It was clear. We were honored and fortunate to know his wishes. We were all glad we had had "the conversation that mattered."

It was easily decided in that waiting room we would then not allow the health care team to use a ventilator, and we would also not allow them to use CPR. We all agreed, "He will have a good death, a death he had control over."

I then called his primary physician who had been at the hospital after his stroke and had since gone home. On the phone I shared how much our family appreciated his relationship with my father and how we had decided not to implement any "heroics" measures at this time, due to my father's condition and the fact he had told us, over and over again, to allow him to die with dignity when the time came, with no technology used to keep him alive. The physician was very kind and compassionate. He shared with me how our father was a truly wonderful man whom the physician had come to appreciate over the years. He also shared how he too had been told by our father "not to use technology when the time comes to keep me alive." The physician then stated, "I too agree with the decision your family has come to, as it was always your father's wishes."

The physician then stated, "Since your father can speak a few words at this time, however, you will need to ask a nurse to go into his ICU room and document his wishes when you ask him so we have it charted." I knew that was the law, as that's what "autonomy" and personal rights were all about. I agreed. I thanked him again for all he had done and thanked him for his relationship and care of our father. I then went to the Family Waiting Room to relay to my family the telephone conversation with the physician and take the next step, to go into his room to ask our father about his wishes so the nurse could document them.

We, his three adult children, walked into his ICU room. I went to the right side of my father's bed, and my sister and brother went to the left side of the bed. The nurse was literally at the foot of the bed with my father's chart in her hand. She had the chart in one hand and her pen in the other. I sat on the bed next to my father and asked him the question we all had talked about, year after year, and we knew what he wanted, but now, sitting on his bed I had to ask him one more time. I indicated the nurse was here and I needed to ask him his wishes about any kind of advanced life support.

I said, "Dad, we have talked about this many times before, but with the nurse here, we need to know from you while you can still speak, what would you like us to do if you continue to go downhill? If you need any type of mechanical life support?" He stated as clear as a bell: "DO ANYTHING YOU CAN TO KEEP ME ALIVE!"

All I could think at that exact instant was: "What?" In one instant we went from allowing him to die with dignity, what he had always talked about, to the prospect of having him hooked up to machines. It meant our family might have to make more decisions in the future if the goals of care being hoped for did not work. I again repeated in my mind those words . . . "DO ANYTHING YOU CAN TO KEEP ME ALIVE." And we did.

He lived for the next 7 years—7 years that were filled with rehab therapists, speech therapists, swallowing concerns, memory loss, new living arrangements, and (at times) hired health care providers. During these years as a family, we learned a great deal about life, about loss, about our father, and about ourselves.

The 7 years after his stroke were not all easy. Many days and weeks were terrible, and my father's quality of life was not the best. But he chose to be alive. His fear, and whatever else he was thinking that very moment in that ICU, we will never understand, but we respected his wishes, and the health care team respected them. He was alert enough to make his own decision, yet not aware of the "unintended consequences" of his decision if he would have had to be ventilated. If he would have needed CPR to "keep him alive."

These 7 years were not the best of years for our father or our family, but they taught me a great deal about family, about having the EOL discussions early on and often, and also about how life can change in an instant.

THE CHALLENGE OF PLANNING FOR END OF LIFE

Today, things are different. Advance care planning (ACP) and health care directives have arrived on the scene. Today there are laws requiring hospitals to ask patients if they have a health care directive.

However, the laws have not, by themselves, transformed how we deal with EOL decisions. The laws don't require health care providers to take any action beyond anything more than asking the question, "Do you have a health care directive?" If the patient does have a health care directive, they are then asked: "Is it already in the medical center system?" If it is in the system, providers must determine if the documents can quickly be found, and ascertain whether it is a current health care directive or an old one. If the patient does not have a health care directive in the medical center chart, no further action is required by the hospital. The hospital has asked the legally required question, and no further follow-up is required.

This needs to change. This legalistic, formulaic way providers routinely deal with matters of life and death does nothing to stimulate meaningful ACP conversations among families. Having advance directives (ADs) is a start, but having ADs stored in a file at home, or in a safety deposit box, does not substitute for ongoing meaningful conversations about living and dying, hopefully conversations that have taken place far in advance of a medical crisis.

In this chapter I share some ideas, based on my years of practice as a social worker and grief therapist, on how professionals can help facilitate families to have conversations that matter. This chapter isn't about "The 5, 10, 20, or 25 questions health care professionals should always ask patients and families with whom they work." Rather, it's about the stories—each family's story—and how that influences how they will cope with illness, crisis, and death.

OUR EVOLVING FAMILY STORIES

I have been married to the same person for over 36 years. We met hitchhiking in Australia and have had deep, intense discussions over the years. Like other couples and families, our discussions always start out hoping "the day of needing to use our health care directives will be in the far future."

In our early years my wife and I bought a home that needed some fixing up. We agreed we would replace the wallpaper in the kitchen with new wallpaper. We thought: just head to a local home center, run in, and quickly agree on the wallpaper we want to buy.

Yikes, our "perfect relationship" underwent a bit of emotional bantering for a while until we finally came to an agreement on what we really wanted for our kitchen. What does it mean to appreciate where the other person is coming from when she says, "This is what I would like to have!" It was only wallpaper, but it generated within each of us a passion for what we thought we wanted and for what each of us thought was good, for not only ourselves, but also for the other.

Conversations about EOL and ACP choices do not need to be postponed until they are initiated in a medical setting. Why wait until the crisis happens? As individuals, and professionals, can you open the dialogue within your own family? Can you also think of having the conversation that matters over and over again? Can you engage in ongoing communication about EOL care and ACP with your loved ones and with your patients?

Conversations about EOL are not one-time events. They evolve. Communication about EOL care and ACP evolve as we grow older. Conversations about EOL care and ACP evolve as each of us define and redefine the values that give meaning to our quality of life. Take a moment to consider what values were important to you when you were 18, 20, or 25 years of age. Are those same values important for you today, or have you redefined what is important to you now? Have you had important discussions, conversations that matter, with your loved ones? Or have the topics of EOL care and ACP felt to be too difficult to discuss? Have you discussed with anyone your EOL care and ACP, and the values and desires you would want to guide them, including those who mean the most to you? Or have you avoided the conversations that matter most?

As happened for my father and my family, life can and does change in an instant. Being prepared, having things discussed far in advance of a crisis, provides for earlier opportunities to share our values and prepare those we love to represent us clearly.

DEALING WITH DARK EMOTIONS

Miriam Greenspan, in her book *Healing Through the Dark Emotions: The Wisdom of Grief, Fear, and Despair* (Greenspan, 2003), defines the "dark emotions" using three words: grief, fear, and despair. She talks about the importance of exploring these "dark emotions." As a result of such exploration, we can gain "wisdom" and insight that allows us to make better decisions and live a fuller life. Most people put off having conversations about their quality of life and about their values and EOL wishes. As a result, when the crisis happens, they have not yet had those meaningful discussions. In my work, I hear over and over again, "I wish we would have talked about it before the crisis happened."

Life-threatening events happen not only to older adults, but unexpected, life-changing events also occur in the lives of young adults. Crises—car or sports accidents, strokes, and so on—happen to 18- and 20-year-olds. Unexpected events do not happen only to those who are actively anticipating EOL realities. Examples of EOL/ACP choices that may need revision over the years are decisions related to organ, tissue, and eye donation. Have you shared your own thoughts regarding organ or tissue donation?

REFLECTIONS ON LIFE AS WE WORK WITH OTHERS

I taught for over 23 years, starting in 1989, a required 8-week course, 2 hours each week, for 54 second-year medical students. The course, *The Psycho, Social, Spiritual Aspects of Life-Threatening Illness,* was not intended for students to complete an exam by "remembering five points," or answering multiple choice questions. My goal was to provide students opportunities to appreciate, along with becoming physicians, that in the future some of them may have their own family or be in an intimate relationship. Each year students had chances to make many of the same decisions their future patients and families would be deciding.

On the first day of the class the students were given a Minnesota Health Care Directive to complete by week #8. They were to "have the discussion" with their spouse if married, their partner or fiancée, and also with their own parents. Not only were they given a health care directive to complete, but the first day of class, each student was also "diagnosed" with a terminal illness they would die from exactly 1 day after taking the final exam—that was an exact prognosis! They were going to die and had only weeks to live. They contemplated who to talk with and what to say. They were asking the same questions that those they would be caring for in the future would be asking, "What do I need to do now before my final days, my final hours?"

Each of the students also had various assignments to complete while they were "dying." Writing a letter to the most important person in their life, to be read after they died, was one example. Each week I would remind them, "You only have X number of weeks left to live."

In addition to each student "dying" over the length of the course, one third of the class each year, along with attending the classes and doing the required assignments, followed a real-life terminally ill person (known as a "friend," not a patient) and that person's family. They spent at least 1 hour a week in the person's own home, or wherever the person with his or her terminal illness was living. I would also meet with this particular group of students every 2 weeks to process the experience.

When it came to asking their dying "friend" about his or her health care directive, it became clear it was more than just having someone witness or notarize a document. Students learned the difficulties of having conversations that many "friends" had never had previously. The definitions of "quality of life" had changed from what the definitions might have been in previous years when the dying persons were more fully capable in the physical or cognitive aspects of their lives.

THE IMPORTANCE OF CULTURE

Each family has its own culture, values, fears, and history that cannot be discovered through what can be witnessed on the surface. Instead, like icebergs, each patient's and each family's real stories lie below the surface. The family in front of you is not *your* family, not the family you may have worked with yesterday; nor will it be the family with whom you will spend time tomorrow. Each individual, each family, has its own unique constellation, its own distinctive fingerprint.

Wisdom comes from exploring our cultural traditions, our rituals within the family. It comes from exploring what we are afraid to ask. It comes from making lists of questions to ask health care professionals who can explain what terms like "intubate," "peg," and "withdraw" all mean. When we have knowledge, we make better decisions. We make better choices. Unlike choosing wallpaper, with EOL choices, we often do not get the chance for a "return" or "re-do." There can be permanent unintended consequences from our decisions.

MOBILES AND SHATTERED GLASS

I believe strongly in the usefulness of metaphors in working with patients and their families. One helpful metaphor is the family system as a mobile. I ask the patient/family to imagine a mobile: colorful objects hanging in balance, generally pleasant to the eye, and fun to play. But a mobile is delicate and can be broken if hit too hard. I remind families some mobiles hang outdoors, some hang indoors, and some can be created in our own minds.

I encourage them to imagine a family mobile with each member in their family making up the "parts:" spouses, partners, children, parents, grandparents, aunts, uncles, relatives, significant others, and friends. I remind them that even those individuals who were once part of the family mobile and have died continue to maintain a weight on the mobile, perhaps lighter, but still a weight that needs to be counterbalanced. I remind them some weights can, after death, be the heaviest parts of the mobile.

Each family and every mobile is unique. As professionals, we need to remind ourselves that families need to be assessed and assisted based not on our perception of the mobile and how the parts are related, but rather on how it is described and perceived by those on the mobile. Many mobiles are based on relationships far beyond bloodlines. Listen to the stories—the stories below the surface; the stories that remain unspoken.

Imagine a family mobile with all of its parts constantly changing and in process. The parts change constantly prior to a family member's diagnosis of an illness, during the chronic phase of the illness, and if things do not go well, as the family member dies.

Often a family member of a person in crisis will say, "I just want our family to be like it was before"—but this is not possible. When one person on a family mobile is diagnosed with an illness—regardless of the prognosis—the person, and the family mobile, will never be the same.

To mix metaphors: "Who are the 'plate spinners' on this family mobile?" If we think of the Ed Sullivan television show of years ago, we can visualize the person on the stage running around, trying to keep numerous plates spinning, while yet still reaching for more plates to spin. Who are the individuals on the mobile who spin all the plates, choose to spin none or only a few, or are not engaged by other members comprising the mobile to spin plates?   *Families + Changing roles w/chronic illness/*

How, as professionals, can we help families share the load, divide the *death* responsibilities for spinning the plates, or adjust to role changes, which I believe is one of our major tasks? Each of the parts (family members) will have different needs. Through an interdisciplinary approach we have a much better chance of helping families share the plate spinning. With our support, hopefully, each part can be empowered to spin something, even if only for a little while.

Talking about and completing a health care directive in advance can truly help members comprising the family mobile to navigate their mobile balancing act. With meaningful conversation, in advance of medical crises, each part of the mobile can develop meaningful understanding, so if things do deteriorate, each member knows what the patient wants.

As mobiles evolve and take on new shapes, there are always winds that affect their directions. Sometimes the winds are very strong, while other times they are light and barely exist, yet blow when families and friends are not expecting them. Although each part of the mobile will respond to a diagnosis in his or her own way, some more openly than others, do not expect each "part" to not have changed shape in some way. Helping patients and their families complete a health care directive during anticipatory mourning, or review what is in place, provides a wonderful "mobile opportunity." The mobile, as mentioned before, will never be exactly the same! *prepare A.D. w/ families...*

After a diagnosis, due to openness, sharing, flexibility, and seeking new ways to cope, most family mobiles regain a new way of balancing. However, a few mobiles get severely banged around and find it more difficult to find a new way to maintain their balance. The question as professionals we want to continue asking ourselves about the mobile is, "How do the 'parts' relate?" We know the independent parts that make up mobiles are unique, yet these same parts need to remain interdependent as they balance the family constellation. When I was young and my mother was diagnosed with cancer, she was the part with the illness. She was the part that was affected directly, but in turn each of us in the family, each of the other parts, were also affected.

Each family mobile, and the individual weights of the mobile, change after a diagnosis. How the balancing will take place is based on many factors. What is the quality of the relationship between the parts? What are the roles within the family? What are the family rules and expectations, and the family strengths and weaknesses? What developmental milestones have been achieved, or not, by the family? What are the immediate and long-term needs of the family? What is the family's communication style and how flexible are its members? What are the ages of the parts of the family mobile? What are their cultural and ethnic origin, spiritual or religious beliefs, and financial resources? What constitutes their primary and secondary world views of their illness? Have they considered plans for a funeral, memorial service, cremation, or burial? What choices have been made regarding organ or tissue donation? Where are members of the family mobile living geographically? Finally, what are their previous experiences with death and loss?

We can learn a great deal by asking just two simple questions. First, we ask the patient to share how he/she dealt with their last crisis. Then, we ask about how the family coped with the last crisis. These questions will provide insight regarding how they will cope during this current crisis, and elicit which tools in their toolbox have or have not been helpful? What you see is not always obvious. It is vital to explore what is below the surface.

To mix metaphors yet another time, life will always have a different window through which to look. When a window is broken, the glass, even if glued back together, will never be the same again, no matter how hard one tries. As professionals who work with patients and families, we know that when significant events take place in people's lives, they will never be who they were before. Major transition points shatter the glass. Being diagnosed with and living with an illness or dealing with the dying process is constantly shattering and creating new windows for individuals and their families.

It is through constantly changing windows that the families with whom we work perceive the world. Some individuals and families think they can quickly find all the pieces and glue them back together as they were prior to being diagnosed with an illness. Others learn some of the glass will always be blurred. Life-changing events challenge our individual and family coping skills and force us to re-examine our priorities.

COPING WITH THE REALLY BIG STORM

Living in Minnesota, with snow a huge part of the winter lifestyle, we are often told by the TV and the National Weather Service weather persons, "A BIG winter snow storm is coming! A really, really big snow storm." You think to yourself as they stand in front of some "blue screen" and point their fingers and click the advance button on the images on the TV set, "Will it really arrive, and how big is BIG?" You also think to yourself, should I get gas for the snow blower just in case it does arrive, or can I wait until it arrives, hoping the roads will be plowed and the snow and wind will not be so bad that I can't go get gas for the snow blower?

Life can also be like that. We don't know when the "BIG storm in our lives" will arrive. For some of us, regardless of our ages, it may be soon and sudden, for others it may be further down the road. But the "storm is coming." It will hit our family, our mobile. The question is, "Did we prepare for it, or did we assume it really won't happen to anyone in my family, or to me?"

Families are constantly changing during their normal life cycles and stages, and any therapeutic interventions and strategies must look at all the parts, at the entire mobile, not just the person with the illness. Again, at what stage of this illness is the idea of a health care directive introduced to the patient, or has the discussion between health care provider and the patient not yet taken place, as it might be seen as too premature or too negative during a time of fighting for curative care? However, we buy car, home, and life insurance, hoping not to use them. We study the best plans at the time and then proceed to purchase what is needed for our family and our immediate and future needs. Can we afford not to talk about a health care directive early on in our relationships with health care professionals? Can we afford to continue hoping that a sudden, traumatic accident or illness will not take place?

STEWARDSHIP, JUSTICE, AND PROFESSIONAL ETHICS

Health care professionals also need to be realists in the area of ethics related to stewardship and justice. From an ethics perspective, the principle of justice is described as the moral obligation to act on the basis of fair adjudication between competing claims. As such, it is linked to fairness, entitlement, and equality. In health care ethics, this can be subdivided into three categories: fair distribution of scarce resources (distributive justice), respect for people's rights (rights-based justice), and respect for morally acceptable laws (legal justice) (Gillon, 1994). Ethical stewardship on the other hand refers to principles and morals that guide an individual or an organization, and generally refers to management, particularly of others' finances, goods, or household.

Because my father stated, "Do anything you can to keep me alive," should the health care system have gone along with his or our family requests if he would have needed additional care, and especially "non-beneficial" care? He was fortunate: he did not need to be ventilated, and in turn our family was not placed in the situation to make the decision later to withhold technology or to have a do not resuscitate (DNR) order written.

What would the health care establishment have done if they knew any additional treatments were non-beneficial for our father? Would the health care professionals have felt they could/should say no, or would they have been too concerned about legal issues to meet our father's and our family's EOL request?

So, the question of what would be nonbeneficial treatment should also be part of the patient/family dialogue. Health care professionals and health care systems today are clearly at the point where they will no longer just nod their heads and agree to extend non-beneficial treatments. Rather, providers are refusing to provide additional treatments if these treatments are truly non-beneficial.

PERCEPTIONS OF SUFFERING AT THE EOL

Even when EOL discussions are held with patients and families, for many patients the physical and psychological concerns can become overwhelming. My father clearly demonstrated with his "DO ANYTHING YOU CAN TO KEEP ME ALIVE" that being alive, regardless of his quality of life, was at that moment in time more important than dying. Opposite my father's decision to stay alive, there are patients who at some point on their dying journey not only no longer want curative treatments, but do not want to wait for death. They want control over their death. They want control over when they will die.

I received recently an e-mail from one of my clients whom I first saw 21 months ago, shortly after her son's suicide. Then, only 3 months after her son's death her husband was diagnosed with cancer. I saw her as a client at least monthly over those 21 months. Her e-mail read, "My husband killed himself a few hours ago. He shot himself and I am mad at him, but neither I nor my daughter blame him due to all the suffering he has endured over his last eighteen months with cancer."

Also, recently I received a phone call from an adult son who said, "my best friend and co-worker, my dad, shot himself due to his suffering." When the son came in for counseling, he told me the father had left next to his body a piece of paper with a quote from palliative care physician and author Ira Byock's (2004) *Four Things That Matter Most.* He had marked a check mark next to each of the four statements: "I forgive you. I hope you forgive me. I love you. It's OK to die!" Both of these individuals who killed themselves had cancer.

Both of these individuals had family mobiles with various parts or family members who loved them, and both had health care directives. These individuals were not merely statistics, they were real persons with real lives, continuing an ongoing presence on their family mobiles.

As professionals we need to remind ourselves trying to help and support mobiles maintain perfect balance all the time will not happen. Life and its daily events create change. Thoughts and feelings create change. Cataclysmic events such as suicide cause massive change, but it is during the process of balancing that families ideally learn to adapt.

Whatever our professional involvement may be with families who are trying to cope with a life-threatening, chronic, or terminal illnesses, we need to see ourselves as a team of folks helping and supporting them, not as the Lone Ranger who can do it alone. No one on the interdisciplinary team is the right person, at the right time, for every patient. Each of us needs to remind ourselves in our professional roles that we are not on the patient's mobile, but we are, instead, looking at the patient and the family mobile from a clinical distance.

THE PROFESSIONALS' OWN STORIES

How do we as professionals individually cope with our own "stories," our own family mobiles, and our own personal views of past shattered windows? Like the families with whom we work, we too need to see our lives as always evolving, as always changing. We need to be aware of our own fears and prejudices, our own conscious and unconscious thoughts, and our own attitudes and responses to the people with whom we work. We too, like the families we encourage to explore their "dark emotion," need to look at our own fears and challenges on our life journey.

We too at some point may be asked the same question as those arriving in emergency departments: "Do you have a health care directive?" What is good for those we work with is also very good for us. Planning far in advance and having conversations that matter are important for not only your patients and their families, but also for yourself.

Professional caregivers need to remember that each family mobile is made up of parts, yet not just any parts. These parts are not statistics, nor "the colon cancer in room 401," "the TBI in Neuro," or the "challenging family" in the waiting room. These parts, full of stories and lives lived, still have hopes and dreams. They are connected and interconnected to family members and friends, to their own life networks.

As we remind the families we work with that their mobile will never be exactly the same again due to the illnesses they are dealing with, we also need to remind them, and ourselves, it is through efforts to create change, take chances, and have the conversations that matter—conversations that move us forward, as individuals, and as families, toward deeper understanding of each other's values and beliefs—that we can help guide and better provide ACP and EOL care.

REFERENCES

Byock, I. (2004). *The four things that matter most: A book about living*. New York, NY: Free Press.

Gillon, R. (1994). *Principles of health care ethics*. New York, NY: John Wiley & Sons.

Greenspan, M. (2003). *Healing through the dark emotions: The wisdom of grief, fear, and despair*. Boston, MA: Shambhala.

CHAPTER 12

Advance Care Planning and Nursing Home Residents and Families: Lessons Inspired by TV Game Shows

Mercedes Bern-Klug
Jane Dohrmann
Patrick A. Dolan Jr.

[handwritten note: Do residents find these discussions disturbing or intrusive? Upsetting?]

If there is any setting where end-of-life (EOL) discussions should be expected, appreciated, and embraced, it is in long-term care settings, in particular nursing homes. Not all nursing home residents face imminent death, but the vast majority of long-term care nursing home residents suffer from advanced chronic conditions and are in advanced older adulthood. Indeed, about half of nursing home residents are age 80 or older at the time of admission (Buchanan, Rosenthal, Graber, Wang, & Kim, 2008). The advanced illness and age increase the chance of dying. Using data from the Health and Retirement Study (HRS), Kelly et al. (2010) reported that of the HRS respondents who died as nursing home residents, the mean length of stay was just over a year (13.7 months) and that two-thirds of HRS respondents who died in the nursing home did so within a year of admission. Lengths of stay vary widely. Data from the 2004 National Nursing Home Study indicate the median length of stay on the day the survey was administered was 463 days, although 20% of residents had been there less than 3 months and 25% for more than 3 years (National Center for Health Statistics [NCHS], 2008, Table 12).

BACKGROUND

Of the 2.4 million 2009 U.S. deaths, about one in five (21%) occurred in nursing homes (CDC, 2012). Data from death certificates indicate that 278,837 persons aged 85 or older died in a nursing home in 2009, accounting for over a third (38%) of all deaths of people aged 85 or older. These figures underrepresent the amount of death experienced by nursing home residents, because the numbers exclude residents who die en route to the hospital or while hospitalized. For example, data from the HRS indicated that 23% of respondents who were nursing home residents died in a hospital (Kelly et al., 2010). Although persons aged 85+ account for a plurality of nursing home deaths, it is important to note that 191,831 persons between the ages of 65 and 74 died in nursing homes in 2009, as did close to 36,000 persons under the age of 65 (CDC, 2012). Most people who die in nursing homes are older adults, but not all. If we focus on deaths of persons with dementia, we find that about two thirds of dementia-related deaths occur in nursing homes (Volicer, 2005).

The Role of Contemporary Nursing Homes

While dying is not uncommon in nursing homes, in some respects it has been obscured. Since the changes in hospital reimbursements, brought about by Medicare's prospective payment in the 1980s, the core mission of U.S. nursing homes has become less clear. Some of this confusion can be attributed to the pronounced growth in proportion of "skilled" beds that provide post–hospital care (e.g., subacute or rehabilitation) and are reimbursed at a higher rate, with higher profits than long-term care beds. In fact, the national average daily Medicare skilled care reimbursement rate was $412.42 per day in 2008, compared with the national average Medicaid reimbursement for long-term care of $164.68 per day (Eljay, 2012). In 2009, the actual cost of providing care to Medicaid residents exceeded Medicaid reimbursement by $16.79 per resident per day according to the Eljay Report, 2012, prepared for American Health Care Association (AHCA). People who are admitted to nursing homes for skilled care typically remain less than 3 months before being discharged back home. In some cases, skilled care residents remain in the nursing home, where their level of care converts from short-term rehabilitation to long-term care. For the rest of this chapter, "long-term care" residents include all residents who are not in the nursing home for sub-acute care or short-term rehabilitation. Within a nursing home, then, important missions compete for preeminence. Do nursing homes mainly provide short-term rehabilitation? Long-term care? Care for the dying? How an organization answers this question profoundly influences the culture of the organization. An emerging mission is the provision of excellent palliative care, along with both short-term rehabilitation and long-term care. So far, the industry has yet to fully embrace a palliative care mission, despite the fact that the majority of residents meet the criteria for palliative care put forth by the National Consensus Project for Palliative Care (2009), due to having a progressive chronic condition, a life-threatening illness, or a serious or terminal illness. *A AB Palliative Care*

The goal of palliative care is to prevent and relieve suffering and to support the best possible quality of life for patients and their families, regardless of the stage of the disease or the need for other therapies. Palliative care is both a philosophy of care and an organized, highly structured system for delivering care. Palliative care expands traditional disease-model medical treatments to include the goals of enhancing quality of life for patient and family, optimizing function, helping with decision making, and providing opportunities for personal growth. As such, it can be delivered concurrently with life-prolonging care or as the main focus of care (National Consensus Project for Quality Palliative Care, 2009, p. 6).

Resident Health and Functional Status Characteristics

Nursing homes provide a wide range of services, meeting a proliferation of resident needs. Geriatrician Robert Kane groups nursing home care into five categories: rehabilitation and subacute care; chronic physical, but not mental, disability; dementia; permanent vegetative states; and terminal illness (Kane, 1996). Complicating matters is the fact that many residents require several categories of care. Furthermore, each category encompasses multiple subdivisions. For example, some with dementia are bed bound. Some persons with dementia are chronically ill, while others (or the same person at a different time) are terminally ill.

In the recent past, care needs of long-term care residents have steadily increased. Over the past decade, as more alternatives to nursing homes (in particular assisted living) have become available, some people have avoided nursing homes entirely (e.g., by utilizing the hospice waiver they can remain in an assisted living facility as they approach the EOL), and others have postponed entry into a nursing home. It has become increasingly important for people entering nursing homes to engage in advance care planning (ACP). The federal government has instituted a care planning system in American nursing homes that, if used properly, can facilitate ACP.

Federal Laws Related to Advance Care Planning in Nursing Homes

Most nursing homes (88%) are certified to receive both Medicare and Medicaid (NCHS, 2006, Table 1). As a condition of retaining Medicare/Medicaid certification, nursing homes must comply with federal regulations.

Two statutes are directly related to ACP: the Omnibus Reconciliation Act of 1987 (OBRA, 1987) and The Patient Self-Determination Act (PSDA) of 1990. The PSDA requires health care facilities (including hospitals and nursing homes) to notify patients upon admission that they have the right to have an advance directive (AD; see Chapter 1). As part of the admission process, nursing home residents are to be asked if they have an AD. The nursing home must include copies of the document in the medical charts of those residents who present them. The nursing home is responsible for informing patients without ADs that they may make such documents, and the facility must provide basic information about ADs.

In 2004, the National Center for Health Statistics (NCHS) collected data on the prevalence of ADs among nursing home residents. They found that 18% of residents had a living will in their chart, and just over half (56%) had a do not resuscitate (DNR) order (Jones, Moss, & Harris-Kojetin, 2011). The presence of either of these forms of ADs varied by age and race. Older residents and white residents were most likely to have an AD in their medical chart.

While the PSDA is focused on the presence of a document (the directive), the OBRA mandates minimum care plan processes for Medicare-and/ or Medicaid-certified nursing homes. The law requires that all residents of a Medicare-and/or Medicaid-certified nursing home have an individualized care plan. To develop the care plan, the Centers for Medicare and Medicaid Services (CMS) require certified nursing homes to use a standardized assessment tool, the Minimum Data Set (MDS). The current version, MDS 3.0, collects data on hearing, speech, and vision; cognition; mood; behavior; preferences customary routines and activities; functional status; bladder and bowel; diagnoses; health conditions; nutrition; skin; medications; special treatments; and use of restraints. Information from the MDS is to be used by the interdisciplinary team to develop a care plan. The staff is expected to invite the resident to the quarterly care plan meeting, and the resident may ask that the family be included. We found no nationally representative data that describe the extent to which residents and/or family are present at care plan meetings, but anecdotal evidence suggests that family attendance is uncommon. Furthermore, it is unclear how fully residents and family members are informed about changes in the care plan when they do not attend the meeting.

Not only is it uncommon for residents and family members to attend care plan meetings, physicians do not usually attend either. As a result, key perspectives are missing from the mandated meetings. The absence of the resident, family, and physician voices diminishes the possibility of a comprehensive care plan being developed and fully communicated, and therefore confounds efforts to get all necessary parties on the same page.

The Social Support System of Nursing Home Residents

Most nursing home residents (79%) are visited in the nursing home at least weekly, and family members comprise 82% of visitors (the most frequent visitor [52%] is the resident's adult child) (My Inner View, 2010). It is not uncommon for residents to receive weekly or monthly phone calls (or increasingly electronic communication) from family members living far away. The notion that families usually abandon their members after admission to nursing homes is a myth. It is, however, a fact that some residents outlive their support systems and many (53%) are widowed (NCHS, 2008, Table 12). The members of the residents' "circle of support" (family, friends, worship community, etc.) are often called upon to participate in medical decision making with or on behalf of the resident. With approximately half of residents cognitively impaired (AHCA, 2012, Table 12), the role of family and friends as surrogate decision makers becomes all the more important.

WHAT CAN WE LEARN ABOUT ACP IN THE NURSING HOME FROM TV GAME SHOWS?

With this broad overview of nursing homes in mind, we can use TV game shows as analogies to highlight key challenges faced by those engaged in ACP in nursing homes. The television game show can be used heuristically to encourage discussion of the rules governing the experiences of dying or serving as a surrogate. The concept of a "game" underscores the role of chance. Residents can know what their preferences are, yet sometimes land in unexpected situations. We focus on three popular, recent U.S. game shows. Readers unfamiliar with the shows are invited to view actual episodes online, as the rules of the games are briefly sketched, rather than thoroughly described.

Jeopardy®: The Importance of Asking the Right Question

As they play *Jeopardy*, "America's Favorite Quiz Show," contestants are presented with answers, and to score points, must come up with appropriate questions. The game board is divided into columns naming various topics (e.g., history, current events, sports, or even "Potent Potables"). Under each topic are a series of answers, whose correct questions earn increasing amounts of money. The contestant selects a topic and a dollar amount. The host reads an answer, to which the contestant must give the *question* to score points. By way of example, in the case of this chapter, if the answer is "health care agent" then the contestant is to provide a question, to which "health care agent" would be the correct answer. A contestant might say something like, "What is the name for a person making health-related decisions on behalf of an incapacitated adult?"

In *Jeopardy*, the board provides the answer and the contestant the question. The U.S. health care system has developed the answer, "ACP." It behooves people involved in health care to consider all the important "questions" to which ACP is the response. It is common to think of the question as "what means can adults use to communicate their medical wishes in the event they become incapacitated?" In turn, "communicate their medical wishes" is sometimes reduced to two questions: Who should be appointed as surrogate decision maker and what medical interventions are to be pursued or avoided? Often, preferences related to decisions about CPR and the use of artificially administered nutrition and hydration are discussed. These are important issues. Yet a more complete question to the answer "ACP" would underscore the importance of knowing the residents' goals of care—in other words, "What is it they hope medical care can help them achieve?" *Beyond the POLST...*

The Importance of Knowing Goals of Care

Confusion about goals of care jeopardizes the residents' quality of care. A clear understanding of the goals of care guides decision making about specific medical interventions. Residents' values and beliefs drive their goals of care. Their social history, medical history, and experiences of the health care system condition their expectations. Their goals may change over time as their lives and conditions change, and their understanding of their condition changes. It is crucial to conceive ACP as a process rather than an event, in part, precisely because people change their minds about their goals of care. Because of the central role that goals of care play in ACP, it is imperative to begin engaging in ACP conversations well before people suffer cognitive decline.

When nursing home residents become unable to communicate and engage in medical decision making, a clear understanding of the goals of care can guide decision makers. Health care agents inform and remind the health care team of the residents' goals, as care plans are developed and carried out. The quality of medical care lies, in part, in the extent to which the care delivered is consistent with patient preferences. If we don't know what the patient (in this chapter, the nursing home resident) prefers, how do we know if we are providing patient-centered care?

Kaldjian, Curtis, Shinkunas, and Cannon (2009), surveying the literature published between 1967 and 2007, concluded that the following six categories account for the vast majority of goals of care: (a) cure; (b) longer life; (c) function/quality of life/independence; (d) comfort; (e) achieve life goals; and (f) support for family/caregivers. The set of six goals of care categories can be used to organize a discussion among residents, health care agents, and staff. The residents' goals of care should be reviewed whenever their condition changes, at every quarterly care plan meeting, and whenever residents or families wish. Residents, family members, and staff should discuss under what conditions residents would want to change their goals of care. In other words, are there changes in health status, prognosis, or other factors that would prompt residents to change their goals of care? Knowing this answer could help the health care agent, in the event the resident becomes unable to communicate.

Understanding and accepting the residents' goals of care cannot provide all the answers ahead of time; nor can they provide a detailed map for surrogates to follow in all situations. A grounding in residents' goals of care frames the discussion of possible interventions and the ends toward which the interventions aim. An ACP process that includes a thorough discussion of goals of care can be likened to the resident providing the health care agent with a compass, a tool to help point them in the right direction. Because for many residents suffering multiple advanced chronic conditions, there is no one clear road map to cover all possible medical scenarios in the indefinite future. Even though it is not realistic to have the resident weigh in on all possible future medical decisions, there are decisions about key medical interventions that should be discussed. For example, knowing whether the resident would like CPR attempted in the future is important, as well as the resident's preferences related to the use of a tube to provide nutrition and preferences related to pain and symptom relief.

There is a mechanism that many states have adopted to document the scope of desired treatment for people approaching the EOL. The mechanism is a Physicians Orders for Life-Sustaining Treatment (POLST). In 1991, Oregon introduced POLST (see Chapter 6), and it is now a recognized medical standard of care in nursing homes and hospices in many parts of the country to ensure that goals of care are reviewed and then converted into medical orders. The completed POLST form is to remain with residents when they transfer settings. POLST forms document physician orders regarding attempting CPR, tube feeding, and the level of medical interventions in the event of a medical emergency. Currently, a dozen states have endorsed POLST programs and 18 are developing programs (POLST, 2012). Wisconsin's Gunderson Lutheran Medical Foundation's, "Respecting Choices" model of ACP includes POLST when working with persons with advanced chronic illness (http://respectingchoices.org/).

A part of ACP involves appointing a surrogate decision maker. When conducting this planning, staff and residents must recognize the enormous responsibility imposed on people when asked to make medical decisions on behalf of a loved one who is not able to communicate. The surrogates' feelings need to be taken into account as part of the ACP process. Many of the models designed with ACP as the answer are aimed at facilitating decision making and the communication of the patients' specific wishes. This is necessary but not sufficient, in part because of the complexity of the circumstances that surrogate decision makers may face.

It is time to recognize that surrogates can suffer emotional, psychological and spiritual harm, when, responsible for ensuring that their loved one gets the care wished for, they see the plans fail, in some cases through no fault of their own. Part of the ACP process should be an opportunity for the nursing home residents to clarify that they do not hold the agent 100% responsible for the outcomes. Some family members serving as surrogate decision makers will be relieved to hear comments such as, "I don't hold you responsible for the fact that I am mortal," "I'm not completely sure myself what I would want 2 or 3 years from now, or if the situation were completely different," "I appreciate you staying with me on this part of my life's journey," or " I deeply value your peace of mind, and thank you for contributing to mine by being willing to serve as my surrogate." Persons facilitating ACP conversations should be mindful of the importance of recognizing this opportunity to include the conveyance of these messages, as well as goals of care and intervention preferences. Another benefit of conceptualizing ACP as a process and not an event is to be able to continue to support the health care agent. *Sum o gate Health care agents*

If the *Jeopardy* answer is the "ACP process," it is time to consider broadening the question to include the feelings of the surrogate. Ideally, the process helps the agents to feel empowered to represent the wishes of the residents, without overstating their responsibility for outcomes. The best question then may be, "What is a process by which adults can communicate their goals of medical care, provide guidance on specific interventions, and communicate their appreciation to surrogates for being part of the process, in the event they lose the ability to communicate in the future?" As mentioned earlier, Kaldjian et al. (2009) determined that one of the most commonly reported patient goals of care is to support family members. Considering the emotional needs of the surrogate decision maker can be a form of addressing the residents' goals of care. Following the example of Jeopardy, it is time to broaden the question to recognize the emotional impact of this responsibility on surrogates, when the answer is "ACP."

Wheel of Fortune®: Don't Count on Controlling Everything

Another popular TV game show is *Wheel of Fortune. This show* requires both luck and skill. To win, contestants must solve a word puzzle. The puzzle is revealed letter by letter. To earn a chance to guess a letter, the contestant must first spin a giant wheel. The wheel is separated into wedges, each wedge representing a different outcome. For example, one wedge may say "lose a turn" while another wedge may say "win a trip to Paris," and another lists a cash prize. When the contestants get enough money, they can buy a vowel to help solve the word puzzle. Luck enters the game when the contestant spins the giant wheel; luck affects where the wheel lands and, therefore, whether the contestant will get the chance to "buy a vowel" or attempt to solve the word puzzle and win the game. Contestants know what they would like to land on; they have their preferences, but cannot count on landing on a certain wedge. Contestants cannot advance unless they happen to land on a wedge that allows them to continue. Luck affects the amount of playing time and the chances of winning.

Selecting the letters to play (one consonant or vowel at a time) is part luck and part skill. Contestants know that in the English language certain letters are more common than other letters. Furthermore, the word puzzle also involves familiarity with American culture as well as skill in guessing answers based on incomplete information. Furthermore, the person who correctly solves the word puzzle and wins the round may not be the person who correctly guessed most of the letters. Each contestant is constrained by the luck and skill of the other players.

Lessons from *Wheel of Fortune* can apply to ACP. Residents may communicate what sort of an EOL experience they prefer, which interventions they are willing to endure, and which they wish to avoid. Yet, residents don't control on which wedge the wheel will stop. We can take this one step further by saying that the wheel residents face will have different wedge options, depending on the dominant health condition the resident faces. Lunney, Lynn, and Hogan (2002) categorize EOL trajectories among older adults into three groups: organ failure, cancer, and neurologic conditions including frailty. Nursing home residents whose overall health status is dominated by organ failure face different wedges than residents whose overall health is primarily affected by advanced cancer. Every time the wheel spins, the only certainty is that it will eventually stop. Despite the preferences of the player, the circumstances surrounding where the wheel stops are uncertain. In the medical decision-making context, uncertainty is rarely explicitly discussed, which can lead residents and their health care agents to believe they have more control than they do.

In many cases, having the discussions and completing the paperwork does contribute to the delivery of the type of care desired. In other cases, however, despite the best efforts of the residents and health care agents, the EOL care delivered is inconsistent with the preferences communicated. How can that be? There are many reasons that even if residents express their wishes, residents do not receive the care desired. Three reasons will be discussed in this chapter: (a) the complex medical characteristics of nursing home residents; (b) the communication challenges posed by the nursing home setting; and (c) the lack of a seamless health care system.

Complex Medical Characteristics of Nursing Home Residents

Most nursing home residents suffer multiple chronic conditions. The sheer number of conditions complicates prognoses and can increase care needs. Furthermore, not only do most nursing home residents suffer multiple chronic conditions, these conditions are frequently quite advanced. The combination and severity of conditions complicates residents' health status, prognoses, and decision making. This "ambiguous dying syndrome" (Bern-Klug, 2004) complicates the timing of adjusting goals of care, and makes it difficult to get everyone to agree when a nursing home resident should be considered "dying." As different people understand medical situations in different ways, even people having what they consider the best interests of the resident at heart develop different ideas about what amount and type of care should be pursued. Confusion occurs, and the interested parties must work hard to make sure everyone is pursuing compatible goals.

Communication Challenges in the Nursing Home Setting

Nursing homes are complex systems. It can be difficult to keep all the interested parties, family members, staff members, physicians, and residents current with respect to residents' health status, prognoses, and care-related preferences, so that everyone can make decisions with roughly the same information, especially when the decision is needed quickly, and even more so when the decision is needed outside the regular business day. The staffing challenges in the nursing home industry make this particularly difficult.

Most nursing homes in the United States are understaffed, both in terms of the number of staff members and their training (National Consumer Voice for Quality Long-Term Care, 2012). The measures nursing homes take to deal with staffing issues have varying implications for residents who are not capable of communicating their wishes. For example, some nursing homes deal with staffing shortages by hiring temporary nurses from an agency. Staff who are not familiar with the nursing home setting in general, and with the culture and protocol of the specific nursing home to which they are assigned, are ill prepared to function effectively as a part of a team. Their lack of institutional memory and knowledge of individual residents and staff not only lessens their individual ability to function effectively in the moment, but can also complicate the jobs of permanent staff.

In addition to not having a sufficient number of well-trained nurses available, most nursing homes do not have a licensed independent provider such as a physician, physician's assistant, or an advance practice nurse present. When serious medical events occur, staff phone a physician, usually the resident's personal physician or the facility's medical director, and relay information about the resident's status. The physician determines the next step. If staff perceive a situation as an emergency, they call 911, usually for an ambulance and transport to the ER. Although staff may frequently attempt to contact the resident's family, they do not always succeed before a decision is required. Resident preferences communicated through a POLST form can be useful here.

Lack of a Seamless Health Care System

Lack of a seamless health care system complicates continuity of care. If the nursing home resident remains in the nursing home for all care then the resident and the family interact with one system mainly. The moment a resident transfers to the ER or to the hospital, the resident and family must deal with a different system, with different rules, protocols, people, professions, financial charges, reimbursement systems, accommodations, and expectations. In a word—different cultures. It is not uncommon for a 911 call to undermine carefully made plans, especially as the resident approaches the EOL. Health care agents face circumstances they attempted to prevent, in a setting, for example an ER, they attempted to avoid. They realize that the situation does not correspond with the resident's wishes. What can be perceived as "bad luck," or lack of skill on their part, is actually the result of systemic problems, beyond the control of individual health care agents.

Let's Make a Deal®: The Importance of Recognizing an Opportunity

The TV game show *Let's Make a Deal* also involves luck and skill. The host circulates among the members of the studio audience and selects a contestant. Once the contestant is selected, the grand prize of the show is revealed. For example, the grand prize could be an expensive vacation or a new car. Contestants must estimate the price of some consumer items, and if they do so accurately, they are presented with three doors on the stage numbered #1, #2, and #3. An individual contestant chooses a number and what lies behind the door is revealed. The prizes behind the doors vary from undesirable joke prizes to items of value, and behind one of the doors is the grand prize. Once contestants select a door, they have the option of keeping the prize or trading for a chance at what lies behind one of the two remaining doors. A better prize may lie behind one of the two remaining doors, yet there is also the chance for a prize that is much less desirable.

In terms of ACP in the nursing home, we can consider nursing home residents and their surrogates the studio audience. We can think of the doors as leading to various medical outcomes, including the course of the residents' deaths. Residents do not control when their names are called. They cannot be certain what is behind the doors, but they have some ideas, and they know that some contents are more desirable than others. Resident satisfaction with outcomes depends on having clear ideas of the goals of care, and these clear ideas have value when residents understand their prognosis, especially as the EOL approaches. Suppose door #1 is pneumonia, and #2 is renal failure, and #3 is congestive heart failure. Does door #1 constitute an opportunity to avoid #2 and #3? Choosing the correct door can reduce pain and suffering for the residents. Some people, for a variety of reasons, find some deaths preferable to others.

ACP exists to explore these issues. While dying and death are first and foremost the resident's experience, the quality of a loved one's death has emotional, psychological, and spiritual consequences for surviving decision makers. In the event that a peaceful doorway to death presents itself, residents, families, and staff have the option to consider accepting that doorway to death, in the hopes of sparing residents more painful or undignified deaths later. Once the resident is considered to be at the EOL, some residents and decision makers value the cessation of suffering over the extension of life.

Individual, cultural, or religious beliefs influence residents to value various deaths differently. Some deaths include more pain and suffering than others. As part of a comprehensive ACP process, residents should be well informed about the possible ways in which different conditions can affect their dying process. For example, people with chronic obstructive pulmonary disease die differently than people with diabetes, cancer, or Alzheimer's disease. Most lay people do not realize how differently people die (Nuland, 1994). Once individuals, families, and health professionals acknowledge mortality, a different kind of discussion will ensue. Once proxy decision makers understand that even though they may be able to postpone their loved ones' deaths for a few hours or maybe days, they can't prevent the eventual death. They must decide if and when to end attempts to extend life, and when to refuse further interventions other than those designed to ease symptoms, and do so in ways consistent with the residents' values and beliefs. When do they stop choosing new doors? Some residents may wish to spare caregivers and family members the sorrow of a protracted death, or they may wish to avoid pain. Other residents and family members value keeping the person alive as long as possible.

For some, the only appropriate choice is the choice to stave off death for as long as possible. The quality of the death is less important than putting it off. Residents and surrogates will choose any door that offers the possibility of delay. Being alive is the goal. Health care agents may feel compelled by personal, religious, and cultural values and beliefs to keep their loved ones alive as long as possible. To choose otherwise is to be left feeling responsible for the death of family or friends. Shortening a person's life violates their understanding of their responsibility. They resist all attempts to implicate themselves in the hastening of the death of a person they hold dear. An ACP process that facilitates discussions about values and beliefs can afford the resident, surrogate decision maker, and staff to better understand the influences on decisions about goals of care and specific interventions. These discussions can contribute to building understanding, and care commensurate with resident preferences.

ASSETS OF THE NURSING HOME SETTING

Most of this chapter has been devoted to challenges. It would be wrong to end without recognizing some of the assets and strengths of the setting. First, most families remain involved, indeed quite involved, with a family member who lives in a nursing home. In most cases, the families constitute strengths on which to build, especially during planning care for residents who are not able to communicate wishes. Second, two assets already in place that serve residents and their surrogates can be strengthened: the PSDA and the federal requirement for quarterly care plan meetings.

During the admission process and before the quarterly care plan meetings mandated by law, residents (when cognitively able) and the families should be encouraged to attend quarterly care plan meetings, either in person or through some electronic accommodation. If the resident and family cannot attend quarterly, a special effort should be extended to include them at least annually. Unless residents and/or surrogates opt out, these invitations should come in writing. Whether residents or the surrogates attend or not, they should receive a written summary of the care plan, signed by the staff person to be contacted for questions, objections, or further discussion. Each care plan should include the resident's goals of care, and should explicitly address how the care plan supports the resident's goals of care.

In addition to the strengths listed above, there are two other important assets available to nursing home residents: hospice care and the commitment of the nursing home staff.

Hospice

Medicare covers hospice care when residents are eligible (see medicare.gov). Medicare beneficiaries can receive hospice in their own home, in a hospice setting, or in a nursing home. When nursing home residents receive hospice, they are entitled to all the care the nursing home usually provides as well as care from hospice staff and volunteers. This translates into a support team that specializes in medical, spiritual, and emotional care and support at the EOL. Hospice teams consist of the residents, families, nursing home staff, the residents' physicians, the hospice medical director, hospice registered nurses, hospice aides, social workers, spiritual counselors, music therapists, volunteers, and bereavement counselors. Care is provided by a team specializing in assessing and addressing pain and symptom management. Invoking hospice can mean access to medicine and equipment not otherwise available, for example a more fully featured hospital bed. Plans for care are determined by goals of care. While nursing homes have residents as their target recipients, the hospice model constitutes the unit of care as patients together with their families. For example, family members of nursing home residents enrolled in hospice can access counseling, assistance with decision making, spiritual support, and bereavement care. In addition, the caseload for hospice workers is much lower than for nursing home workers, so hospice staff and volunteers are able to spend more time with residents. In addition, hospices employ health professionals (nurses and social workers) with higher levels of education than are available in many nursing homes.

Although the percentage of nursing home residents who receive hospice services before death has been steadily increasing from 14% in 1999 to 33% in 2006 (Miller, Lima, Gozalo, & Mor, 2010), hospice benefits remain underutilized. One third of hospice users in general are enrolled in hospice for less than seven days before death, even though the benefit is for anyone who has a terminal illness and is expected to live for 6 months or less (National Hospice and Palliative Care Organization, 2012). Families often say, "If only we had known what hospice provides, we would have contacted them earlier." At admission, if appropriate, and during any care planning, nursing homes should inform residents and their families of this option.

The Importance of Nursing Home Staff

Staff members have the power to greatly improve the experience of living and dying in a nursing home. ACP for nursing home residents must build on the strengths of the staff. Those residents who enter having already established an ACP process should share their goals and plans with the staff. The staff is responsible for documenting these goals and preferences in the residents' medical chart and revisiting them regularly. However, not all newly admitted residents have embarked on ACP prior to admission. Therefore, every nursing home should have a few staff members (preferably nurses and/or social workers) who have been specially trained to conduct ACP discussions with residents and, if the resident is willing, with family. The discussions and decisions resulting from the planning sessions must be documented for other staff to benefit. The goals of care should be reviewed as part of the quarterly care plan meetings.

Unlike in the hospital setting, nursing home staff interact with residents and families over extended periods of time, over weeks, months, and years. Trust, mutual respect, and affection often develop. In some cases, the nursing home staff members know aspects of the residents' day-to-day life better than the families. Especially in the case of residents with severe cognitive impairment, the knowledge held by the staff combined with that held by the family can enable the team to develop an appropriate care plan that enhances the resident's quality of life, and when the time comes, quality of death.

Trusting and supportive relationships among residents, family, and staff constitute assets when medical crises emerge, and decisions must be made. Anything that the stakeholders in nursing home care can do to facilitate supportive relationships among residents, staff, and families should be pursued. Licensed social workers in nursing homes have many skills that can help strengthen the social environment in the nursing homes, for example, skills in interpersonal communication, crisis management, team building, decision making, advocacy, dealing with grief and loss, and facilitating groups.

SUMMARY

Nursing home settings are socially and medically complex settings that can challenge even the most steadfast surrogate decision maker. Staff, many of whom lack advanced training and adequate support, frequently overwhelmed due to understaffing, are expected to care for residents with a broad variety of medical, emotional, and mental health issues. Nursing home residents and families are affected by the culture of the facility and that of other health care providers, such as hospices and hospitals. Staff should understand that each transfer or change of status has the potential to become a crisis to residents and their families, in part because each transfer includes a change in culture, which takes time and effort to learn. People are seldom prepared for the culture clashes among hospice, hospital ERs, nursing homes, and other institutions of the health care system. These clashes can be interpreted as, and sometimes they constitute, poor quality care.

TV game shows present lessons that health care professionals can apply to nursing home residents and surrogates. When defining the concept of ACP, it is important to emphasize goals of care as well as recognize that health care agents can be profoundly affected (for good or ill) by their role. Uncertainty must be factored in. The complexities of residents' conditions must be recognized and accounted for. The complexities and the uncertainties of the health care system as a whole and individual institutions within that system must be stressed.

Readers are encouraged to use these well-known games to help stimulate discussions and communicate options to nursing home residents, families, and staff, and provide the opportunity to explore different scenarios before crises occur. Games related to ACP help to promote discussions that can facilitate the exchange of ideas and knowledge while promoting the sharing of values and understandings, all within the context of uncertainty, a context ever present in the reality of EOL care yet seldom explicitly discussed. While specific television shows were used in this chapter, it would be possible to use game boards and card games as analogies as well. The CODA alliance (www.codaalliance.org) has developed and sells a card game, "Go Wish," to help people think about and discuss what is important to them in the event they become seriously ill. Brenda Barnes (2009) has published a book targeted toward adult children who may serve as surrogate decision makers for a parent. The book is designed to inform and stimulate conversations related to ACP. The playful title of the book is, *Esther Has a Living Will and Other Fairy Tales for Adult Children.*

Over the coming decades, as members of the baby boom cohort age and decline, ACP will become more important than ever, particularly in nursing homes. It is projected that half (46%) of the persons who reach the age of 65 in the year 2020 will spend some time in a nursing home, including the 9% who are projected to spend at least 5 years as a nursing home resident (Spillman & Lubitz, 2002).

Nursing homes, more than any other institutions, must be prepared to work with residents who have already begun planning as well as encouraging residents to begin. Once ACP becomes universal in the general adult population, the burden on nursing homes to establish the practice will subside. However, all nursing homes should ensure the presence of staff prepared to assist residents, family, and other staff members; appreciate the need for ACP; and develop the skills to engage in meaningful and productive discussions. We are all in this together.

ACKNOWLEDGMENT

Professor Bern-Klug thanks the Obermann Fellows Program for support.

REFERENCES

AHCA (American Health Care Association). *2012 LTC Stats: Nursing facility patient characteristics report.* Accessed June 24, 2012. http://www.ahcancal.org/research_data/oscar_data/Pages/default.aspx

Barnes, B. L. (2009). *Esther has a living will and other fairy tales.* New York, NY: splash'em.

Bern-Klug, M. (2004). The ambiguous dying syndrome. *Health & Social Work, 29*(1), 55–65.

Buchanan, R. J., Rosenthal, M., Graber, D. R., Wang, S., & Kim, M. S. (2008). Racial and ethnic comparisons of nursing home residents at admission. *Journal of the American Medical Directors Association, 9*, 568–579.

CDC (2012). NCHS, Underlying cause of death 1999–2009 on data available on CDC Wonder Online Database, released 2012. Author generated data.

Eljay, L. L. C. (2012). *A report on shortfalls in Medicaid funding for nursing home care.* Report prepared for the American Health Care Association. Accessed April 7, 2012. http://www.ahcancal.org/research_data/funding/Pages/EljayReportOnMedicaidFundingS hortfalls.aspx

Jones, A. L., Moss, A. J., & Harris-Kojetin, L. D. (2011). *Use of advance directives in long-term care populations.* NCHS Data Brief, #54.

Kaldjian, L. C., Curtis, A. E., Shinkunas, L. A., & Cannon, K. T. (2009). Goals of care toward the end of life: A structured literature review. *American Journal of Hospice & Palliative Medicine, 25,* 501–511.

Kane, R. L. (1996). The evolution of the American nursing home. In R. H. Binstock, L. E. Cluff, & O. Von Mering (Eds.), *The future of long-term care: Social and policy issues* (p. 149). Baltimore, MD: Johns Hopkins Press.

Kelly, A., Conell-Price, J., Covinsky, K., Cenzer, I. S., Chang, A., Boscardin, W. J., & Smith, A. K. (2010). Length of stay for older adults residing in nursing homes at the end of life. *Journal of the American Geriatrics Society, 58,* 1701–1706.

Lunney, J. R., Lynn, J., & Hogan, C. (2002). Profiles of older Medicare decedents, *Journal of the American Geriatrics Society, 50,* 1108–1112.

Miller, S. C., Lima, J., Gozalo, P. L., & Mor, V. (2010). The growth of hospice care in U.S. nursing homes. *Journal of the American Geriatrics Society, 58,* 1481–1488.

My Inner View. (2010). *2009 National survey of consumer and workforce satisfaction in nursing homes.* Author. Accessed July 5, 2012. http://survey.myinnerview.com/publications/whitepapers.php?id=66

National Consumer Voice for Quality Long-Term Care. (2012). *Staffing fact sheet.* Accessed July 20, 2012. http://www.theconsumervoice.org/advocate/staffing

National Hospice and Palliative Care Organization. (2012). *NHPCO facts and figures Hospice care in America,* 2011 edition. Accessed July 8, 2012. http://www.nhpco.org/i4a/pages/index.cfm?pageid=5994

NCHS. (2006). *Nursing home facilities.* Table 1: Number and percent distribution of nursing homes by selected facility characteristics, according to the number of beds, beds per nursing home, current residents, and occupancy rate: United States, 2004. Data from the National Nursing Home Survey. Accessed November 4, 2011.

NCHS. (2008). *Nursing home current residents.* Table 12: Number and percent distribution of nursing home residents by length of time since admission (in days) and mean and median length of time according to selected resident characteristics. U.S.: 2004. Data from the National Nursing Home Survey. Accessed May 2, 2012. http://www.cdc.gov/nchs/nnhs.htm

National Consensus Project for Quality Palliative Care. (2009). *Clinical practice guidelines for quality palliative care* (2nd ed.). Pittsburgh, PA: Author.

Nuland, S. (1994). *How we die: Reflections on life's final chapter.* New York, NY: Knopf.

POLST (2012). *National POLST paradigm programs (map).* Accessed July 7, 2012. http://www.ohsu.edu/polst/

Spillman, B. C., & Lubitz, J. (2002). New estimates of lifetime nursing home use; have patterns changed? *Medical Care, 40,* 965–975.

Volicer, L. (2005). *End-of-life care for people with dementia in residential settings* (White paper). Chicago, IL: Alzheimer's Association.

CHAPTER 13

Watch Over Me©: Therapeutic Conversations in Advanced Dementia

Cory Ingram

Dementias are clinical syndromes caused by various diseases of the central nervous system and characterized by acquired persistent functional decline and intellectual impairments including, but not limited to, memory, executive function, language, and visual spatial skills. Alzheimer's type dementia is the most common primary form of dementia (Mendez & Cummings, 2003). It is a terminal condition with no treatments currently available to cure or reverse the pathophysiology of the disease. In the United States, an estimated 5 million people have Alzheimer's disease, and this number is predicted to increase to 8 million by 2030. It is the fifth leading cause of death among American adults. Recent data from the Centers for Disease Control and Prevention demonstrate that Alzheimer's disease is the sixth leading cause of death of Americans 18 and older and the fifth leading cause for those aged 65 and older (Xu, Kochanek, Murphy, & Tejada-Vera, 2010). The incidence of dementia of all causes rises by age. Approximately one third of all people over the age of 85 may meet criteria for the diagnosis of dementia, and as many as one half have at least a mild impairment of memory and cognition.

As it is a disease of older adults, people with dementia often have coexisting chronic illnesses of various degrees that affect their digestive tracts, hearts, lungs, kidneys, livers, marrow and blood, spine, hands, feet and joints, eyes, and ears. This results in a significant symptom burden and clinical challenge to effectively assess and treat a person's discomforts and distress. A wise clinician draws on the observations of nurses, other health care professionals, and family caregivers in making assessments. Whenever a patient's distress is severe or prolonged, evaluation and direct examination by a doctor is essential.

Dementias are considered to be terminal conditions. Whether a distinct progressive disease (such as Alzheimer's or Pick's) or in combination with other comorbidities (as in the case of vascular dementia), dementias contribute to shortening affected people's lives. In one Dutch study, only 14% of people with dementia survived to an advanced- to late-stage dementia (Koopmans & van Weel, 2003).

The current American health system does not always serve patients with dementia well. A recent study identified that 19% of nursing home decedents with cognitive issues had at least one burdensome transition of care near the end of life (EOL) (Gozalo et al., 2011). Nursing home residents in regions with the highest quintile of burdensome transitions were significantly more likely to have a feeding tube, spend time in an ICU in the last month of life, have a Stage IV decubitus ulcer, or have late enrollment in hospice.

Effectively communicating about advance care planning (ACP) can change and improve care for persons living with dementia. Individuals who engage in ACP are likely to see several specific benefits for themselves and their loved ones. The person with dementia is more likely to have his or her EOL desires known and followed. The person experiences a better quality of life and endures fewer invasive procedures and ICU admissions at the EOL. Families experience less stress and more satisfaction. The costs of care—to families as well as Medicare—are correspondingly less. Advance directives (ADs) have been shown to decrease family conflict and distress, be associated with fewer transfers to hospitals, less death in hospitals and in ICUs, less use of CPR and mechanical ventilation before death, and a higher likelihood that personal EOL wishes will be honored (Caplan, Meller, Squires, Chan, & Willett, 2006).

Whenever possible, ACP should include the completion of formal AD documents. These documents can be emotionally challenging for patients and families to complete, but they can provide family members with clear authority to make decisions for their loved ones and, by clearly conveying the individual's wishes, can alleviate the burden that families may feel in making decisions during future, life-threatening complications of the illness. Care planning that involves patients and their families in collaboration with the patients' physicians and clinical teams is an ongoing process.

This chapter outlines a practical approach to communicating with people with dementia and their informal caregiving network of family and friends. It is intended to be practical and applicable in a variety of settings as a guide for professionals of many disciplines. The Watch Over Me©

approach extends to communication with patients and their families in the process of shared decision making, care planning, and anticipatory guidance for life completion and closure.

PREDICTABLE CAREGIVING NEEDS OF PERSONS WITH DEMENTIA

From the moment the diagnosis is made or even suspected, affected individuals and their families have several predictable needs. They need access to information, and if it is not available in the doctor's office, they need to be referred to sources of reliable information, which may include advice regarding credible online resources. People need support in adjusting to the current and future implications of the illness. Support in this context means more than a compassionate ear. Supportive counseling often entails significant time invested in understanding the particular details of people's lives, values, and perspectives so that professional caregivers can help them understand the impact of the diagnosis and functional prognosis on the person's or family's living situations, plans, hopes, and fears. From the beginning of the illness, it is important to involve patients and their families in an ongoing process of education about their condition and shared decision making to identify patient-centered medical goals and plan for predictable medical decisions and contingencies. This includes having specific crisis management plans.

Such counseling and care planning is central to good care for patients with dementia. Clinicians caring for patients with dementia are encouraged to discuss a full range of topics that impact a patient's physical and emotional well-being. However, at a minimum, physician–patient and family education and care planning must include whether or not to initiate potentially life-prolonging treatments, including CPR, mechanical ventilation, kidney dialysis, and medically administered nutrition and hydration. When trials of life-prolonging treatments are desired, it is helpful for physicians to discuss in advance patients' and families' thoughts about when or under what circumstances the treatments might be withdrawn.

In addition, family members and friends who are, or will soon be, caregivers need training and practical support, as well as information, tips, and resources for their own health and well-being. It sounds reasonable and straightforward, but these basic services are not always readily available and at present such needs may go unmet. The result is unnecessary pain, strain, confusion, and suffering on the part of both patients and those who love them.

Specialist palliative care teams are increasingly available to assist in addressing the needs of both patients and families. Palliative care teams can extend practical assistance in navigating health systems and coordinating care, as well as responding to patients' physical, emotional, spiritual, and social distress and strive to enhance the quality of their daily lives. Palliative care teams and hospice share more in common than in differences. There is, however, one important difference. Palliative care teams provide holistic care to people living with dementia and their families and hospice teams provide palliative care to them when they are dying from dementia. Hospice programs deliver team-based palliative care to people who are dying, including in the very last stage of dementia. Hospice has been shown to benefit both patients and families (Torke et al., 2010). Hospice is typically available to support families in caring for patients in their homes and can also serve patients in long-term care settings in conjunction with facility staff.

In contemporary medical practice, efforts are problem based; basically, the core problems are injuries or illnesses. The goals of medicine are to cure, prolong life, and restore function. Clinicians assess patients and development treatment plans. In the context of dementia, often with significant comorbid conditions, curing and restoring function are out of reach, and alleviating suffering and enhancing quality of life become paramount goals. Since death is inevitable, at some point the best care must extend to ensuring a safe and comfortable dying experience. In caring for people facing the EOL, more medical treatment does not always represent better care.

The trajectory of dementia is without question predictable. Certainly, fluctuations stutter the course. However, the overall trend is that of declining function.

NATURAL PROGRESSION OF DEMENTIA

The tasks of navigating our days and world have been aptly divided into Activities of Daily Living (ADL) and Instrumental Activities of Daily Living (iADL). A checklist or inventory of ADLs and iADLs is essential when staging dementia. A simple approach to remembering the difference is to think of ADLs as everything you do in the morning to prepare yourself for the day, such as: bathing, dressing, transferring, toileting, grooming, and feeding oneself. Everything you do to navigate the world *after you are ready for the day* are identified as iADLs, such as: managing finances, transportation, medication, communications, laundry, housework, shopping, and cooking.

As with the inventory of ADLs and iADLs, the simplification of a range of conditions into stages can be useful in understanding patients' experiences in, anticipating and preparing for pertinent issues and problems. Reisberg et al. (1989) defined seven stages of dementia.

In Stage I, there are no clinical symptoms. Stage II is characterized by a person complaining about forgetfulness. In Stage III, other people typically begin to notice a person's functional deficits. A hallmark of Stage IV is the impairment of one or several iADLs with preservation of ADLs. Due to disorientation and progressive loss of iADLs, people in Stage V appear well dressed and ready for the day. However, they are disoriented and unable to perform most iADLs; hence, Stage V is often described by the saying "All dressed up and nowhere to go." Stage VI is marked by incontinence, an inability to recognize loved ones, and wandering. It can be thought of as the "Velcro" stage in which people tend to cling to others, particularly in dementia facilities or nursing homes. In Stage VII a person is dependent in ADLs and can only speak a few words. The patient is dependent on others for mobility such as rotation in bed and transfer for toileting and wheelchair. Most time is spent in bed, unable to effectively communicate with others.

EOL care in dementia can be thought of as spanning Stages V, VI, and VII and may take place over many months or several years. However, Stage VII is when the patient is dependent in ADLs and clearly approaching the EOL predominantly from dementia. Unfortunately, at present it is only in the later substages of Stage VII, when the affected person is unable to ambulate or speak more than six words in a day, that an individual with dementia meets Medicare eligibility criteria to receive hospice care.

THE FAMILY JOURNEY

Whenever one person receives a serious diagnosis, a family experiences the subsequent illness. Virtually every patient with advanced dementia has a family, whether it is a family by blood relations, marriage, or friendship. For an elderly person with advanced dementia, family can be thought of by the phrase "for whom the person matters." Operationally, family are the people who visit, call, and physically care for the patient, which often includes their long-time nurses, aides, and housekeepers.

Physicians and clinical teams can support each family member and guide a cohesive process of making decisions and providing care. Family members who are children, parents, or siblings of the person with dementia can be expected to have discernible styles of relating to one another— and making decisions—that have been formed by history and culture. An understanding of the family system can help in counseling patients and family members in coping and on the caregiving system throughout the illness. The dominant personalities and decisional style of a family often become apparent over time. There may be *insiders* and *outsiders* in a family's patterns of conversing, making decisions, or providing care. Distance, time, and financial resources may all contribute, but a family's history and its members' personalities also contribute to the ways people approach these difficult situations. Clinicians can astutely take note of these family characteristics, without judging which members of a divided family are right or wrong. Observations of a family's style, which may vary by culture, are valuable in counseling people who are struggling not only with treatment decisions, but also with the physical, emotional, and social strains of dementia. Skillful counseling can identify sources of strength within families and guide family members in coming to agreement and, correspondingly, avoid conflict.

Having someone they love become seriously ill naturally makes people feel emotionally vulnerable; it evokes worry, anxiety, and fears. Supportive counseling for a family member of a patient with advanced dementia can start by "stating the obvious": We have found that it puts family members (including a patient's close friends) at ease and builds a therapeutic alliance to say aloud that it is apparent how much they love and are worried about the person who is our patient.

Similarly, during family meetings for the sake of making decisions, when differences of opinion are voiced—or tempers flare—between family members, it is often helpful to explicitly acknowledge that despite disagreements, everyone present loves the person who is ill, and therefore, everyone present is hurting. Clinicians can add that people come to these decisions differently—and we may or may not be able to come to an agreement about whether and for how long to use specific treatments—but each one is trying to do what they consider right and best for the person.

A family's journey from pre-diagnosis through the diagnosis, changes in plans and shifts in roles through chronic care, shared care, institutionalized care, and ultimately through the EOL care and into grief will be as unique as a fingerprint. Yet within the unique, personal experiences of every patient and family there are predictable challenges, decisions, and dynamics that every family is likely to encounter (Caron, Pattee, & Otteson, 2001).

When an elderly mother or father becomes affected with dementia, adult children commonly feel conflicted about making decisions, sometimes against the parent's wishes. It may be a decision to no longer allow the person to drive or use the stove.

I have found it helpful to present these challenges as developmental stages within the lifecycle of a family. During adolescence, parents often need to enforce limits for the safety and well-being of the teenager, even when it makes the young person angry and causes a scene. To do otherwise would be irresponsible. When dementia robs a parent of the ability to safely drive or use a stove top, it is only responsible for the children who were once those teenagers to set limits, even if doing so makes one's mother or father angry—and causes a scene. Most families eventually come to realize this on their own, but anticipatory guidance by a clinician can facilitate the process, avoiding a lot of confusion and guilt feelings along the way.

OPPORTUNITIES FOR DECISION MAKING AND ADVANCE CARE PLANNING

Figure 13.1 represents a paradigm shift from the regular problem-based approach to caring for seriously ill people with multiple medical problems to a model to incorporate goals based on care, attention to symptoms, and healing. Inherent in this model is that the best care possible for seriously ill people is not found in the sum of the treatment options for each medical problem, but rather in the treatments that best represent a person's goals and values. This is particularly important in advanced dementia where more medical care and more medical treatments may actually lead to increased suffering, loss of independence, and decreased quality of life.

WATCH OVER ME: THERAPEUTIC CONVERSATIONS

The rest of the chapter will serve to provide a practical framework where you can take the academic foundations of dementia staging, the family journey, and anticipatory guidance and apply them practically to conversations around ACP for people with dementia. I encourage practitioners to take bits and pieces and use them to serve their patients. We often find ourselves in various settings in which this framework will need to morph into a different form to serve that setting. I hope that the framework and practical examples of syntax and vocabulary will assist in the conversation. Remember, our contact with the patient and family is a therapeutic intervention.

FIGURE 13.1 Concurrent Problem-Based and Goals-Based Care.

Diagnosis	Treatment	Goals	Symptoms	Healing
Dx 1 →	Tx 1		Sx 1	ACP
Dx 2 →	Tx 2		Sx 2	Independence
Dx 3 →	Tx 3	G 1	Sx 3	Safety
Dx 4 →	Tx 4	G 2	Sx 4	Communication
.	.		.	Legacy Development
.	.		.	Tasks of Life Completion
Dx X →	Tx X		Sx X	Attention to the Whole Person

Healing: Increasing quality of life in the face of declining function, increasing symptoms and approaching end of life.

ACP, advance care planning.

The guiding principles listed below are in a particular sequence. However, the sequence and use can vary depending on the clinical encounter. Figure 13.2 gives an overview of Watch Over Me.

Prepare

Therapeutic conversations with patients and families living with dementia start prior to sitting down with the patient and family. Preparing for a conversation seems intuitive. However, it does take time, and experientially the time invested pays off during the conversation. Using a structured tool to review a person's chart can help to gather the information that will prepare one well in leading the conversation. Trust is foundational to the therapeutic ACP conversation, and knowing the pertinent background information prior to entering into the conversation will help bolster one's confidence as well as patient and family trust. In some circles, this chart review tool is called a rounding tool. When reviewing the medical chart, it will become overwhelmingly apparent that the attention to the medical detail often outweighs attention to the social, emotional, and personal experience of an illness such as dementia.

FIGURE 13.2 Watch Over Me®: Therapeutic Conversations in Advanced Dementia.

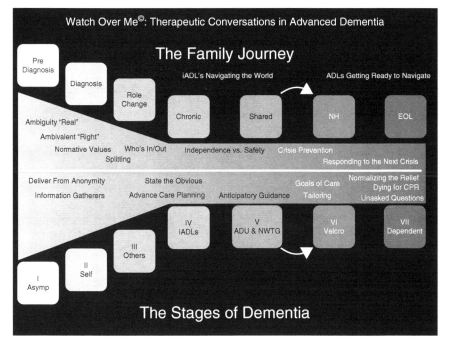

ADL, activity of daily living; ADU & NWTG, all dressed up and nowhere to go; iADL, instrumental ADL; EOL, end of life; NH, nursing home.

Create the Space

Think of the space for the conversation as a physical and emotional space. I often look for a private and quiet physical space that is unlikely to be interrupted. I check to make sure that a box of tissues is present in the room and that there are enough chairs present for everyone to sit and interact with one another. The emotional space takes time to create as well. Some of the practical factors about creating the emotional space start from the first introduction. I let them know who I am and what role I serve. I introduce other team members and medical learners I am teaching and ask for permission for their observation. When we are all seated, I like to make sure I know who is present and what their relationship is to the patient and each other, so I ask everyone present to introduce themselves. If other clinicians from disciplines are present, we make sure to introduce them and their roles in the conversation. I often thank them for taking the time to meet with us and reflect briefly on the importance of coming together to talk about caring for their loved one. Their loved one may be present; however, often in persons with advanced dementia lacking decisional capacity, the meeting may serve to only upset them. Creating the space of the conversation from an emotional standpoint continues throughout the conversation. The foundations of the conversation are formed largely in the next two sections on agenda setting and delivering the patient from anonymity.

Set the Agenda

After introductions, I often find it helpful to reflect briefly on why we have come together for the conversation and invite input at this time from anyone present as to what they were hoping we would talk about. The inherent pitfall is getting off on a tangent from the start. The clinician needs to lead this conversation.

In my experience, failure to identify the agenda up front leaves some family members less engaged, as they are waiting on a moment to talk about their agenda item. I typically give some sense of when I will cover the agenda items identified and ask them to remind me if I forget. I make certain to write the agenda down as they name the topics. Anytime a group of people gets together to talk about ACP with health care professionals, there is some degree of uncertainty, eagerness, and anxiety that agenda setting seems to defuse.

Deliver the Person With Dementia From Anonymity

With the agenda set, I comment that we have collected a good list of things to cover. I may also add in a few agenda items myself. However, I typically don't jump right into the agenda items. First, there is an opportunity to reflect on the personal aspect of why we are all coming together. There is a person, and his or her life at the center of the conversation, so there is an opportunity to deliver that person from anonymity. This largely represents a social history that has been removed from a bulleted item in the medical chart to an expanded thoughtful review of the person's social history at the front of the conversation to acknowledge who the patient is as a person. Asking for permission to talk openly is important. As we know, people living with serious illness want to talk about ACP, but at the same time, they want sensitivity to when they are ready to talk (Wenrich et al., 2000)

State the Obvious

Stating the obvious is as easy and as hard as it may seem. This is something I learned during my palliative care fellowship from Dr. Ira Byock and adapted to persons with dementia and their families. Stating the obvious is nothing other than simply stating the obvious. What is the obvious thing to say when meeting with patients and families living with dementia? *Stating* the obvious is contrasted with *asking* the obvious. A pitfall to stating the obvious is that as the conversation facilitator you make an assumption that the obvious is the obvious. In fact, you may be wrong, but I would not let that prevent you from stating the obvious. In delivering the patient from anonymity the conversation almost always culminates in a history that outlines the family transitions from pre-diagnosis to diagnosis, to role change, chronic care, shared care, institutionalized care, and to EOL care. Paralleling this is the history of loss of iADLs and ADLs and the progression from Stage I to VII. You may be tempted to ask the obvious, such as, "How did that make you feel when your mother needed your assistance with bathing?" Or this question of the obvious, "Are you concerned your mother is wandering the neighborhood when you are at work?" The response to asking the obvious is often a single-word answer and an unspoken message of disbelief that you just asked the obvious. In contrast, just state the obvious: "I can't imagine how difficult it must be to worry about your mother's wandering and her safety."

Stating the obvious gives you an opportunity to contextualize, honor the person with dementia and the caregiver, and provide a healing space for a reflective response from the family. An example of stating the obvious is founded in common themes of the family journey and the stages of dementia. During the progression of dementia people experience ambiguity and ambivalence to the diagnosis and progression. In fact, not all caregivers will be on the same page with knowing if this is real and if they are right in their interpretations. Equally inherent in the disease journey is the balance of independence and safety. Typically, caregivers value their loved one's safety over his or her independence, and the patient often values independence and may lack sufficient insight in the disease process to understand concerns for safety. The concept of contextualization is simply laying a foundation upon which to state the obvious.

Determine Understanding of Illness

Commonly, persons engaged in a conversation for ACP for a loved one with dementia may not have a full grasp of the illness or complex of illnesses. Often dementia is not seen as a terminal condition and, therefore, prior to giving information about the illness, it is important to inquire about the person's understanding of illness. Often, the history of the disease progression and the family journey has already been reviewed, and it is still important to inquire about their understanding of the illness today and what their understanding of the future may be. It is common, in my experience, to find persons with a long-lived experience caring for a loved one with dementia who are nevertheless unaware their loved one has a terminal illness that will render him/her unable to communicate, eat, walk, toilet, and live if the disease progresses to its end stage. A pitfall to avoid here is an unnecessarily lengthy review of all the previous testing and medical work-up.

Identify Hope

Hope is inherent to medical care. Hope also changes throughout a dementia journey. Typically, when a person receives a serious diagnosis like dementia, he or she hopes that the diagnosis is wrong. This often fosters the ambiguity and ambivalence experienced by patients and families. Hope shifts to hoping for a cure. However, in dementia, people learn quickly that there is no cure and that there is a paucity of treatment options to slow the progression. Hope shifts again to living as well as possible with the illness to living as comfortably as possible with the illness. At some point in time hope shifts again to represent hope that becomes more difficult to talk about and stands often in direct contrast to the typical goals of medicine. Hope shifts to dying peacefully and hoping that your loved ones will prosper and live well after you have died.

Once again, the sum of the treatments doesn't add up to better care. Treatments need to be tailored when hope is directed toward living as comfortably as possible and dying peacefully. Keep in mind this time where hope resides in dying peacefully may last years. In breaching the subject of hope, I often ask for permission, contextualize, and then ask. This gives family an opportunity to describe where hope is at this time. Far too often people are readily able to describe everything they don't want, almost like a photographic negative. They don't want pain, nursing homes, to be a burden on others, or to use up their financial means, leaving their families without an inheritance. Asking about hope allows them to talk about what they want in the setting of advanced illness.

Normalize Feelings of Relief in Grief

The toll to caregivers has been well described in the literature. The patient gets the disease, and the family lives with the illness. Among the many feelings experienced by caregivers, guilt seems to stand out. Often caregivers find themselves making choices between things on a menu of items they simply don't want. I have yet to encounter a caregiver of a loved one with advanced dementia that hasn't experienced guilt during and after their loved one dies. In fact, in my experience, the guilt is twofold. They feel guilty about the decisions they have to choose from on their loved one's behalf and, secondly, they feel guilty because they know they will feel relieved when their loved one dies. I have yet to find a caregiver with a loved one in late Stage VI or VII that hasn't experienced this new form of guilt. In fact, many have hope directed toward their loved one dying in their sleep.

Tailoring and Anticipatory Guidance

As for many people caring for a loved one with advanced dementia, it is common that as the disease progresses from Stage VI to VII, they will need an increase in services either in or outside of their home in an institution. Independence will give way to safety, and their personal life will be tailored to meet their needs. Family often needs assistance in tailoring the medical life of their loved one, specifically around issues of medical treatments, interventions, and CPR. One example of anticipatory guidance is found in pediatrics, where loved ones are informed about what is next, what to do, and when to call. We apply this same principle in Watch Over Me.

Maximum Conservative Treatment and Care

The vocabulary and syntax used in communicating with seriously ill people and their families is sometimes unfortunate. It is not an uncommon experience to hear care directed primarily toward comfort characterized by discontinuing treatments, stopping the antibiotics, and not feeding mom.

There are, however, more accurate and therapeutic ways of communicating about these very special times of life when a person with advanced dementia in Stage V, VI, or VII needs medical care tailored to represent individual goals and values. I recommend shifting the vocabulary and syntax away from what the patient doesn't receive to vocabulary and syntax representing what the patient will receive. Often perceptions of "there is nothing more we can do" prevail during these stages of dementia, and, frankly, nothing is less true.

The terms "maximum conservative treatment" and "maximum conservative care" are terms that I use to represent the landscape of care options in Stages V, VI, and VII. Maximum conservative care is always part of the care plan. It is the very foundation of the caring of one human being by another. Providing them a clean, warm, safe, comfortable, professional approach to caring well for them—making sure their personal needs of toileting, bathing, dressing, and oral care; social, emotional, and spiritual well-being; and expert pain and symptom management are being carefully and professionally managed. Maximum conservative care may, in fact, be the complete plan of care for a patient with advanced dementia. It may also be accompanied by maximum conservative treatments to include antibiotics both oral and intravenous, surgeries for fractured hips, and medical treatments for chronic illness. The transition from the combined maximum conservative treatment and care to maximum conservative care requires ongoing evaluation of patient function, disease and treatment burden, and modifiable quality-of-life determinants.

Dying for CPR

CPR has no role in advanced dementia, yet our default approach is to offer it to every patient. More accurately, we offer it to their caregivers. In my experience, caregivers feel as though they are making decisions between life and death when asked about CPR. Of course, it is unique that we offer an arguably ineffective treatment to persons who will not benefit from a trial of CPR. People get their information on CPR from the TV rather than medical professionals. The common vocabulary used is similar to that of running out of gas. If your heart stops, would you like us to restart it? It implies the possibility of success. If you run out of gas, would you like me to bring you some? CPR in advanced dementia is different, and the question is really much different. There is clearly something worse than a person dying, and that is the person dying badly. Dementia often gives the caregivers and the local medical establishment adequate time to formulate a response to a person dying with advanced dementia. It is, however, very difficult in good conscience to recommend CPR for persons with advanced dementia. It is hard to identify what is in it for them with unlikelihood of success.

The Unasked Question

The unasked question, as I have coined the term, is the question that never gets asked when a person with dementia has arrived in Stage VII and is unable to speak, eat, or ambulate. I call it the unasked question because the questions that are asked are represented in Figure 13.1 and can best be thought of as questions to determine therapies for identified diagnosis. For example, let's say that Diagnosis 1 (Dx 1) is the inability to swallow. Then the medial question and conversation is: Do you want your loved one to have a feeding tube? The answer will determine Treatment 1 (Tx 1). Yet there remains an unasked and vitally important question. Can you identify it? The unasked question informs the goals for treatment. Only after the goals of treatment have been determined can we determine what disease-specific treatments fit the goals. The unasked question is simply, "If your loved one isn't allowed to die from the natural progression of their disease, what will he or she be allowed to die from?" Of course, that isn't how you ask the question. I suggest that you need to contextualize, ask permission, and then ask the question with adequate foundational contextualization.

This question—what will he or she be allowed to die from—gets at the heart of the matter. It is the unasked question, and in Figure 13.1 it starts to inform goals of care to determine Goal 1 (G1) and Goal 2 (G2). This represents a departure from standard medical care and a paradigm shift toward goals based on care and healing.

APPLYING THE PRINCIPLES OF WATCH OVER ME

Mrs. Petra Snoepwinkel is a 77-year-old retired professor of English literature living with her husband, Hans. Petra, widowed 12 years ago, married her long lost high school sweetheart, Hans, 8 years ago, and by all accounts they had a wonderful time traveling about the world.

Petra's high blood pressure and kidney function worsened to the point where she needed to be on dialysis 3 days a week. She started dialysis 2 years ago, and her kidney specialist is concerned that her quality of life is severely impaired and the burden of dialysis may be outweighing the benefit to Petra and her family. Common to dialysis, Petra develops a very low blood pressure when her blood is removed from her body and filtered through the dialysis machine. She has also suffered through life-threatening infections of the blood stream eight times in the last 3 months. She has been hospitalized each time and almost died on four occasions, requiring machines to support her breathing for several days. Over the last 5 years Petra's dementia has worsened and Hans has covered and cared well for her. Petra is dependent in her ADLs, and she is being sedated with medications to allow her to undergo dialysis. She is in Stage VI dementia, no longer recognizing her husband. She has never completed an ACP document, and Hans wants her to live as long as possible and get the best care possible.

Prepare

During your review of the chart you see that Petra was diagnosed 5 years ago. She had gone to see her local clinician with complaints of forgetfulness and was referred to a specialist. After 4 hours of paper tests, many

(continued)

(continued)

questions, blood tests, and special x-rays of the brain, with Hans at her side, she was told that she had dementia. In just 4 hours her common complaint of forgetfulness had just received an official and devastating name, dementia.

Following the diagnosis, Petra and Hans returned to life as usual. Petra had a diagnosis, but life hadn't changed. Hans focused on his good moments and covered for her deficits. Life was essentially unchanged. She remembered and forgot as much as his friends. She knew his family and friends and everyone in her family had always died from other things such as accidents, heart disease, and strokes. She had no intention of entertaining the diagnosis of dementia. At age 77 Petra was certain that if she had dementia, it would remain a small footnote in this chapter of her life.

Hans and Petra lived in a lovely home in an upscale neighborhood and had enjoyed an active social life until 3 years ago, when Petra wandered off and got lost in the airport in Amsterdam while Hans was in the men's room. Luckily, Petra was quickly and safely found prior to boarding a plane back home to Connecticut. Hans kept this story to himself, but over the next year it became increasingly difficult for Hans to conceal his wife's forgetfulness and changing functioning.

Setting the Agenda

Petra's forgetfulness had worsened and now impaired her ability to complete not only common tasks of daily living but also basic tasks of caring for oneself. Petra could no longer speak on her own behalf and conversations about anything medical upset her and provoked agitated behavior.

Hans had always attempted to have Petra talk about her wishes for medical care due to her diagnosis of dementia; however, she never did. Hans found himself trying to represent her wishes against an ever lengthening list of medical diagnoses and therapeutic options with the love of his life, Petra, losing all functions that she so valued in life.

You ask, "I appreciate you all coming together today to talk about Petra's care. This is really important and I have the time this afternoon to talk to you about a number of things that I identified when reviewing her chart, but first I would ask all of you what you were hoping to talk about today. I want to create a list of topics important to you and Petra's care. So, if you could, maybe just name the topics; we can cover the details as we proceed forward."

(continued)

Deliverance From Anonymity   *(continued)*

You transition with the Snoepwinkel family, "I appreciate the agenda that we have created and I think that we can cover what you all have identified in the time we have today. Prior to coming to this meeting today, I reviewed Petra's medical chart and it may be surprising to you, but it tells me very little about who she is as a person and how you all entered into her life. If it would be okay with you (asking for permission), I would like to take the next 5 or 10 minutes to better understand who Petra is as a person. I don't even know where she was born."

Stating the Obvious

Here is an example: "I appreciate you sharing all that you have about Petra. I can only begin to imagine how challenging your lives have been in the last few years. I can honestly say you and Petra have been through a lot. I want to take a moment to reflect on what you have told me and recognize several key elements that you mentioned that seemed apparent to me. If I have interpreted the details incorrectly, let me know (contextualization). I want to commend you and your family. As I have listened closely and read between the lines, I can only imagine that you and your family have been going through times of questioning yourselves about what you were experiencing with Petra. Wondering, 'Are we right about what we are experiencing and is it really happening?' I heard you describe how as a family you have navigated the difficult role changes that have occurred when Petra lost her ability to manage her finances and go to work. Now her independence is becoming more limited and she is not enjoying or understanding this newfound lack of independence, and at the same time you all are more worried about her wandering off than her independence. I can imagine at several times in the last years you have experienced feelings of guilt in the midst of trying to care well for Petra." Then just remain quiet and let the next steps unfold. You have honored their disease stage, family journey, and emotional experience.

Determine Understanding of Illness

I often contextualize and ask, "As I mentioned earlier, I reviewed Petra's chart and I have a really good understanding of her medical background. I spoke with her neurologist and her nurse at the adult day care to gain a better understanding of how the illness is affecting her on a daily basis. I know that we have covered a fair amount already today, so I do not

(continued)

want you to recount all the medical history, but it is important for me to have a handle on what your collective understanding is of what is going on with Petra in broad strokes, of her medical conditions in an itemized list to make sure that I know where everyone's understanding of her illness is at this time. Would it be okay to do that?" I often ask clarifying questions to determine the appropriate stage of dementia and then explain that to the caregiver.

Identify Hope

It tends to follow along these lines: "I appreciate you reviewing Petra's history for me. It seems as though, and I am not surprised, you have a good handle on the implications of her illness for her life. You all have been through a lot and I commend you on engaging in this conversation today. We have covered a lot [contextualization]. I want to ask you a more difficult question, a question that gets a bit more at the heart of caring for Petra and a question that will help us understand how to provide her the best care possible. Would that be okay? [Ask permission.] In my role, I often take a moment to acknowledge that Petra got this disease, and you and your family are living with the illness. This isn't easy. I know that you recounted Petra's illness and I understand from my review and from your history that she has Stage VI dementia characterized by her inability to control her bowel and bladder, her wandering, and her inability to recognize people she loves. As you noticed, she is coughing after meals, suggesting swallowing problems typical of early Stage VII dementia, known for dependence on others for all her cares, including swallowing, speaking, and ambulation [contextualization and anticipatory guidance]. I can only imagine that you have given thought to how all this might play out, and therein lies the question I what to ask you. Knowing what you know about Petra's illness I can imagine that hope may be difficult to identify at times. However, that is the question that I want to ask. I am wondering what you and your family are hoping for from Petra's medical care at this time, knowing her and having insights into how she would choose to be cared for given her advanced dementia."

Normalize Feelings of Relief in Grief

I attempt to normalize the relief in the following way: "I commend you on caring for Petra all these years. She prepared well and arguably that has been a blessing for you. However, this is still difficult. Often people

(continued)

(continued)

experience all the decisions as a terrible restaurant with a menu of items you don't want. As we reviewed today, you have done a wonderful job in caring for Petra. I have a sense that this may be true for you. As we have been talking today, I listened closely and recognized something similar to many caregivers that I have met with over the years. Perhaps this isn't true for you, and if it isn't, please correct me. I can imagine that this journey has been laden with a fair amount of guilt. In fact, as Petra approaches the EOL, I would not be surprised if you are experiencing guilt in a new way. In the past, the guilt has revolved around decision making and the shifting landscape of your life together. At this time, I can imagine that the guilt may also be found in the anticipated relief that many caregivers experience when their loved ones dies. Is this true for you?"

Tailoring and Anticipatory Guidance

"As we have talked, Hans, it appears as though Petra has Stage VI dementia evidenced by her inability to control her bowel and bladder, her inability to recognize family, and her wandering. I commend you on watching over her and keeping her safe. It seems as though she is demonstrating signs of Stage VII, as she has a very small vocabulary and is only taking a few steps at a time. I think that we can anticipate in the near future she will exhibit more signs of Stage VII. She will likely have difficulty eating and swallowing and her food may go into her lung. She will likely eat and drink less and she will spend more time in bed. I would recommend we talk about how we will respond to these medical problems as they arise so that we have a response that best honors Petra and represents her goals as best we can. Would that be okay?"

Maximum Conservative Treatment and Care

"Hans, I have to say that I can't begin to know how very difficult this must be for you to make decisions on behalf of Petra at this time of life, when she is living every day with two organs, her brain and kidneys, failing. It may seem like there is nothing more we can do. However, there is a lot we can do. I think it would be helpful to talk about how we can best care for Petra. Currently, she is being sedated to receive dialysis treatment that causes her blood pressure to be very low, not to mention the life-saving treatments for the life-threatening blood infections she is

(continued)

(continued)

getting regularly. Her current care would be what I would call full medical treatment. Often, for people who are in this advanced Stage VI of dementia, we start to define other goals of care. Certainly, we will always provide Petra maximum conservative care to keep her safe, warm, and dry, with attention to her symptoms. I am wondering if we should be shifting from full medical treatments to maximum conservative treatments at this time due to her decline and approaching EOL. This would allow us to talk about what treatments match your stated goals for Petra. Would this be okay?"

Dying for CPR

"Hans, I know when Petra was admitted to the hospital the doctors and nurses asked if you wanted her heart restarted if it stopped, and if she quit breathing if you would want us to breath for her. When they asked, I know you consented to her undergoing these procedures. I can only imagine that the questions they were asking felt like you were choosing between life and death. If I am honest with you and if I understand how you have been seeing her declining, then the question isn't about restarting her stopped heart or breathing for Petra. The question isn't about choosing between life and death. If that were the question then we would always choose life. The question is, when Petra dies will we allow her to die peacefully with you at her side, or will you be driven from her side while she dies undergoing an attempt of resuscitation?"

The Unasked Question

"I know that the medical teams have asked you about a feeding tube for your mother, whom you love and for whom you have been caring. I think it is important that we talk about that, but I want to suggest that the decision isn't that simple or only about a feeding tube. This leads me to ask you a very difficult question that gets to the heart of caring for your mother. Is it okay if I ask you a question a bit closer to the heart? I think, as we have been speaking today, that we recognize that your mother is in Stage VII for VII stages of dementia and, honestly, we have recognized that this stage is where people with dementia approach the end of their lives. I know that your mother is no longer eating and in fact is not showing any interest in eating by mouth. I know the doctors have offered a feeding tube, and I want to talk about it but first I need

(continued)

to ask you a question that you might experience as being a bit callous, but honestly, it is a truly caring question that gets closer to the heart of the matter in caring for your mother with advanced dementia. I think we recognize that the natural progression of her disease is resulting in her dying from her disinterest and inability in eating. We can certainly give her a feeding tube. However, that won't change the natural progression of her illness, and it does raise the question that nobody has asked you. A feeding tube will certainly push your mother's frail physical state further, but not make her immortal. Therefore, it raises the question that if your mother isn't allowed to die from the natural progression of her illness, we can push her more, but then what is she going to be allowed to die from?"

In Petra's case, her family wants to continue to sedate her for dialysis while choosing not to treat her next septic episode. They want full medical treatments at a time of life when there is no benefit to identify and harm to the patient will occur. This calls for the unasked question to be asked in yet a different way. "I understand that you want to continue your mother's dialysis treatment and that you understand that without it she would be allowed to die peacefully. At the same time you have decided not to treat her next septic episode. In thinking about this, I have to ask you to acknowledge this very difficult situation, as I understand it. Your mother has a natural way to die peacefully and we are not going to allow that; rather we are going to push her forward to get something arguably worse and then not treat the sepsis? Do I understand you correctly?"

Summary

Mrs. Snoepwinkel is living with multiple terminal illnesses and, arguably, the care planning that a patient and family must navigate will directly impact her quality of life. The decisions made will impact how she lives and dies. There is clearly something worse than her dying, namely dying badly. In addition, her family's well-being and her legacy will be impacted by how her care is directed. Efforts for ACP will likely increase the chance that in the midst of the inherent sadness of the situation, both Petra and her family will be well.

CONCLUSION

Dementia is a terminal illness that most people will encounter in some capacity and role during their lifetime. Watch Over Me offers a framework to counsel patients and families living with dementia. An understanding of the stages of dementia as determined by a person's functional ability determined by iADLs and ADLs will help inform families and patients of their current situation and help to provide insight in to the future. The anticipatory guidance will help the patient and family in their journey as they transition in role, living setting, and EOL care planning. The stages of dementia and the phases of the family journey are practically connected, and Watch Over Me helps professionals to counsel patients and families as they navigate and make medical treatment and ACP decisions to help them live well in the face of a functionally debilitating disease like dementia.

REFERENCES

Caplan, G. A., Meller, A., Squires, B., Chan, S., & Willett, W. (2006). Advance care planning and hospital in the nursing home. *Age and Ageing, 35*, 581–585.

Caron, W. A., Pattee, J. J., & Otteson, O. J. (2001). *Alzheimer's disease: The family journey*. Plymouth, MN: North Ridge Press.

Gozalo, P., Teno, J. M., Mitchell, S. L., Skinner, J., Bynum, J., Tyler, D., & Mor, V. (2011). End-of-life transitions among nursing home residents with cognitive issues. *The New England Journal of Medicine, 365*(13), 1212–1221.

Koopmans, R. T. C. M., & van Weel, C. (2003). Survival to late dementia in Dutch nursing home patients. *Journal of the American Geriatrics Society, 51*(2), 184–187.

Mendez, M. F., & Cummings, J. L. (2003). *Dementia: A clinical approach* (3rd ed.) Philadelphia, PA: Butterworth Heinemann.

Reisberg, B. G., Ferris, S. H., de Leon, M. J., Kluger, A. A. Franssen, E. E., Borenstein, J. J., et al. (1989). The stage specific temporal course of Alzheimer's Disease: functional and behavioral concomitants based upon cross-sectional and longitudinal observation. *Alzheimer's Disease and Related Disorders, 317*, 23–41.

Torke, A. M., Holtz, L. R., Hui, S., Castelluccio, P., Connor, S., Eaton, M. A., et al. (2010). Palliative care for patients with dementia: A national survey. *Journal of the American Geriatrics Society, 58*, 2114–2121.

Wenrich, M. D., Curtis, J. R., Jr., Channon, S. E., Carline, J. D., Ambrozy, D. M., & Ramsey, P. G. (2000). Communicating with dying patients within the spectrum of medical care from terminal diagnosis to death. *Archives of Internal Medicine, 161*(6), 868–874.

Xu, J. Q., Kochanek, K. D., Murphy, S. L., & Tejada-Vera B. (2010). Deaths: Final data for 2007. *National Vital Statistics Reports, 58*, 19.

CHAPTER 14

On Writing One's Own Advance Directive

Joe Jack Davis

Death is a friend of ours, and he that is unwilling to entertain him is not at home.

Francis Bacon

Imagine that you are stung by wasps and have an anaphylactic reaction. You stop breathing and have no pulse. A bystander performs cardiopulmonary resuscitation (CPR) until an aid crew arrives and takes over. You are transported to an ER where your heart fibrillates. Electroshock returns the heart to a normal rhythm. After you stabilize, the doctors suspect that you might have suffered a serious brain injury. You may have suffered some heart damage also.

You are transferred to the ICU for close observation and monitoring. Your ability to speak is uncertain. You have sustained severe brain injury with small chance for recovery. Several days later your heart fibrillates again. An emergency code is called and a response team gathers and prepares to shock your heart again. Do they or don't they perform CPR?

How the above scene plays out probably depends more than anything on your age and overall health, and also on whether you have an advance directive (AD).

If you are a young person, you may never have conceived your death or living with severe disabilities. You might consider doing everything, enduring everything, to survive, to extend your life, even if it means being dependent on others for help with the activities of daily living.

If you are older, if you have lived a rewarding, active life, you might pre-fer to die from fibrillation than survive in the story above. Without an AD that expresses your preferences, without a person who knows your wishes clearly and speaks for you, resuscitation will be attempted. If successful, you risk lingering in the ICU with brain damage and a fragile heart. If you survive to be discharged from the hospital, you will be severely disabled with lifelong dependency on caregivers. For the person who has decided that he will refuse any heroic measures that would keep him alive, an AD is his best assurance that his wishes will be honored. Otherwise, physicians are going to do everything possible to extend that person's life, with no con-sideration for how much additional suffering their efforts may cause.

Longevity is the usual goal of U.S. medicine, not quality of life. You are your own best advocate. A strong AD and Designated Power of Attorney for Medical Affairs (health care proxy) are your best assurances of getting what you do or do not want with respect to medical care.

As a general surgeon whose career spanned four decades, I cared for many critically ill and dying patients. Often the family of such a patient would ask me to "do everything" for their loved one, ignoring the over-whelming odds against their relative surviving surgery or recovering and achieving a quality of life close to the one enjoyed previously. I often won-dered what I would have heard from my patient had I been able to have the same conversation with her. Some of these patients recovered from surgery with terrible disabilities and lifelong dependencies. Some never regained consciousness, dwindling in the ICU to the hiss of the ventilator and the impersonal beeping of other life-support apparatuses until some-one directed that the machines be discontinued.

I knew a person diagnosed with multiple myeloma, a cancer of the blood system with a survival rate of 3 or 4 years at best with conven-tional treatment. He chose to improve his odds with a stem cell transplant, which required intensive chemotherapy to destroy his cancerous blood cells. Unfortunately, after the above preparation for transplant, with his immune system significantly impaired, he acquired a fungal infection, which caused respiratory collapse. He ended up in the ICU on a ven-tilator, more tubes piercing his body than is imaginable and being fed intravenously. He stayed that way for almost 2 months, after which his wife, at her wits end wondering what was right for her husband, said, "Stop!" The respirator was discontinued, and he died without ever taking another breath. As astonishing as it might seem, this patient had no AD, as if he never contemplated that he might die from his disease. He had not talked to anyone about his preferences, including his wife and his doctor. Everyone involved was in the dark about what to do when things started going wrong. His death was ugly. Every doctor I talked to who witnessed his dying whispered to me, "Please, promise me, if you ever find me that way, you'll help me to die."

The treatment goal of most doctors in the United States is to extend the life of their patients. Yet, for themselves, doctors approach their time of dying differently. Perhaps because they have fewer unrealistic expectations about what modern medicine can accomplish, doctors typically get less treatment, rather than more, when death beckons. It is not that they do not want to live; their goal is to die well, peacefully, and with dignity. Most doctors want to die at home, which most can achieve with the help of hospice. Doctors strive not to die in a hospital hooked to machines, cared for by strangers.

My experiences with many bad deaths prompted me to write my first AD, which has undergone multiple revisions as I have aged. I know for me what constitutes a quality lifestyle and what does not, enabling me to know how I would, or would not, want to live, and also how I would and would not prefer to die.

I learned that a good death is probably attainable, something that can be fostered. Communication is key—what we do or do not want if our life is threatened—expressed orally *and* in writing to our closest loved ones and our care providers, especially our physicians. In addition, we should choose a health care proxy to answer for us, to stand up for us, if we are unable to speak for ourselves. The person we choose should have a clear understanding of our wishes. It was not unusual in my own family to have discussions about death around the dinner table; consequently, for us as a family, the subject of death is not an uncomfortable one, which is not true for most people in American society.

When I was asked to contribute to this book, I recognized the opportunity to offer some clarity to those wanting an AD but not knowing where to begin. Even I find that the language in templates is confusing, the questions regarding clinical situations obscure. I could see that if I presented my own AD as an example, defining terms and explaining specific clinical situations, perhaps I could make the completion of one's own AD less daunting and perhaps more tailored to one's own personal wishes. For the person wanting a ready-made document, the best one in my opinion is offered for free, online, at the Compassion and Choices website (www.compassionandchoices.org). This particular AD is combined with the form for designating a health care proxy, which is convenient.

What follows is a copy of my own AD with a discussion of its contents:

ADVANCE DIRECTIVE FOR JOE JACK DAVIS, MD

Having thought about what constitutes a good life and a good death almost from the time I began managing patients, I know without doubt that Quality of life, not Quantity, is what is most important. Certainly it is better to have lived

(continued)

ADVANCE DIRECTIVE FOR JOE JACK DAVIS, MD   *(continued)*

life passionately, enjoying the entire length, width, and breadth of it, than to have simply lived the longest life possible. I know that I have successfully achieved this. Quality to me has to do with thinking, seeing, hearing, smelling, touching, feeling, tasting. Quality is being able to talk, to participate in a conversation, contributing to the subject by being focused and interested. Quality is about writing, expressing my opinions and sharing my thoughts. Quality is about reading, enjoying good writing, and sharing my opinions about both with others. Quality is recognizing my loved ones and friends, being able to express my love for them and feel theirs in return. Quality is having the ability to experience Nature in a joyful way. When my condition, physical or mental, becomes impaired with little or no chance for recovery, when I am unable to experience the quality things I mention above, then I will want to die. If I am able to think and speak for myself, I will make and voice these decisions for myself. If I am unable to act on my own behalf, I hope there is someone who knows me well enough to make the decisions for me. To that person, I want to say in advance, "Thank you. I am grateful that someone loves me and understands me enough to carry out my wishes."

Now I will consider my body, system by system, and declare my wishes to my loved ones, my physicians, and to paramedical persons:

Let us start with the central nervous system. If I suffer severe and probably irreversible brain damage, or am rendered quadriplegic, I do not want to live. Do not start life support. This includes CPR, ventilator support, IV fluids, nutrition, and surgery. Allow me to die from such pathology. If I suffer hemiplegia plus aphasia that is likely irreversible, I would not want to live. If I am able to think, you will see me starve myself to death after such injuries. If I develop dementia, hopefully I will be able to deal with my situation early enough, which means choosing an early exit while I am still capable of ending my own life. If I fail, I will have failed myself. I consider progressive dementia or a vegetative state the ultimate examples of lingering, worse than death. If I develop either and am unable to experience Quality as I have defined Quality above, please enable me to die. Do not feed me, hydrate me, or medicate me. If I am lingering as the result of brain pathology and develop any condition that calls for heroics, please do not initiate them; allow the problem to cause a natural death.

If I have heart failure or stoppage due to a sudden cardiac event (MI, arrhythmia), attempt resuscitation with CPR and/or defibrillation. If CPR is successful, and if my cardiac condition is determined fixable (and I am with intact brain function), I would want the problem fixed. If my heart problem is irreparable and/or I am brain damaged after the event, then allow me to die without further treatment.

If I develop respiratory failure that is more than likely irreversible, or will require a breathing machine for longer than four weeks, reverse any paralyzing agent that has been used to facilitate breathing support. Tell me what is happening, then pull the breathing tube and unplug the machine. I will try to say goodbye to my loved ones before I die. I consider dying on a ventilator a bad death.

(continued)

ADVANCE DIRECTIVE FOR JOE JACK DAVIS, MD *(continued)*

If I cannot eat with little hope of eating again, I do not want nutritional support. Do not put a feeding tube in me. Do not start IV nutritional support. If an IV is already running, give only enough fluid to allow administration of medications to make me comfortable. Allow me to die from no food or fluids, which is what I would do if I was coherent. Starvation with dehydration will cause renal failure. All are relatively painless conditions and good ways to die.

If my kidneys fail in a way that is likely irreversible, I do not want to be dependent on dialysis. Do not allow this. Allow me to die in uremia.

If I suffer major burns, let's say 50% or greater of total body, full-thickness burns which would render me a Burn Unit patient for months or longer, do not put me through the resuscitation, including ventilator and IV support. Without resuscitation, respiratory failure and/or kidney failure would occur and result in a natural death, which would be merciful. Recovery from severe burn injury takes years, and perhaps never happens, with physical and mental pain that I do not want to experience. I consider life following such a burn the opposite of Quality.

If my mind isn't affected but I'm subject to one or more of the above situations, no one will be faced with answering for me. I feel confident that I will be decisive and make logical decisions that will hasten my death. I have dealt with patients afflicted with problems in all these areas many, many times; I know the problems first hand. I have witnessed way too many bad deaths. I have also witnessed too many people existing in the shell of their body, unable to care for themselves, unable to participate in life. I refer to this as Lingering. Resuscitation and care under these circumstances is not extending life; this represents preventing a good death.

I have lived a great life, a long life, with and around wonderful people. Any of the pathologic situations I've mentioned above make Quality as I've defined it unattainable. When the Quality is gone, with little or no chance for reversal, it is time for me to die. I want to Die Well, on my terms, at the right time. I'll write it one last time: Quantity is not important to me.

_____   Witness: _____

Joe Jack Davis
September 4, 2012

_____

DISCUSSION OF THE ABOVE ADVANCE DIRECTIVE

Bad Death/Dying Poorly

For me a bad death is one in which the process of dying is turned over to the medical team, almost guaranteeing that the dying occurs in a hospital or care facility, the final care provided by strangers in an alien environment. More and more people in this country are choosing to die at home, but still the great majority die in a hospital or nursing home. Care in this scenario commonly involves machines, the time of the dying dependent on someone else's decision. Dwindling too often describes this clinical picture. When dying would be merciful, prolongation of our existence (this is not life) is impersonal and lacking dignity. Unfortunately, this is what most U.S. doctors are trained to do. Often, their efforts to extend life results in additional suffering. Most of us would not choose to die this way.

Good Death/Dying Well

Paramount to my definition of dying well is dying without pain and not alone. Further improvement would include being surrounded by family and friends and dying in familiar surroundings (especially home). Icing on the cake would be getting to settle any differences with those in attendance, to say "I love you," and to say "goodbye."

Can a patient die well in a hospital? The answer is "yes" if most of the above conditions are met for the patient. Marie was such a patient, a lovely 90-year-old lady who fainted following persistent lower intestinal bleeding. The usual investigative procedures and tests failed to identify the site of bleeding, which could have been anywhere in the intestines. Her attending physician and her gastroenterologist wanted me to operate to stop the bleeding, ignoring the possibility that I might not be able to find the source. I explained the options to Marie and her family, none offering a guarantee of success. Marie told me she had lived a good life, and as one of the few survivors left from her generation, she was not interested in heroics. Marie declined exploratory surgery and further transfusions, having learned from me that she would die comfortably from blood loss. I could guarantee her that she would experience no pain. Her family supported her decisions. The other doctors resigned from her case, but not before criticizing Marie and documenting that they felt I was wrong not to push her to have surgery. Twelve hours later Marie died peacefully and comfortably in her sleep with her loved ones at her bedside. Her entire family was grateful that she had not had an operation. Her story exemplifies dying well.

Heroic Support

The list commonly includes IV fluids, nutrition, mechanical ventilation, drugs such as heart and blood pressure stimulants and antibiotics, CPR, dialysis, and surgery. If a person is adamantly against the nonsurgical life support mentioned above, then that same individual should also refuse emergent/urgent surgery that would be considered life saving. Surgery would too often prove fatal without the other heroic support. For instance, many patients following anesthesia need short-term ventilator support.

Similarly, patients whose food intake has been marginal before surgery will need nutritional support afterward if unable to resume eating promptly.

Today, with modern transport systems that get patients to the hospital quickly, and with excellent doctoring and nursing care, patients are surviving graver and graver catastrophes that not that many years ago would have been fatal. This says nothing about the quality of life of the survivors, many doomed to live with horrible disabilities and lifelong dependencies.

For the individual who has decided that he would refuse any heroic support that might delay his dying, he would do well to avoid going to the hospital or dialing 911. Both agencies are in the business of resuscitation and of extending life.

Nutritional Support

When a patient is hospitalized with a life-threatening illness or injury, very quickly he will need nutritional support to avoid the complications of a starvation state. If that patient cannot eat, nutrition can be given directly into the gastrointestinal (GI) tract via a tube, or through a special IV. Either way is labor intensive and expensive, each with its own advantages and complications. Nutritional support is usually discontinued when a patient is able to eat. If the patient is getting ventilator support, nutritional support is indicated early, the intent being to minimalize muscle wasting and the time spent on the ventilator. Eating is one of life's sublime pleasures. If I have no prospect of being able to eat again, I do not want a tube placed into my gut to keep me alive. If I'm coherent, I will state this. If unable to speak for myself, I want someone to refuse nutritional support for me.

Arrhythmia

Arrhythmia implies abnormal heart rhythm. It usually refers to ventricular fibrillation or tachycardia, both of which result in ineffective pumping action and cessation of blood flow. It is usually fatal unless normal rhythm is restored.

Ventilator/Respirator/Mechanical Ventilation/Breathing Machine

A ventilator is a bellows that breathes for the patient who cannot breathe for himself. Mechanical ventilation requires a breathing tube in a patient's airway and care in an ICU. Usually such a patient is paralyzed with drugs to maximize the benefits of the machine. A breathing tube is a soft, plastic tube about a foot long. Such a tube can damage a patient's vocal cords if left in place longer than 3 or 4 weeks. After that, the patient needs a tracheostomy, a tube surgically placed into the airway below the vocal cords through the lower neck. With either of these breathing tubes in place, a patient is unable to speak. Most patients with respiratory failure eventually breathe on their own and are disconnected from the ventilator. In worst circumstances, patients need a ventilator the remainder of their lives (Steven Hawking, Christopher Reeves). If I am on a ventilator for longer than 4 weeks with little chance of getting off, I want the paralyzing drugs stopped so that I have the opportunity to awaken, have the breathing tube removed, and say goodbye to my loved ones.

Dialysis

Without kidneys one builds up toxins in the blood that in a week or so will lead to coma and painless death. Dialysis involves an artificial kidney machine that "cleans" the blood of toxins. Acute kidney failure can be transient, requiring only short-term dialysis. Unremitting, chronic renal failure requires lifelong dialysis. A dialysis session usually takes several hours to complete, after which the average patient is "wasted" the rest of that day. The typical patient has to repeat dialysis three times a week. Chronic dialysis patients are often some of the sickest and most fragile of patients, requiring their own specialist (nephrologist) for care.

CPR

CPR is performed when a victim has no heartbeat and/or stops breathing. This involves blowing a large breath of air into the victim's lungs, followed by heavy pressure applied to the breastbone with the heel of one's hand (hard enough to compress the underlying heart and force blood out of the heart chambers, mimicking the pumping action of the heart). CPR extends thousands of lives annually and has become the standard procedure in hospitals and nursing homes when patients have cardiac or respiratory arrest (unless there are orders stating otherwise). CPR can also involve electrically shocking (defibrillation) the heart to convert an ineffective heart rhythm into one that works. The better the overall health of the patient, the more likely CPR is to be successful. However, CPR has a dismal track record when used in chronically ill or terminal patients. The number of these patients who eventually leave the hospital is infinitesimally small. If I have an unexpected cardiac and/or respiratory arrest as an isolated event (I have no prior pathology in either of these organ systems), then I want CPR. However, if I am critically ill or terminal when I arrest, I do not want CPR. Death due to either circumstance would be a natural and good way to die.

Terminal Condition

If a person has only 6 months or less to live in the eyes of two physicians, his condition is called "terminal."

Brain Injury/Pathology

The brain pathologies to which I refer leave you severely compromised cognitively, unable to live independently. Stroke, brain hemorrhage, and head trauma are examples (e.g., Terri Schiavo). I consider a vegetative state a condition far worse than death.

Hemiplegia

Hemiplegia refers to the paralysis of one entire side of the body.

Progressive Dementia

For example, Alzheimer's.

Aphasia

Aphasia is the inability to speak.

High Spinal Injury

Severe spinal injuries of the neck cause quadriplegia (paralysis of all four limbs) and occasionally respiratory failure. These injuries are permanent and leave the victim severely disabled. Evacuation of bladder and bowel no longer occur naturally. These patients are at high risk for infection (pneumonia, urinary tract) and for skin breakdown (bedsores). Life span for them is usually significantly shortened (e.g., Christopher Reeves). At my age, I do not want to live with this degree of incapacity.

Severe Burns

For purposes of discussion I chose 50% or greater of the total body surface area burned full-thickness (third degree). Burns of this severity are associated with very high mortality rates and even greater complication rates. Recovery requires emergency resuscitation, months spent in a Burn Unit, many operations to restore skin coverage and preserve limb function, and often requires lifelong physical therapy. Pain control issues are huge. Survivors often say they would never have wanted resuscitation had they known what they were in for at the beginning. If I am the unfortunate victim of a burn this bad, I would prefer to die, which would occur anyway without heroic support. If I am able to speak for myself, I will refuse resuscitation, asking only for pain relief while waiting to die.

Bad things happen to good people—meaning you and me. Any of us could have a life-threatening problem tomorrow. Does it then not make good sense to have a document that clearly states what we want done if we are in a medical crisis? Does it then not make good sense to talk with our loved ones about what we would want, what they would want, if any of our lives were threatened by some pathologic condition? Does it then not seem prudent to name someone who knows us well to speak for us if we are unable to speak for ourselves? In the introduction above, the reader will find ample information for writing one's own AD. The time is right. Do it!

PART III

Implementing Advance Care Planning: Model Programs

Introduction

Leah Rogne

It is clear that just giving individuals the legal right to make choices about end-of-life (EOL) care has not been enough to shift how we deal with dying, death, and care. As health care providers and communities have had more experience with advance directives (ADs) and with individuals who find the whole process of dealing with EOL daunting and confusing, many communities have developed focused programs to provide public education about death and dying and to provide user-friendly tools for advance care planning (ACP). Drawing on lessons learned from the disappointing results of the SUPPORT Study (The SUPPORT Principal Investigators, 1995) and other efforts to promote ADs, model programs have moved from a forms-focused approach to a broader ACP approach, taking care to provide community awareness programs, support systems, and a variety of resources to help individuals understand their options, explore their choices, and (perhaps most important) learn how to communicate with their families, friends, and health care providers about their values and desires about how they would like to live until they die.

This part features four model programs that have drawn on research, the experience of others, and their own experience to develop effective advance planning initiatives. Research and experience have led them to develop strategies for dealing with common barriers for the public, for health care providers, and for meeting the needs of special populations. All of these programs emphasize the central role of communication in ACP and provide resources to support people to lift the veil of silence around issues related to death and dying, and help community members communicate effectively about their wishes about their care during EOL. Two programs are statewide coalitions, and two are model local/regional initiatives. (See Chapter 22 in this volume for other programs and resources focused on ACP and EOL care.)

In Chapter 15 Linda A. Briggs, associate director of the acclaimed initiative Respecting Choices® at the Gundersen Clinic of LaCrosse, Wisconsin, outlines how the Respecting Choices three-step model of ACP addresses some of the key barriers to effective planning for EOL care. Focusing on the importance of understanding, reflection, and discussion among practitioners, patients, and family members and the facilitation of conversations appropriate for patients in various stages of wellness and/or illness, Respecting Choices has succeeded in transforming its community to the extent that by 1996, 85% of decedents had ADs and, more important, 98% of patients' wishes were honored at EOL. Briggs discusses how Respecting Choices has been replicated in other communities and emphasizes the importance of effective training of facilitators, organizational commitment, and the infusion of conversations about EOL throughout the community as well as within health care institutions.

Chapter 16 features a statewide initiative, the Take Charge Partnership of Pennsylvania. Partnership founders Margaret L. Stubbs, Jolene Formaini, Cynthia Pearson, and Dena Jean Sutermaster describe the development of the partnership, which got its start in the late 1990s as a part of community awareness and action project associated with the Public Broadcasting Service's television series on death and dying, *On Our Own Terms: Moyers on Dying.* The authors describe how the all-volunteer partnership has provided community outreach and resources to foster action that makes a difference in how individuals, families, and communities deal with EOL issues. Actions have included a series of 26 regional forums to discuss the television series and to lay the groundwork for local action, the development of an online resource bank, and a series of public service announcements. The partnership has developed a robust web-based education system that provides short videos (free of charge) and online discussion guides on ACP, the reality of caregiving, hospice and palliative care, and managing pain. An especially innovative approach has been a web resource called "Empower Others." This tool is directed toward a variety of individuals who interact with the public, such as members of religious and community organizations, barbers and hairdressers, health care workers, tax preparers, employers, counselors and therapists, educators, and trainers and coaches. It communicates the idea that you don't have to be an expert to talk about EOL matters and provides these community members with resources to initiate important conversations when appropriate. Stubbs and her colleagues provide helpful tips on how to build what they call a "proactive, agentic" grassroots organization on a shoestring budget and how to prioritize outreach efforts that can make an immediate difference in the community.

In Chapter 17, Judy Citko, executive director of the Coalition for Compassionate Care of California, outlines key successes of the statewide group. The Coalition's groundbreaking initiatives on EOL care in nursing homes succeeded in developing a system to reduce unnecessary nursing home-to-hospital transfers at EOL and showcased promising practices to provide high quality care in nursing homes for those nearing EOL. Citko describes how the Coalition's workgroup created a guide to EOL nursing home care that is explicitly tied to federal nursing home regulations as a way of gaining adoption of and legitimacy for the recommended new way of dealing with EOL in a long-term care facility. Citko also outlines the Coalition's work to promote the use of Physicians Orders for Life-Sustaining Treatment (POLST) as a way to deal with some of the shortcomings of traditional ADs, and discusses its efforts to create a system that empowers persons with developmental disabilities to direct their EOL care. Finally, she describes the Coalition's work to create a process that assures that EOL conversations take into account the variety of cultural and spiritual beliefs that prevail in our increasingly multi-cultural society.

Finally, in Chapter 18, project implementation coordinator Cari Borenko Hoffman outlines the ACP initiatives of Fraser Health Authority in British Columbia, Canada. By creating engaging education programs for the public and for practitioners, and by working with a network of other organizations in the province and throughout Canada on education, outreach, and policy, Fraser Health has fostered effective conversations about EOL care among patients, families, and providers, resulting in a dramatic increase in the proportion of people in its service region having ACP documents. Fraser Health drew on the Gundersen Clinic's Respecting Choices® model and put a particular emphasis on involving physicians in planning and feedback to increase physician attention to the goals of ACP for their patients and families.

REFERENCE

The SUPPORT Principal Investigators. (1995). A controlled trial to improve care for seriously ill hospitalized patients: The study to understand prognoses and preferences for outcomes and risks of treatments (SUPPORT). *Journal of the American Medical Association, 274,* 1591–1598.

CHAPTER 15

Respecting Choices®: An Evidence-Based Advance Care Planning Program With Proven Success and Replication

Linda A. Briggs

With the passage of the Patient Self-Determination Act (PSDA) in 1991, leaders from health care organizations across the United States scurried to set policies and practices in motion to demonstrate compliance with the letter of the law. The admission assessment question, "Do you have an advance directive?" was launched at nearly every health care organization across the country. Forms and brochures were created to inform patients about their rights to have an advance directive (AD). Now, nearly two decades later, this typical approach to the completion of ADs has proven ineffective: the prevalence of completed documents remains low, but even when completed, they are often unavailable, unknown to the treating physician, or too ambiguous to guide clinical decision making (Fagerlin & Schneider, 2004; Tonelli, 1996; Wu, Lorenz, & Chodosh, 2008). Furthermore, ADs may be ineffective in preventing unwanted life-sustaining treatment at the end of life (EOL) (Kass-Bartelmes, Hughes, Rutherford, & Boches, 2003; Lorenz et al., 2004; Teno et al., 2004).

Health care leaders in the community of La Crosse, Wisconsin, took a decidedly different approach to compliance with the PSDA—one more aligned with the spirit of the law and intended to help individuals maintain

TABLE 15.1
Prevalence, Availability, and Consistency of Advance Directives in
La Crosse County After the Creation of an ACP System in '91–'93

	LADSI*	LADSI**	P VALUE
	Data Collected in '95/'96; N = 540	Data Collected in '07/'08; N = 400	
Decedents with ADs No. (%)	459 (85.0)	360 (90.0)	0.023
ADs found in the medical record where the person died No. (%)	437 (95.2)	358 (99.4)	<0.001
Treatment decisions found consistent with instructions	98%	99.50%	0.13

ADs, advance directives; LADSI, La Crosse Advance Directive Study One

SOURCE: *Hammes and Rooney (1998). **Hammes, Rooney, and Gundrum (2010).
Copyright: 2011 Gundersen Lutheran Medical Foundation, Inc.

autonomy over future health care decisions. The La Crosse approach began with the question, "What assistance do individuals need to plan ahead for future health care decisions?" To best answer this question, the program focused on communication strategies and informed decision making. This approach has clear and convincing evidence that it works. Following implementation of this comprehensive AD model, an evaluation of all adult deaths in La Crosse County over an 11-month period from April 1995 until March 1996 reported that 85% of decedents had an AD; of these ADs, 95% were found in the medical record at the time of death, and 98% of the time there was evidence that patients' wishes were honored (Hammes & Rooney, 1998). Ten years later, these stellar outcomes were maintained and improved (see Table 15.1), thus demonstrating the impact of a well-designed system for sustaining person-centered outcomes (Hammes, Rooney, & Gundrum, 2010). Over the years, this system has become known as advance care planning (ACP) and the proven program as Respecting Choices.

This chapter explores why the Respecting Choices approach is different from typical AD approaches and the reasons why it has worked when other approaches have failed. It describes the key elements for building a successful ACP program and provides examples of how Respecting Choices faculty have assisted in replicating this model in other communities, cultures, and organizations around the world.

HOW IS THE RESPECTING CHOICES APPROACH TO ADVANCE CARE PLANNING DIFFERENT FROM THE TYPICAL APPROACH TO ADVANCE DIRECTIVES?

The typical approach to ADs has focused on completion of a standard, legalistic form and in compliance with the PSDA or other regulatory guidelines. This focus has resulted in a series of yes and no questions on admission (e.g., "Do you have an AD?" and "Would you like more information?") and, unfortunately, created impersonal and ineffective practices regarding information presented to patients and the quality of their interactions with health care providers. "Just get it done" is often the mantra for busy professionals or others who do not feel comfortable having—or do not feel prepared to have—ACP discussions. More importantly, this approach ignores the need to address the multiple barriers to engaging individuals and their families in the planning process. While many Americans are knowledgeable about the importance of ADs, they remain unmotivated to participate due to personal beliefs, misunderstandings, perceptions of how difficult the activity may be, or the belief that it can wait for a future time (Eiser & Weiss, 2001; Sahm, Will, & Hommel, 2005; Schickedanz et al., 2009). Health care providers also remain uncomfortable and unskilled at having ACP discussions (Christakis, 1999; Scherer, Jezewski, Graves, Wu, & Bu, 2006; Yedidia, 2007). The perceived lack of time and reimbursement for ACP activities are further impediments to provider-initiated quality conversations (Legare, Ratte, Gravel, & Graham, 2008; Weiner & Roth, 2006).

The Respecting Choices approach is different. It assumes that conversations are the key to successful planning, that time and resources will be needed, and that health care providers will require communication skills training. Several characteristics of the Respecting Choices approach to ACP help overcome the barriers to participation in planning discussions, improve the decision-making process, and produce a more effective written plan.

THE GOALS OF ADVANCE CARE PLANNING ARE DEFINED

The success of any program is measured by whether it achieves its stated goals. When the goals of ACP are narrowly defined (e.g., increase the incidence of completion of ADs), then only narrowly defined strategies will be designed to meet this goal. Although it is desirable for the planning process to result in the completion of a written plan that is consistent with statutory and regulatory requirements, the Respecting Choices approach has more comprehensive goals:

1. Assist individuals in making informed health care decisions.
2. Assist in the selection and preparation of a qualified health care proxy.
3. Honor informed decisions.

To gauge the achievement of these far-reaching ACP goals, one must do more than count the number of ADs completed. To accomplish more specific goals, communication strategies are designed to provide planning assistance to individuals and their families at multiple encounters, to include chosen health care agents in discussions, and to assist agents in understanding their loved ones' preferences. In addition, systems are created to ensure that plans are available and actionable across the continuum of care to achieve the goal of honoring individuals' informed health care decisions.

ADVANCE CARE PLANNING IS PERSON-CENTERED

The initial development of the Respecting Choices program was prompted by multiple stories of patients whose goals and values for future health care were unknown. These stories included individuals who could no longer communicate their preferences for future medical care due to sudden injury or complications from advanced illness. Families, physicians, and other health care providers felt the impact of this void on bedside decision making. Families were stressed morally, ethically, and physically with the uncertainty of making decisions for a loved one. Personal narratives provided the framework for designing an ACP system that has kept the individual's perspective front and center.

Person-centered interviewing skills form the core of Respecting Choices ACP facilitation. These skills are the vehicle through which to explore the individual's experiences, fears, religious or cultural beliefs and goals for living well, among other variables. This assessment forms the basis for crafting an individualized approach to planning.

Person-centered ACP is focused on engagement and not merely education. Educational efforts to increase understanding of the importance of ADs have been successful yet have not had a significant impact on participation in the ACP process. In a 2005 Pew Research Center survey on ADs, 84% of respondents were aware of the importance of their rights to make life-sustaining treatment decisions (www.pewtrusts.org/news_room_detail.aspx?id=23572). The missing link for many individuals is motivation. Consistent with Prochaska's stages of change model, motivational strategies assist in moving individuals from precontemplation (no interest in taking action) to action (participation and making changes) (Prochaska & Velicer, 1997).

Respecting Choices uses a variety of strategies to motivate individuals to participate in planning and helping them understand the components of a well-designed planning process.

THE PROCESS OF ADVANCE CARE PLANNING INVOLVES UNDERSTANDING, REFLECTION, AND DISCUSSION

Most individuals who complete a written AD are well intentioned. They are hopeful that the plans will guide others in making health care decisions consistent with their preferences. Unfortunately, they are unaware of the obstacles that may prevent their good intentions from being realized. They are often left with a false sense of security that the mere completion of a document will accomplish their intent. While the terms "AD" and "ACP" are often used interchangeably, the distinction between them could not be more important. The typical event of completing an AD does not ensure informed decisions will be made, or that they will be followed. In a study of bereaved family members where 70% of loved ones had completed an AD, significant gaps were found in the type of EOL care they received (Teno, Gruneir, Schwartz, Nanda, & Wetle, 2007).

Without adequate and ongoing discussion, typical ADs are incapable of providing the level of individual choice, comfort, and control in the last weeks, months, or years of life that most desire. In the absence of a quality planning process, individuals who complete ADs (and their families) often experience frustration and disappointment when conflicts arise over treatment decisions. In fact, the original title of the La Crosse program, "If I Only Knew," represented a common theme from families who faced difficult health care decisions for a loved one without adequate knowledge or understanding of their loved one's goals, values, or beliefs (Colvin & Hammes, 1991). This uncertainty leaves its mark on families required to make substitute decisions. Research has demonstrated that ACP interventions have a positive impact on family members, who report less stress, anxiety, and depression than those not receiving assistance (Detering, Hancock, Reade, & Silvester, 2010; Wright et al., 2008).

The Respecting Choices solution to "If I Only Knew" situations was to help patients verbalize their goals, values, and beliefs well before a medical crisis, and to help loved ones be better prepared. While current authorities recognize the need to move from the mere completion of an AD document to a process of communication, a common definition for this process does not exist. This lack of clarity on the components of an effective ACP process has led to several unfortunate consequences:

- It is assumed that anyone can initiate ACP discussions, regardless of the quality of their communication skills or preparation.
- Without agreement on the content of ACP discussions, standardized training programs cannot be developed, and providers do not gain consistent facilitation competencies.

- Without a competently trained workforce, a consistent and reliable ACP service cannot be delivered or reimbursed.
- With wide variation in the delivery of ACP services, the ultimate goal of honoring individuals' informed decisions cannot be achieved.
- Research studies define ACP differently (or not at all), making the ACP intervention difficult to replicate and refine.

Respecting Choices defined the components of the ACP process from the outset of the program as follows: *ACP is a person-centered, ongoing process of communication that facilitates individuals' understanding, reflection, and discussion of their goals, values, and preferences for future health care decisions.* This definition has guided the training of ACP facilitators and the organization of the ACP team, has produced a competent and reliable ACP service, and has stimulated ongoing quality improvement activities. Below I discuss each of the components and outline how each plays an integral role in the ACP process.

Understanding

Understanding involves more than providing information on how to complete a legal or statutory document. Individuals need to understand why ACP is important for all adults, the consequences of not planning, and what is involved. For example, in choosing a health care agent, individuals need assistance in understanding the qualities necessary for this role, related responsibilities, and strategies for discussion. Consistent with the principle of informed consent, individuals need information on the decisions that they are being asked to make. Individuals with advanced illness and more complex decisions need specific information to understand their relevant treatment choices and the concomitant risks, benefits, and alternatives. Not only do individuals need adequate information to make informed decisions, they desire it. A recent EOL survey found that 75% of individuals are concerned about not having adequate information about treatment decisions (Regence Foundation, 2011). As people live with advanced illness and decisions become more complex, the desire for accurate and useful information increases (Pfeifer, Mitchell, & Chamberlain, 2003). When patient understanding of treatment options is not embedded in the planning process, individuals are forced to make uninformed decisions at often inappropriate times. Consider the standard question that many patients are asked on admission to a hospital or long-term care facility: "Do you want cardiopulmonary resuscitation (CPR) if your heart or breathing were to suddenly stop?" It is asked as a yes or no question, sometimes by an unqualified individual (e.g., an admissions clerk). Can you imagine being asked this question? What information would you desire before making this decision? Would you want to know the success of CPR in restarting your heart and breathing? Would you want to know what your physician would recommend based on your medical condition? Would you want to know the complications of CPR or the alternatives? You would likely need time to gather this information and weigh the facts against your personal goals, values, and beliefs. This process of understanding is critical to making informed decisions and consistent with the familiar informed consent process used for making any serious medical decision, such as whether to undergo a recommended surgery or procedure.

Reflection

Information and understanding are key components of an effective planning process, but individuals also make informed decisions based on personal values, goals, and beliefs (e.g., religion, culture). Individuals need time and assistance weighing these personal variables against the factual information provided. Without time for reflection, individuals may make decisions that, although based on accurate information, are inconsistent with personal values. Consider the individual in a nursing home who is contemplating the CPR decision. Initially, the individual is interested in attempting CPR; however, in further conversation the individual expresses the additional goal of NOT returning to the hospital. The goal of not being hospitalized is in conflict with the choice to attempt CPR because transfer from the nursing home to the emergency department is inevitable. When patients have multiple and conflicting goals such as these, their goals must be clarified and prioritized through a skilled facilitation process. To ensure adequate time for reflection, the planning process must begin well before a medical crisis and be individualized to the patient's expected illness trajectory.

Discussion

Once understanding is increased and time for reflection is allowed, individuals often value talking to others who will be helpful in personal decision making. Discussions with their physicians, religious advisors, other family, and most importantly their chosen health care agents, must take place prior to completion of a written document. Selecting and preparing a qualified agent is paramount to ensuring that future decisions will be consistent with the individual's goals, values, and beliefs. During one ACP discussion, the author learned that a patient with advanced kidney failure had decided he did not want CPR. Unfortunately, only his renal dialysis staff was informed of this decision. He had not discussed this decision with his health care agent (in this case, his son) or with other family and close friends. He was unaware of the importance of preparing his family and friends to honor his decision and to anticipate what actions were appropriate. This CPR conversation opened the door for further understanding of his goals and preferences and better preparation for his loved ones.

In summary, the Respecting Choices approach to the ACP process of understanding, reflection, and discussion is distinctly different from the typical approach, which is focused on completion of an AD.

A STAGED APPROACH TO ACP

ACP is not a one-size-fits-all conversation. The common practice of assuming that one planning session and one document will suffice over the lifetime of an individual is unrealistic and impractical. Why would planning for a healthy adult look similar to the specific planning for a person with advanced heart failure? Why would we expect individuals to have the capacity to project themselves into a future state of chronic illness (e.g., advanced heart failure) and make informed decisions about what they would or would not want at some point in the future?

Over the years, Respecting Choices has developed a staged approach to planning called First®, Next™, and Last Steps™ ACP (Figure 15.1). This

FIGURE 15.1 Stages of Advance Care Planning Over the Lifetime of Adults.

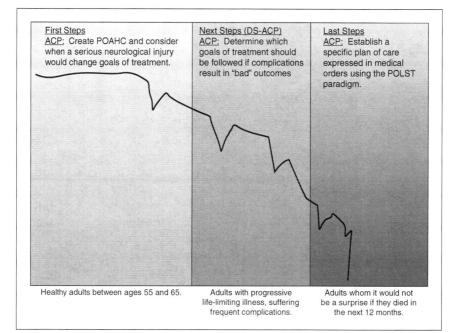

ACP, advance care planning; DS-ACP, disease-specific advance care planning; POAHC, power of attorney for health care; POLST, physician orders for life-sustaining treatment.

SOURCE: Copyright: 2011 Gundersen Lutheran Medical Foundation, Inc.

staged approach integrates planning as a dynamic process sensitive to the changing needs and goals of individuals as they move from a healthy state to one of progressive decline. This approach makes practical sense to patients when ACP is woven into the fabric of routine care over the lifetime of an individual and throughout the multiple venues of care.

First Steps ACP is intended for all adults, but specifically for those older than 55 or 60 years. It is focused on helping individuals appreciate the importance of planning as a routine component of quality health care and to normalize the conversation. The specific goals of First Steps ACP are to assist in the selection of a qualified health care agent; identify any personal, religious, or cultural beliefs that may affect future decision making; identify goals of care for a severe neurologic injury; and complete a power of attorney–type of AD. This stage of planning can be integrated into routine practices in many ways, such as through annual wellness appointments, illness-specific support groups, faith community ministries, and senior center health services. As the name implies, planning will need to be revisited over time and as goals and values change.

Next Steps ACP is a specific planning process for patients who have advanced illness and are experiencing a decline in function, complications, or more frequent clinical encounters. Qualified health care professionals working as part of the patient's health care team invite patients to revisit their ACP goals in light of their changing illness trajectory. The Next Steps conversation also makes sense to patients who realize they are getting sicker and desire information about future options. Through an in-depth person-centered interview, individuals are given an opportunity to discuss their current illness progression and to understand potential complications and related treatment options. Moreover, fears, experiences, hopes, and gaps in information are identified and addressed. Individuals are assisted in clarifying their goals in selected "bad outcome" situations that provide guidance for future decision making. Delivered in the outpatient setting while the patient's illness is well managed, this intervention includes the chosen health care agent who, through active participation in the planning discussion, becomes better prepared to make future health care decisions if necessary. This dyadic interview opens the channels of communication between patients and loved ones, strengthening relationships for ongoing discussions and decision-making abilities (Briggs, 2003). In randomized, controlled studies of this intervention with patients with advanced illness, the Next Steps ACP intervention increased understanding of treatment choices between patients and their agents, decreased decisional conflict, and was highly satisfying (Detering et al., 2010; Kirchhoff, Hammes, Kehl, Briggs, & Brown, 2012).

Last Steps ACP is intended for those individuals whose death in the next 12 months would not be a surprise, such as frail elders living in long-term care or those in hospice. This stage of planning is highly specific and timely because complications from advanced age or illness are anticipated and emergency responses are necessary. Informed treatment decisions are made proactively by the patient or by his/her designated surrogate and converted to medical orders signed by a physician so they can be followed throughout any venue of care. To meet the needs for Last Steps planning, the La Crosse community implemented the Physician Orders for Life-Sustaining Treatment (POLST, 2012) program in 1997. Sixty-seven percent of individuals who die in the La Crosse community have completed a POLST medical order form (Hammes, Rooney, Gundrum, Hickman, & Hager, 2012). Through ACP discussions, families and health care providers have clear direction on the types of emergency treatments patients desire, thus decreasing decision-making uncertainty and unwanted interventions.

The staged approach to planning has many practical benefits for patients and health care providers alike:

- It integrates planning decisions over the course of an individual's life, helping them make health care decisions that are timely and appropriate to their stage of illness.
- It does not ask or require individuals to complete a checklist of specific treatments that they would or would not want at some hypothetical point in the future. Rather, it integrates planning as a component of routine care at appropriate intervals and revisited as a person experiences advanced illness and its progression over time.
- It acknowledges that goals and values may change over time.
- It accepts that patients will need more specific guidance in making clinical decisions as they live with advanced illness.
- It allows for the selection and training of qualified individuals who will be prepared to facilitate ACP discussion for different stages.
- It provides for the creation of increasingly specific written plans to guide clinical decision making as illness progresses.

WHY HAS THE RESPECTING CHOICES APPROACH TO PLANNING WORKED WHEN OTHER APPROACHES HAVE FAILED?

When the leaders of the La Crosse ACP initiative began their work, they created a vision that went far beyond the goals of the PSDA. They made a commitment to design a comprehensive and coordinated program that would be integrated into routine practices across the continuum of care and embedded in community venues where people socialize, receive services, and pray. To accomplish the goals of ACP (i.e., assist in making and honoring informed health care decisions) they realized that systems would need to be created to reliably deliver ACP services and communicate informed health care choices across the continuum of care. There were no magic bullets or quick fixes. A system would need to be designed that would need ongoing evaluation and improvement. They decided to start small and build success over time.

The result was the creation of an ACP microsystem. Clinical microsystems have formed the core of many health care programs aimed at shaping professional behavior, satisfaction with care, effectiveness, safety, and cost (Nelson, Batalden, Godfrey, & Center for the Evaluative Clinical Sciences at Dartmouth, 2007). Specifically, this ACP microsystem was constructed to identify and honor individuals' informed health care preferences as a component of quality health care services.

The Respecting Choices ACP microsystem has four key (and interrelated) elements that have been tested in large and small communities. Strategies to build each element must be identified and addressed (Hammes & Briggs, 2011). In attention to any one of the key elements creates gaps that will impact the achievement of ACP goals.

Key Element #1: Designing Systems to Support Advance Care Planning

Effective systems that are hardwired into the routines of care help busy professionals do the right thing and increase the chances that the goals of ACP will be achieved.

Key ACP systems must include the following:

1. A uniform AD document that assists in clarifying individuals' goals and values and is clinically useful.

2. A team approach to ACP where referrals are made to the most qualified individual as needed.

3. An effective and efficient medical record system for entering, storing, retrieving, and transferring documents, as well as capturing the essence of ACP discussions.

Respecting Choices ACP consultations with organizations and communities around the world have consistently uncovered gaps in these key systems—some underdeveloped and others nonexistent. For example, AD documents are often confusing and lack sufficient specificity to guide clinical decision making. These documents may be poorly understood and supported by health care providers. Multiple documents may exist in a single community, adding to the confusion for consumers as well as for health care providers. While most communities have individuals who are responsible for helping others to complete a written AD, inadequate resources exist to provide individualized assistance in helping people understand their treatment options (and related benefits and burdens) or weigh information against personal goals and values. While electronic medical storage systems are currently in development, the challenge of document portability and update remains.

Once key systems are adopted by an entire community rather than a single health care organization, widespread progress can be made and consumers will receive common and consistent messages about the importance of ACP and individualized assistance in planning. Written plans are created that are useful for clinical decision making, understood by health care providers, and available as needed. Now, the goal of honoring individuals' informed decisions becomes possible.

Key Element #2: Advance Care Planning Facilitation Skills Education and Training

The growing recognition of the need to include communication as part of the ACP process is evident in such reports as the AD and ACP Report to Congress (Wenger, Shugarman, & Wilkinson, 2009). Respecting Choices has taken a leadership role in defining the skills necessary to have quality ACP discussions and assist individuals in making informed health care decisions.

A core element of the Respecting Choices program is the creation of the role of the ACP facilitator (Briggs, 2012). The ACP facilitator demonstrates competence in assisting individuals in making informed health care decisions through a customized planning process. The facilitator is trained to competently deliver a consistent and reliable planning service to all patients across the continuum of care. ACP facilitators are often non-physicians who work as part of the patient's health care team, making referrals as needed and helping physicians provide focused assistance to their patients. The non-physician model for ACP facilitators does not exclude physicians from taking an active role in the planning process because many patients seek guidance from their personal doctor. The ACP facilitator helps patients identify knowledge gaps, fears, and questions for their physicians, which serves to enrich the patient–physician relationship. While physicians also need to develop effective ACP communication skills, Respecting Choices acknowledges that it is unrealistic to believe that physicians will have adequate time to provide a consistent ACP service to all who need it without the support of another team member.

The value of the role of the ACP facilitator becomes evident to physician colleagues who have tested this model through pilot projects and personal evaluation. In the words of one palliative care physician, "This conversation...forms part of the initial establishment of a relationship with persons with advanced illness. As such, it serves to help educate, set expectations, and guide the subsequent supportive care system" (Klemond, 2012, p. 91).

Consistent with the staged approach to ACP, facilitators identify which certification training (i.e., First, Next, or Last Steps) is most appropriate for their background, experience, and level of ACP responsibility. Specific communication skills are identified for each training program, providing an opportunity for individuals with varying backgrounds to participate in the ACP service. For example, First Steps facilitators may be nurses or social workers from outpatient clinic settings, community volunteers from senior centers, or chaplains and parish nurses from faith communities. To competently assist with Next or Last Steps planning, facilitators typically need health care experience, knowledge of advanced illness, and opportunities to work integrally with the rest of the health care team. Next Steps ACP facilitators are typically experienced registered nurses who work as care coordinators or navigators for patients with complex needs, or social workers from renal dialysis or cancer centers who have other related responsibilities with patients with advanced illness. Last Steps facilitators are often palliative care practitioners, nurses and social workers from long-term care venues, or home and hospice providers.

Respecting Choices ACP facilitator training programs have a long and rich history of success in achieving baseline competency and producing standardized curricula that are reproducible through train-the-trainer instructor certifications. This standardized approach to facilitator training is effective, satisfying, and ensures the preparation of an ACP team that works together to deliver a reliable ACP service across all stages of planning.

Key Element #3: Community Engagement and Education

To educate individuals on ACP, many programs develop brochures, pamphlets, and presentations focused on the completion of ADs. Such single-modality strategies are often ineffective at changing behaviors (Lorenz et al., 2004). The American public has been well educated in the purpose of ADs. In a 2005 Pew Research Center survey, 84% of respondents were aware of their rights to complete a document that would direct future medical care (Pew Charitable Trusts, 2012). This level of AD knowledge has not dramatically changed the incidence of completion of written plans. Education alone is rarely sufficient in changing behavior.

Respecting Choices recommends a multifaceted approach to ACP education by including engagement strategies intended to promote dialogue, create a meaningful experience, and motivate people to participate in the planning process. Suggested strategies include:

■ Integrating social marketing ideas, such as branding (i.e., selecting a name and logo for the ACP initiative), to improve recognition throughout a community. In La Crosse, the branding is called "Making Choices" and includes an attractive starfish logo that is used on all written materials, educational fliers, and promotional activities.

■ Using stories of others' experiences with health care decision making in written materials and video examples to emphasize common themes and motivate people to learn more.

■ Developing focused materials to help people with different components of the ACP process, such as an information card for health care agents that describes their role and responsibilities.

■ Customizing information for targeted populations, such as for religious groups or support groups for specific illnesses (e.g., heart failure, cancer).

■ Recruiting representatives from diverse groups in the community to communicate the importance of ACP and to develop culturally sensitive messages.

In addition, community engagement involves developing effective partnerships with key stakeholders, such as religious groups, attorneys, and senior advocates who can assist in disseminating the concepts of the ACP process and make referrals as needed for quality planning assistance.

Key Element #4: Continuous Quality Improvement

All successful programs are nurtured, monitored, and improved over time. ACP programs demand the same investment. Attention to ongoing quality improvement is one of the most important elements in achieving ACP program goals. As new systems, processes, and materials are designed or revised, they are tested through small and focused pilot projects prior to widespread dissemination. There are many reasons to start small and build support incrementally:

■ The initial systems that are created will not be perfect and will need testing to make improvements before wider distribution.

■ Individuals trained as ACP facilitators will need time to integrate new skills into their roles. Starting small will help make this workload more manageable as they increase their competence.

■ Newly formed ACP teams will need to learn to work together, establish referral systems, and assess the effectiveness of the individualized implementation plans.

■ Data are needed to demonstrate the effectiveness of and satisfaction with the new program to increase engagement and speed dissemination.

Respecting Choices has developed a quality improvement framework called *The Five Promises* (Figure 15.2) to guide organizations or communities in developing a comprehensive ACP program. This framework can be used

FIGURE 15.2 The Five Promises.

Promise #1: We will initiate advance care planning conversations with individuals about their preferences for future medical care.

Promise #2: We will provide appropriate ACP assistance as requested.

Promise #3: We will make sure plans created are clear and communicated to those who need to know.

Promise #4: We will store and retrieve these plans so they are available wherever needed.

Promise #5: We will follow these plans as appropriate when individuals can no longer make their own decisions.

to assess the quality of current efforts, assist in the design of specific strategies to meet each promise, and identify related outcome measures.

CAN THE RESPECTING CHOICES MODEL BE SUCCESSFULLY REPLICATED?

In 1999, Gundersen Lutheran Medical Foundation, Inc. made a commitment to support development of a national Respecting Choices program to provide consultation and education to other communities, organizations, and countries interested in replicating the Respecting Choices model. This program has spread internationally, producing several stories of successful replication.

The Respecting Patient Choices program (www.RespectingPatient Choices.org.au) in Australia is modeled after the La Crosse program. Respecting Choices faculty provided extensive consultation and education to help the Australian leaders customize the key elements described above to address the diverse needs of this country. Through a commitment to quality improvement and research, the Respecting Patient Choices program has documented success and has become a national model for implementation in Australia. This program has established standards of practice for documentation of advance care plans, common education and engagement materials, training of facilitators (called ACP counselors), and secured funding for ongoing dissemination, media resources, and research. In 2012, they published the results of a randomized controlled trial of the Respecting Choices–based ACP facilitation intervention in medical inpatients aged 80 years and older. Patients who received the intervention were significantly more likely to have their wishes known and followed than those in the control group (Detering et al., 2010). Patients and families in the intervention group were also more satisfied with their overall hospital experience than were those in the control group. Additionally, family members of patients who died in the intervention group experienced significantly less stress, anxiety, and depression than control group family members. These outstanding research outcomes are reflective of a well-designed system that was monitored and improved over time.

Implementation of the Respecting Choices program is also occurring in the metropolitan communities of Minneapolis/St. Paul in Minnesota. Under the leadership of the Twin Cities Metro Society, 40 members of the Twin Cities health care communities agreed to adopt the Respecting Choices model and collaborate in developing consistent materials (e.g., common documents and education materials), facilitator training, and community engagement (Wilson & Schettle, 2012). These health care leaders agreed not to compete in the area of ACP, collaborate during implementation, and invest in resources to continue dissemination. Among the many outcomes this initiative has achieved is the development of a community engagement campaign in partnership with Twin Cities Public Television that includes listening sessions and an interactive website (http://www.honoringchoices.org). While complete geographic implantation will take several years, leaders have established credibility and expertise to assist other communities across Minnesota in adopting the principles of what the Twin Cities group is calling Honoring Choices Minnesota.

The Respecting Choices Next Steps ACP stage of planning has been replicated with successful outcomes in such health care systems as Allina Hospitals and Clinics, Minneapolis, Minnesota, and for adolescents with HIV/AIDS. Allina Hospitals and Clinics have adopted and implemented a comprehensive ACP program that includes all stages of planning. In particular, the leaders of this initiative have demonstrated the positive outcomes of the Next Steps ACP intervention for heart failure patients, reporting a high rate of completion of a disease-specific planning document to guide future decisions resulting from advanced illness. Heart failure patients who died during the study period were more likely than nonparticipants to use hospice services (Schellinger, Sidebottom, & Briggs, 2011). This study demonstrated important lessons in implementing the Next Steps intervention into clinical practice and gaining support for further dissemination.

The Respecting Choices Next Steps intervention has been successfully replicated in an adolescent population with HIV/AIDS. In a randomized, controlled pilot study, researchers from Children's National Medical Center in Washington, DC reported on the feasibility and acceptability of the family-centered intervention with mostly black, medically stable adolescents with HIV/AIDS and their parent/guardian (Lyon et al., 2009). Compared with the control group, the intervention group demonstrated a significant increase in parent/guardian understanding of their loved one's preferences. Intervention adolescents reported feeling better informed and supported than did their counterparts in the control group. The further investigation of these pilot results is being studied in a randomized, controlled trial funded by the National Institutes of Health.

At Gundersen Health System, the Next Steps ACP intervention has been integrated into a novel program for patients with advanced illness called Advanced Disease Coordination (ADC) (Klemond, 2012). In an effort to more effectively identify and coordinate the complex needs of patients with advanced illness, the ADC program links the unique and related services of ACP, care coordination, and palliative care. The goals of this program are to establish and maintain relationships with patients and families over their final months to years of life, providing timely and appropriate access to needed resources.

SUMMARY

The Respecting Choices ACP evidence-based program can be successfully replicated in diverse communities and cultures. The four key elements of a successful ACP microsystem—designing systems, training and education of ACP facilitators, community engagement strategies, and ongoing quality improvement—are effective principles for customizing an effective ACP program. These principles alone, however, will not yield success. Creating and sustaining a comprehensive ACP program as described requires significant commitment of leadership, human and financial resources, and practical plans for ongoing dissemination. Effective leaders integrate ACP into the strategic vision of the organization, building the infrastructure for long-term success.

Organizational leaders who make this commitment face significant challenges. Those who are successful share a common belief that building an effective ACP program is simply the right thing to do and are willing to invest resources to remove barriers to implementation. Leaders understand that patients and families find ACP highly satisfying and crucial to ensuring that they receive care consistent with their goals, values, and preferences. Successful outcomes are reflected in the stories of those whose lives are touched by ACP interventions.

In the words of one health care agent who participated in an ACP planning discussion with his father, and subsequently used this information to make health care decisions when his father was incapacitated by a severe stroke,

> The conversation was eye-opening for me. With a third party present, I learned things I never knew about my dad.... During the conversation with the facilitator, she asked a lot of questions.... She stuck to the facts.... At no point was there any pressure to choose one option or another.... The choice was

his; the facilitation just provided the road map. In the end...the decision was not up to us; our father made it very clear what he wanted in advance. (Loomis, 2012, p. 154)

These stories are now common in the La Crosse community, and "If I only knew" situations are rare. The comprehensive Respecting Choices approach to creating a sustainable ACP program is worth the investment. This approach has demonstrated evidence that the ultimate goals of ACP are achievable: *to know and honor individuals' informed health care decisions.*

REFERENCES

Briggs, L. (2003). Shifting the focus of advance care planning: Using an in-depth interview to build and strengthen relationships. *Innovations in End-of-Life Care, 5*(2), 11–16.

Briggs, L. (2012). Helping individuals make informed healthcare decisions: The role of the advance care planning facilitator. In B. J. Hammes (Ed.), *Having your own say: Getting the right care when it matters most* (1st ed., pp. 23–40). Washington, DC: CHT Press.

Christakis, N. A. (1999). *Death foretold: Prophecy and prognosis and medical care.* Chicago, IL: University of Chicago Press.

Colvin, E. R., & Hammes, B. J. (1991). "If I only knew:" A patient education program on advance directives. *American Nephrology Nurses Association Journal, 18*(6), 557–560.

Detering, K., Hancock, A., Reade, M., & Silvester, W. (2010). The impact of advance care planning on end of life care in elderly patients: Randomized controlled trial. *British Medical Journal, 340*, 1–9.

Eiser, A. R., & Weiss, M. D. (2001). The underachieving advance directive: Recommendations for increasing advance directive completion. *American Journal of Bioethics, 1*(4), W10.

Fagerlin, A., & Schneider, C. E. (2004). Enough the failure of the living will. *Hastings Center Report, 34*(2), 30–42.

Hammes, B. J., & Briggs, L. A. (2011). *Building a systems approach to advance care planning* (1st ed.). La Crosse, WI: Gundersen Lutheran Medical Foundation.

Hammes, B. J., & Rooney, B. L. (1998). Death and end-of-life planning in one midwestern community. *Archives of Internal Medicine, 158*(4), 383–390.

Hammes, B. J., Rooney, B. L., & Gundrum, J. D. (2010). A comparative, retrospective, observational study of the prevalence, availability, and specificity of advance care plans in a county that implemented an advance care planning microsystem. *Journal of the American Geriatrics Society, 58*, 1249–1255.

Hammes, B. J., Rooney, B. L., Gundrum, J. D., Hickman, S. E., & Hager, N. (2012). The POLST program: A retrospective review of the demographics of use and outcomes in one community where advance directives are prevalent. *Journal of Palliative Care, 15*(1), 77–85.

Kass-Bartelmes, B. L., Hughes, R., Rutherford, M. K., & Boches, J. (2003). *Research in action issue #12: Advance care planning: Preferences for care at the end of life* (March 2003, Pub No. 03–0018 ed.). Rockville, MD: Agency for Healthcare Research and Quality (AHRQ).

Kirchhoff, K. T., Hammes, B. J., Kehl, K. A., Briggs, L. A., & Brown, R. L. (2012). Effect of a disease-specific planning intervention on surrogate understanding of patient goals for future medical treatment. *Journal of the American Geriatrics Society, 58*(7), 1233–1240.

Klemond, T. (2012). Hope for the future with a human touch: Advanced disease coordination. In B. J. Hammes (Ed.), *Having your own say: Getting the right care when it matters most* (pp. 87–98). Washington, DC: CHT Press.

Legare, F., Ratte, S., Gravel, K., & Graham, I. D. (2008). Barriers and facilitators to implementing shared decision-making in clinical practice: Update of a systematic review of health professionals' perceptions. *Patient Education & Counseling, 73*(3), 526–535.

Loomis, G. (2012). One of the most important conversations we had. In B. J. Hammes (Ed.), *Having your own say: Getting the right care when it matters most* (1st ed., pp. 152–154). Washington, DC: CHT Press.

Lorenz, K., Lynn, J., Morton, S., Dy, S., Mularski, R., Shugarman, L., . . . Shekelle, P. (2004). *End-of-life care and outcomes.* (Evidence Report/Technology Assessment No. 43: AHRQ Publication No. 01-E058). Rockville, MD: Agency for Healthcare Research and Quality.

Lyon, M. E., Garvie, P. A., McCarter, R., Briggs, L., He, J., & D'Angelo, L. J. (2009). Who will speak for me? improving end-of-life decision-making for adolescents with HIV and their families. *Pediatrics, 123*(2), e199–e206.

Nelson, E. C., Batalden, P. B., Godfrey, M. M., & Center for the Evaluative Clinical Sciences at Dartmouth. (2007). *Quality by design: A clinical microsystem approach.* San Francisco, CA: Jossey-Bass.

Pew Charitable Trusts. (2012). *More Americans discussing—and planning—end-of-life treatment: Strong public support for right-to-die.* Retrieved from http://www.pewtrusts.org/news_room_detail.aspx?id=23572

Pfeifer, M. P., Mitchell, C. K., & Chamberlain, L. (2003). The value of disease severity in predicting patient readiness to address end-of-life issues. *Archives of Internal Medicine, 163*(5), 609–612.

Physician Orders for Life-Sustaining Treatment (POLST). (2012). *Physicians orders for life-sustaining treatment paradigm.* Retrieved from www.polst.org.

Prochaska, J. O., & Velicer, W. F. (1997). The transtheoretical model of health behavior change. *American Journal of Health Promotion, 12*(1), 38–48.

Regence Foundation. (2011). *Living well at the end of life: A national conversation.* Retrieved from http://syndication.nationaljournal.com/communications/NationalJournalRegenceToplines.pdf

Sahm, S., Will, R., & Hommel, G. (2005). Attitudes towards and barriers to writing advance directives amongst cancer patients, healthy controls, and medical staff. *Journal of Medical Ethics, 31*(8), 437–440.

Schellinger, S., Sidebottom, A., & Briggs, L. (2011). Disease-specific advance care planning for heart failure patients: Implementation in a large healthcare system. *Journal of Palliative Medicine, 14*(11), 1244–1230.

Scherer, Y., Jezewski, M. A., Graves, B., Wu, Y. W., & Bu, X. (2006). Advance directives and end-of-life decision making: Survey of critical care nurses' knowledge, attitude, and experience. *Critical Care Nurse, 26*(4), 30–40.

Schickedanz, A. D., Schillinger, D., Landefeld, C. S., Knight, S. J., Williams, B. A., & Sudore, R. L. (2009). A clinical framework for improving the advance care planning process: Start with patients' self-identified barriers. *Journal of the American Geriatrics Society, 57*(1), 31–39.

Teno, J. M., Clarridge, B. R., Casey, V., Welch, L. C., Wetle, T., Shield, R., et al. (2004). Family perspectives on end-of-life care at the last place of care. *JAMA, 291*(1), 88–93.

Teno, J. M., Gruneir, A., Schwartz, Z., Nanda, A., & Wetle, T. (2007). Association between advance directives and quality of end-of-life care: A national study. *Journal of the American Geriatrics Society, 55*(2), 189–194.

Tonelli, M. R. (1996). Pulling the plug on living wills. A critical analysis of advance directives. *Chest, 110*(3), 816–822.

Weiner, J. S., & Roth, J. (2006). Avoiding iatrogenic harm to patient and family while discussing goals of care near end-of-life. *Journal of Palliative Medicine, 9*(2), 451–463.

Wenger, N., Shugarman, L. R., & Wilkinson, A. *ADs and advance care planning: Report to congress.* Retrieved December 3, 2009 from http://aspe.hhs.gov/daltcp/reports/2008/ADCongRpt.htm

Wilson, K. S., & Schettle, S. (2012). Honoring choices Minnesota: A metropolitan program underway. In B. J. Hammes (Ed.), *Having your own say: Getting the right care when it matters most* (1st ed., pp. 41–56). Washington, DC: CHT.

Wright, A. A., Zhang, B., Ray, A., Mack, J. W., Trice, E., Balboni, T.,...Prigerson, H. G. (2008). Associations between end-of-life discussions, patient mental health, medical care near death, and caregiver bereavement adjustment. *The Journal of the American Medical Association 300*(14), 1665–1673.

Wu, P., Lorenz, K. A., & Chodosh, J. (2008). Advance care planning among the oldest old. *Journal of Palliative Medicine, 11*(2), 152–157.

Yedidia, M. J. (2007). Transforming doctor-patient relationships to promote patient-centered care: Lessons from palliative care. *Journal of Pain & Symptom Management, 33*(1), 40–57.

CHAPTER 16

The Take Charge Partnership "Just Talk(s) About It:" A Model for Sustained Grassroots Activism

Margaret L. Stubbs
Jolene Formaini
Cynthia Pearson
Dena Jean Sutermaster

The Take Charge of Your Life Partnership began operation in 2000. Our earliest meetings were inspired by the community outreach designed by the Bill Moyers team to generate interest in the upcoming Public Broadcasting Services (PBS) television broadcast of *On Our Own Terms: Moyers on Dying* (Moyers, Moyers, O'Neill, Mannes, & Pellett, 2000). Our local Forbes Hospice was one of the national sites for a video conference that provided an opportunity to preview the broadcasts and encouraged community collaboration in planning associated activities. Maryanne Fello, the hospice director, invited individuals from a variety of backgrounds to attend. Some were entrepreneurs; others were palliative care physicians and nurses, hospice care providers and administrators, and area faith leaders. Two of us had no formal connection to health care practice but had cared for dying family members at home and had just published a book on the topic. A representative from our local PBS station, WQED, was also included. We might have dispersed after implementing activities related to the broadcast. But we didn't.

Taking Moyers's call for community action to heart, we decided to meet again to plan a formal organizational structure. At that meeting, in addition to working on promoting the broadcast, we began to wrestle with crafting a mission statement, defining goals, and articulating a vision for future work. Although we have experienced a number of changes to our organization over the years, a guiding principle that has remained from the outset an integral and stated part of our mission is "to educate, support, and empower all people to deal with end-of-life issues." While some aspects of the evolution of our organization are unique, we believe that our process is entirely replicable and hope that our narrative can encourage others to undertake such efforts. Key elements that characterize our effort are taking advantage of opportunities that came knocking; using constraints as opportunities; having a grounding in the individual, practical experiences of lay people; a focus on action; and forming and maintaining relationships with other like-minded, practical activists, including higher-profile champions.

In this chapter, we describe how we evolved into a project-oriented, activist organization working with local and state organizations to improve end-of-life (EOL) care. We focus on how, with funding from the Pennsylvania Department of Aging, we created *Just Talk About It*, a series of 1-minute online videos and study guides covering four subjects identified statewide as most important for the public to learn more and talk about: advance care planning (ACP)/choosing a health care agent; providing care for loved ones; considering hospice and palliative care; and managing pain. Take Charge has been described as "the little engine that could," and we believe our work exemplifies what Margaret Mead meant when she said, "Never underestimate the power of a small group of committed people to change the world. In fact, it is the only thing that ever has."

COMING TOGETHER

When Cynthia Pearson and Margaret (Peggy) Stubbs found themselves at the first community meeting, their book, *Parting Company—the Caregiver's Journey: Understanding the Loss of a Loved One* (Pearson & Stubbs, 1999) had been on the market for about 6 months. It was 10 years in the making, which at times had been discouraging, but, in hindsight, the timing of the book's publication turned out to be very fortunate. Local publicity about the book resulted in invitations for them to talk about it with interested professional and lay audiences. Having spoken at Forbes Hospice, they were invited to attend the videoconference.

Moyers and colleagues' focus on death and dying gave voice to a change in attitudes that had been taking place in the broader culture about the EOL (Moyers et al., 2000). As chronicled by Ariés (1981), care for the dying and burial arrangements had once been an integral part of family life, but over the years, advances in medical technology and funeral practices gradually resulted in the professional management of the EOL. The dying spent their last days in the hospital, not at home; funeral staff prepared the body for visitation at the funeral home, not the parlor at home, and also managed the actual burial. Family members became less involved and less familiar with the dying process and the direct care and associated tasks that might be required.

It was in this context that in the late 1980s, Cynthia and Peggy, friends since the fifth grade who had kept in close touch over the years, found themselves confronting a series of illnesses and deaths among family members and assuming the associated at-home caregiving responsibilities. Cynthia had managed her paralyzed father's care for 2 years before his death. Shortly after that, she lost a brother-in-law to an unexpected heart attack while she was also helping to care for a niece who was dying of brain cancer. Peggy's father had died of complications from surgery to remove an aneurism. Within the next 18 months, she lost her mother to inoperable kidney cancer, and within 3 weeks of that death, her brother, who suffered from mental illness and had been cared for at home by their parents, also died. As they compared notes during these ordeals, they acknowledged that they felt they were wholly unprepared to know what to do in these situations. What they did know was that they felt overwhelmed by the shock and sadness of witnessing the decline of their loved ones in the context of not knowing much at all about the dying process or how to assure that their loved ones got the best care.

At the same time, Cynthia and Peggy's direct involvement in their loved ones' dying was a function of another cultural shift that had begun in the late 1960s and 1970s. A backlash of sorts had formed against the medicalization of natural biological functioning (see Conrad, 1992, 2007). For example, natural childbirth was promoted as an alternative to what critics argued was overzealous medicalization of birthing practice (see Cahill, 2008; Fox & Warts, 1999; Oakley, 1980). Other critics saw the same trend in EOL care (see Hoyer, 1998). Interest in forgoing acute care to provide comfort care for the dying grew in the late 1960s after Dame Cicely Saunders introduced her hospice model of care in England. Eventually, in 1983, legislation in the United States permitted the reimbursement of hospice care under Medicare, in part as a response to the growing demand for less, not more medical intervention at the EOL (Hoyer, 1998). By the early 1990s, more and more people were expressing the wish to die at home, and more and more families wanted to honor that wish (SUPPORT Principal Investigators, 1995). But unlike their nineteenth century ancestors, these well-meaning family members, like Cynthia and Peggy, were not prepared for the tasks at hand.

Writing their book from their perspectives as lay caregivers, Cynthia and Peggy sought to describe the challenging details of caring for dying loved ones at home, hoping to make this "new trend" of home death easier. As participants in the videoconference, they were members of the general public who wanted to honor their loved ones' wishes to die at home, but were hard pressed to know how to do it. At the same time, the palliative care and hospice providers who attended acknowledged a need to educate the general public about what their services actually entailed. People were confused about the meaning of palliative care and hospice. Many understood hospice only as a harbinger of certain death, giving up hope, and "doing nothing." The entrepreneurs who attended were interested in creating and marketing products to help people make decisions of EOL care. All recognized a larger problem: how to engage the public in learning more about death and dying, a subject typically avoided in our death-phobic culture. It was an opportune time for coming together.

ESTABLISHING OUR IDENTITY

The structure imposed by promoting the Moyers broadcast was key to our adopting a collective, concrete, action-oriented perspective. That opportunity gave those of us working in our own ways a chance to rally "round and work together on a very specific, time-sensitive goal with the potential to reach audiences well beyond our own constituencies." The community outreach materials provided by PBS placed a strong emphasis on "building coalitions to affect change" and provided a road map to a number of possible actions to do just that, as well as raise awareness about the broadcast. Thanks to the Moyers team's vision, we saw at that first meeting the value of insuring continued collaboration to keep such activities going on in our region long after the broadcast.

And so, the idea of a regional partnership to further this work began to percolate. At the next meeting, several of us volunteered to draft bylaws for our working group, originally called the End-of-Life Partnership of Western Pennsylvania, and to file for non-profit status. To assist with the filing costs, a local foundation stepped up with a donation, which a local clergy member offered to manage for us through his church until our official non-profit status was conferred. Our idea was that as a nonprofit organization we could eventually receive funding to support collaborative efforts across existing organizations. With volunteer staff and no physical location, our overhead costs would be negligible in comparison to those of other established entities. Although a plus at our beginning, these features of our group would also present challenges for us later on.

At the same time, we worked to implement broadcast-related outreach activities. Our numbers grew as original attendees let others know about the immediate effort. The participation of many volunteers enabled us to plan and staff a range of diverse projects, some of which were to occur well after the broadcast. To serve the broadcast we organized a phone bank to field calls at our local station, and afterward prepared a report of callers' concerns. We compiled a resource directory to support the phone bank volunteers and the community at large, and set up a website to enable public access to the resource guide.

To carry the work into the future and implement our next activity, we partnered with the National Issues Forum (NIF), one of the National Outreach Associates mentioned in the Moyers's outreach materials. This undertaking was especially important in the evolution of our organization. NIF is well known for its encouragement of deliberative dialogue among ordinary citizens in service of providing policy makers with grassroots input during their decision making. Local NIF discussion leaders offered their expertise if our group wished to launch a series of community NIF discussions about the EOL as one of our action projects. NIF had already developed materials, which they had used in other locations to encourage exploration of issues related to death and dying. They could and would provide training for potential discussion leaders. Members of our group, enthusiastic about using the NIF approach, quickly organized to launch the Community Forums project. Forty-seven would-be forum leaders from our group participated in a 2-hour round table discussion as part of a daylong moderator training session at the WQED studios. Potential sites for holding forums ranging from libraries to church basements, to local schools— wherever members of the group had a point of entry—were identified, and invitations to attend were distributed. In all, 26 forums, involving nearly 400 people, were held from just after the initial PBS broadcasts through the end of that year. Following NIF procedures, pre and post questionnaires were completed and analyzed; discussion notes were transcribed, and a summary report, *Western Pennsylvanians Talk about Death and Dying on Their Own Terms* was presented for public review (End-of-Life Partnership of Western Pennsylvania, 2002). The NIF project increased our visibility in the region, and also our credibility in that we were not only raising awareness but also collecting data from and about our efforts on behalf of those whom we most wished to serve—members of the general public. We were pleased that our efforts gave them voice.

With a small grant from another important partner, The American Bar Association (ABA), we implemented our next successful project. The ABA was especially interested in providing information about ACP to senior citizens. Building on the success of our Community Forums project, we were happy to organize community workshops on this specific topic as well. We were advised by our colleagues who worked with seniors that the elderly were not likely to respond with enthusiasm to an EOL or advance directive campaign. So, we chose a less direct, more proactive and agentic approach and named this outreach the Take Charge Campaign. This would prove to be an important paradigm shift for us as we moved forward.

The original structure of our organization included an Executive Committee to manage building the organization. We also named other committees to manage specific tasks. The Education Committee organized guest speakers or suggested group readings. Our Public Relations Committee organized publicity about our projects with local media outlets. Thanks to prompting from some of our entrepreneurial members, we formed an e-Committee to think about how to expand on our web presence. Committees worked at will. At regularly scheduled plenary meetings for the full group, we conducted project-related business in addition to enjoying presentations and discussion of articles. The participation of many volunteers made staffing the range of our diverse projects possible. News of our accomplishments led to our mention in the *Journal of the American Medical Association* (Phillips, 2000) as a grassroots coalition with staying power, among the many that formed as a result of the Moyers outreach. This recognition was an important feature of our identity development. We were characterized as action oriented, working on behalf of the general public, and envisioned as having a future. It was an expectation we were eager to fulfill.

Of course, not everyone stayed with us as time went on. Some of the original participants were primarily committed to education and training within the medical community rather than outreach to the general public. Others affiliated with well-established educational, insurance, or corporate entities eventually started another "organization of organizations" in the region, one with more strategic capacity to shape a regional agenda for improving EOL care. As one of us observed, we were a Volkswagen Beetle compared to their moving van. Although we'd had some successes, we weren't yet commanding a leadership role in the academic or corporate arenas in our region. Although we had hoped to build capacity and garner more credibility and financial support for collaborative projects, we understood that there was work to be done by many, on many levels, and with many target populations. We might have been swallowed up by this turn of events, but instead, we participated as members of the other organization and were pleased to take the role of representing members of the general public, and we continued to implement projects we thought would best serve the public. The constraint of being smaller actually required that we be more selective and very effective in designing and implementing the projects for the audience we wanted most to serve.

ACHIEVING IDENTITY

Now a leaner organization than we were at the outset, in terms of both membership and a more specific purpose, we utilized the services of an organization called the Executive Service Corps (ESC) to help us with strategic planning. This is a group of retired corporate executives in our area who volunteer their considerable time and achieved talent to advise non-profit organizations. With their help, we sharpened our focus, reaffirmed the general public as our target audience, and began to rethink how best to approach the general public. When checking the phone logs, we counted more hang-ups after our name was announced than people asking for us to call them back. In light of how successful the Take Charge Campaign had been, we wondered if perhaps our name, The End-of-Life Partnership, was off-putting to the very group we were trying to reach. It seemed that even people who had sought us out were reluctant to confront the topic so directly, a tendency that we acknowledged, at least intellectually, at our very first meeting.

We had learned from our Community Forums project that participants were eager to talk about issues related to death and dying. Many provided feedback saying they had appreciated the opportunity to discuss and learn about various options. However, far too many also expressed their discomfort and hesitance to talk about these same issues with their own family members. Based on that experience, we were able to acknowledge that while *we* might be comfortable talking directly about death and dying, the people we were trying to reach weren't. Without meaning to, we got caught up in our enthusiasm, and it clouded our vision a bit with respect to thinking about what would really help people warm up to this difficult subject. We decided to change our name to the Take Charge of Your Life Partnership, and redesigned our website to reflect our new proactive, agentic, and yes, backdoor approach, to our work.

We also shifted our attention from the wider variety of projects in which we had been involved to those with the potential to enhance communication about death and dying. We thought that these kinds of projects would prime people to want to learn more about options for care at the EOL, who would, we reasoned, then be more likely to use this new information proactively in formulating their own EOL wishes. Having a smaller membership also contributed to our rethinking the kinds of projects that we could now staff. But again, this constraint served to move us forward and not backward. We began to make the transition from outreach that was exclusively face to face, to a virtual approach via the Internet, which afforded us increasing and cost-effective opportunities to reach the public. We continued to connect to resources at the national level mentioned by Moyers. With a grant from Rallying Points of the Robert Wood Johnson Foundation, we created Take Charge Online, a project that provided information about ACP and other topics via streaming video. Later we were recognized by the same organization as one of three coalitions in the United States to receive an Award of Excellence, making it possible for us to continue with our Internet outreach.

Our accomplishments thus far had been inspired, in part, at an early meeting in September of 2000 with Dr. Joanne Lynn, coauthor of *Handbook for Mortals* (Lynn & Harrold, 1999) and then director of the Rand Center to Improve Care for the Dying and President of Americans for Better Care of the Dying. After this meeting, our modus operandi became "keep on keeping on." Dr. Lynn stressed that the most important thing we could do to help the cause, then at its very beginning, was to string our pearls (of action), one at a time, and to keep them coming. We took her advice to heart.

Our string of pearls grew and our identity as an organization committed to working on behalf of the general public become recognizable at both the national and the local level. As such, and as a result of continued participation in our sister "organization of organizations," the Coalition for Quality at the End of Life (CQEL), as it came to be called, Take Charge was positioned to assist a task force of CQEL members appointed in the fall of 2005 by then Pennsylvania Governor Ed Rendell to make recommendations for improving Pennsylvania's ability to maintain quality at the EOL. For the final report (The Task Force for Quality at the End of Life in Pennsylvania, 2007), which would involve the collaboration of many individuals across the state, members of Take Charge were asked to help write the chapter "Educating the Public." This invitation introduced Take Charge to a much broader audience. Although during the Moyers outreach we had worked with Pittsburgh's mayor and the Chief Executive of Allegheny County to proclaim a "Living Will Month," we had not worked at the state level until our contribution to the Governor's report.

The Governor's report (posted on our website, http://takechargeofyourlife.org/) was extensive. Chapter authors were charged not only with providing accurate information but also with supplying recommendations for action that could involve public–private partnerships. Contributors to our chapter agreed that of the many issues that could be addressed in raising public awareness about the EOL, four stood out as especially important: ACP, the reality of caregiving, clarity about the scope of hospice and palliative care, and managing pain. We wrote about the importance of each and also, as required, provided specific action-oriented recommendations for how to engage the public in thinking about these topics. Our recommendations included:

1. A statewide public education campaign to draw participation from local and statewide media outlets and service agencies, and various elements of such a campaign, was described:
   - Based on our experience, we suggested the campaign be named "The Take Charge Campaign™" or "It's About Your Life™" instead of "EOL Issues."
   - Message development would begin with a focus on the four topics identified in our chapter.
   - Message development would feature storytelling to evoke an emotional response as compared to a report of statistics.

- A series of town meetings, similar to those associated with the Moyers project, could be coordinated by the PBS stations throughout the state.
2. We urged national government and service agencies to provide clients with more information about the logistics of caregiving and help them understand and coordinate available resources.
3. We urged educators at all levels to include a focus on loss and grief into the curriculum.
4. We recommended that individuals "take charge" of their own health care by using a buddy system in which friends agreed to accompany each other to medical appointments and keep track of important records such as a list of medications, insurance information, and the name of and how to contact a designated health proxy.

After the report was submitted, Take Charge continued to generate ideas about what could be done. It was clear to us that a broad-based public awareness campaign would need to be fleshed out over time and would require the coordination of many constituencies, but some of our suggestions could be undertaken in the short term by any inspired groups or individuals. Already inspired, and knowing that it could take a long time at the state level to prioritize not only the recommendations from our chapter, but all of the rest that the other authors had offered, we decided to follow our own advice.

JUST TALK ABOUT IT

In 2007, the Take Charge Board of Directors began to explore the possibility of producing a series of a public service announcements (PSAs) encouraging people to "just talk about it." By this time, video was becoming widespread on the Internet, so we knew that even if we could not get the PSAs on broadcast television, they could be made available everywhere on the web. Although ultimately we envisioned producing videos that would address all the four areas identified as those that the public could most benefit from learning and talking about, we began by developing a single pilot video on ACP. Our choice was based in part on research showing that when individuals and families have discussed their values and wishes in advance, they fare better when a crisis occurs (Prendergast, 2001). In developing the pilot, we also created a process that laid the foundation for future work. The first effort was largely a labor of love and volunteer effort. Board members created the story line, and local producers from the Greater Good Productions completed the script and then cast, filmed, and edited the video. The pilot video was shown to CQEL members and officials at the state Department of Aging, whom we had met through our work on the Governor's report, to learn what interest there might be in partnering to produce the whole series. The series would present three videos each on the topics we highlighted in the Governor's report: ACP, the reality of caregiving, clarity about the scope of hospice and palliative care, and managing pain.

While the path to state officials had been laid by our participation in the Governor's report, several people championed our cause. Nora Dowd Eisenhower, then Secretary of the Pennsylvania Department of Aging, led us to Ivonne Bucher, then Chief of Staff and Director of the Office of Community Services and Advocacy at the state Department of Aging. Ms. Bucher stressed how important it was that our messages appeal to a diverse audience. At the local level, we appreciated the advice of Mildred Morrison, head of the Allegheny County Area Agency on Aging, who also stressed a focus on diversity and helped us navigate the application for and implementation of a state grant. Without the expertise and commitment of these women to serve the public, our series would never have seen the light of day.

Our *Just Talk About It* videos were truly a community project. The videos featured many of Pittsburgh's finest actors along with students from Point Park University and Chatham University who participated in the production. Since Take Charge did not have a county contract, which we needed to accept the funding, Chatham University, where Peggy taught, served as our fiscal agent. Members of CQEL served as advisors to the content at several pre-screenings. The project also benefitted from access to filming locations granted by Forbes Hospice, the Western Pennsylvania Hospital, and Chatham University.

Once the videos were complete, they were posted on our own and the Department of Aging's website (www.portal.state.pa.us/portal/server.pt?open=512&objID=3950&&PageID=455360&level=2&css=L2&mode=2). Our intent had always been that access to the videos would be free of charge, but both we and the Department of Aging realized that an online tool kit to accompany the videos would be useful to people, whether they were viewing as individuals or wanted to use the videos to *Just Talk About It* in a group setting. As a result, the Department of Aging again provided financial support for the development of free online discussion guides (in large and smaller print), which included background material for group leaders as well as specific "take charge" actions that groups or individuals could implement. All of the project materials were available for the public on both our own and the Department of Aging's websites by November of 2010.

Although we lack capacity at present to track the effectiveness of our videos, including enhancing conversations about the EOL, serving as a motivator for naming a health care proxy, or drafting an advance directive, feedback from public screenings has been positive. When viewed recently within a caregiver education and support group led by one of our board members, a middle-aged female caregiver reported a successful outcome in utilizing one of the videos as a conversation starter with her 83-year-old father. She stated:

> My dad is from that generation where you don't talk about things that are uncomfortable. I have been trying to get him to sign a living will for the past two years but he is too stubborn to even listen. He has been surprisingly supportive of my participation in the caregiver support group, and after each session he is eager to find out what I "learned." Last week, after I saw those *Just Talk About It* videos in our session, I decided to show him *instead* of tell him what I learned. He gets such a kick out of the computer, even though he has no idea how to use it! After we watched the first video (*A Family Way*), he completely identified with the stubborn reluctance of the man in the scenario who had no intention of talking about or signing a living will. Then, after he had a good chuckle about how they were a lot alike, he said, "Well, I guess if that guy can look into it, so can I. Bring me the papers and help me figure out what I'm supposed to do. Now what else are you learning in that class of yours?"

This is one example of how the videos can reach one person at a time. On a larger scale, the videos and discussion guides are being used within various group situations, including those facilitated by health care providers. The University of Pittsburgh Medical Center (UPMC) used the *Just Talk About It* materials in multiple health care facilities during their 2012 National Health Care Decisions Day outreach to staff and the community.

THE CONCLUSION...TO OUR BEGINNING

We believe that we were fortunate to start our organization at a time when national attitudes about EOL care were changing and when the Internet was becoming a growing force. Though we did not become the coalition to maintain local collaboration, we were able to carve out our niche at that table and as a result have continued to benefit from personal connections with others in the region and in the state toward a common effort. It was advantageous to have to rein in our vision and to concentrate on actions we could accomplish for the audience we thought we could best serve. Once we achieved that identity and clarity of focus, we just kept on thinking of things to do and doing them as we could.

At the same time, we do recognize that there are challenges to our continuing work. One challenge is that we are small. This helps to keep us on focus, but how will we attract others to continue the work? We have had minimal difficulty implementing our projects via partnerships with people in the broader community, but we see the need to articulate a strategy to ensure that Take Charge is sustainable in the future. And we are older—certainly wiser as well! We recognize a responsibility to help ensure that younger activists will carry on long after we leave our positions as the organization's leaders.

A second challenge is that although grant money has and may again provide a stipend for people who implement a specific project, we are an all-volunteer organization. While this helps to keep costs associated with our organization down (e.g., we have no overhead and so do not have to budget for indirect costs), people do tire, and life circumstances change. Looking for grant opportunities takes time. We are fortunate that we currently have people who have some knowledge of how to do this and the time to do it. In addition, new projects can be expected to call for skills that we may not have.

Another challenge we have is getting the word out about our projects, including *Just Talk About It*. In particular, we need a constant presence in and tracking of social media. While we have taken advantage of student interns, this is a stopgap method of using this platform to its full extent in promoting what we do. A related challenge is to find ways to reach those who have no access to a computer or Internet services. Community meetings such as those initiated as part of National Healthcare Decisions Day can help, but getting people to those sessions, for all the reasons we have discussed, is still no easy task.

In spite of these challenges, we don't dwell on potential negative outcomes. If we had done that 12 years ago, our organization would have been paralyzed. So we will continue to undertake new projects and persist with another round of strategic planning. For example, as a result of a recent strategy session within the Take Charge Board, we have launched another community outreach project, *Empower Others*, on our website (http://take-chargeofyourlife.org/empower-others.php). This project is intended to reach anyone who interacts with individuals in the community, for example, members of religious and community organizations, barbers and hairdressers, health care workers, attorneys, tax preparation consultants, employers, counselors and therapists, educators, trainers, and coaches. By familiarizing ordinary citizens with our resources, we hope to help people realize that you don't have to be an EOL expert to talk with others in the community about these issues and, thus, empower them to start a conversation. Because the resources are free of charge and easy to use, anyone can make a difference by having a personal conversation, directing others to our website, or copying and pasting our short informational pieces into newsletters, flyers, and church bulletins. Supportive materials have been made available online to assist those who are willing and able to provide presentations in small group settings such as those within church communities, health care organizations, college classes, and caregiver support groups. Both the personal conversations and community presentations are strategies specifically intended to reach those who lack computer access.

Empower Others is just one more pearl to add to the others we've cultivated since we first began. What happens next will grow out of what we've already done, if the past is prologue. We intend to keep stringing our pearls, to stay focused on the practical, on what can be done, and then do it. We have no doubt that the positive energy we enjoy from working together will sustain Take Charge well into the future as it does in the present. It may sound naïve, but our best advice to others interested in easing the burden of managing the EOL is to keep doing what you want to do—put one foot in front of the other and keep going.

REFERENCES

Ariés, P. (1981). *The hour of our death*. New York, NY: Oxford University Press.

Cahill, H. A. (2008). Male appropriation and medicalization of childbirth: An historical analysis. *Journal of Advanced Nursing, 33*(3), 334–342. doi: 10.1046/j.1365–2648.2001.01669.x

Conrad, P. (1992). Medicalization and social control. *Annual Review of Sociology, 18*, 209–232. doi: 10.1146/annurev.so.18.080192.001233

Conrad, P. (2007). *The medicalization of society: On the transformation of human conditions into treatable disorder*. Baltimore, MD: John Hopkins University Press.

End-of-Life Partnership of Western Pennsylvania. (2002). *Community forums project report: Western Pennsylvanians talk about death and dying on their own terms*. Retrieved from http://takechargeofyourlife.org/media/eolpreport.pdf

Fox, B., & Warts, D. (1999). Revisiting the critique of medicalized childhood: A contribution to the sociology of birth. *Gender & Society, 13*, 326–346. doi: 10.1177/08912499013003004

Hoyer, T. (1998). A history of the Medicare hospice benefit. In J. K. Harrold & J. Lynn (Eds.), *A good dying: Shaping health care for the last months of life* (pp. 61–69). Binghamton, NY: The Haworth Press.

Lynn, J., & Harrold, J. (1999). *Handbook for mortals: Guidance for people facing serious illness*. New York, NY: Oxford University Press.

Moyers, B. D., Moyers, J. D., O'Neill, J. D., Mannes, E., & Pellett, G. Public television (Firm), & WNET (New York, NY: Television Station). (2000). *On our own terms—Moyers on dying: A death of one's own*. United States: Public Affairs Television, Inc.

Oakley, A. (1980). *Women confined: Towards a sociology of childbirth*. UK: Martin Robertson.

Pearson, C., & Stubbs, M. L. (1999). *Parting company—The caregiver's journey: Understanding the loss of a loved one*. Seattle, WA: Seal Press.

Phillips, D. F. (2000).End-of-life coalitions grow to fill needs. *Journal of the American Medical Association, 284*(19), 2442–2444.

Prendergast, T. (2001). Advance care planning: Pitfalls, problems, and promise. *Critical Care Medicine, 29*(2 Suppl), N34–N39.

SUPPORT Principal Investigators. (1995). A controlled trial to improve care for seriously ill hospitalized patients: The study to understand prognoses and preferences for outcomes and risks of treatment. *Journal of the American Medical Association, 274*, 1591–1598.

Task Force for Quality at the End of Life in Pennsylvania. (2007). *End-of-life care in Pennsylvania: Final report and recommendations.* Retrieved from http://takechargeofyourlife.org/

CHAPTER 17

The Coalition for Compassionate Care of California

Judy Citko

Care toward the end of life (EOL) is deeply entwined with culture. This was the stunning conclusion of SUPPORT (Study to Understand Prognoses and Preferences for Outcomes and Risks of Treatment) (1995) (The SUPPORT Principal Investigators, 1995), a 10-year multi-million dollar study designed to improve EOL decision making and reduce the frequency of a painful and prolonged dying process. The results of the SUPPORT study stunned the health care community because the carefully designed interventions were shown to have had virtually no impact on the patient experience.

One of the most insightful explanations of SUPPORT pointed to the realization that our experiences at the EOL are connected to culture (see Lynn, Arkes, et al., 2000; Lynn, De Vries, et al., 2000). Culture is the broad concept that encompasses the knowledge, beliefs, behavior, values, goals, and practices shared by a group of people, a field of study, an individual institution, or all of humanity. Often, we're not aware of the culture in which we operate because it feels so natural. At the EOL, our experiences are connected to the culture of individual providers at the bedside, the health care institutions in which they work, our health care system at large, and society in general.

That's why a coalition is well suited for changing care practices and patient experiences at the EOL. A coalition can bring together a broad range of individuals and organizations to bring to light that which is unseen, co-create a vision of a better future, and ultimately change cultural norms.

The Coalition for Compassionate Care of California (CCCC) exists for these reasons. The Coalition exists to work on multiple levels simultaneously—including working on the level of professionals, institutions, public policymakers, and consumers—to change the culture of death and dying.

This chapter provides a brief background on the Coalition's history, achievements, and lessons learned. It is an example of what can be achieved through collaboration. We hope that it will inspire you to go out and create change in your sphere of influence.

BRIEF HISTORY

The Coalition for Compassionate Care grew out of a community-based project in Sacramento, California conducted by the Center for Healthcare Decisions (CHCD). In the mid-1990s, CHCD engaged more than 1,000 individuals in a series of public discussions about EOL care. These discussions occurred in two clusters—discussions among clinical staff from a variety of disciplines and discussions in community settings among local citizens. This endeavor sparked local hospitals to make tangible changes in their policies and processes for caring for seriously ill patients.

The success of CHCD's work led to the 1997 convening of a statewide group of health care professionals, long-term care associations, state agencies, and consumers to propose ways to improve EOL care for residents of California's nursing homes. Early on, it became clear that in order to influence nursing homes, the task force needed to be a statewide body. This group produced the ECHO Recommendations, discussed below. As the task force was finishing up its work, the Robert Wood Johnson Foundation (RWJF) announced its Community–State Partnership Initiative, which was designed to establish and support statewide efforts to improve EOL care. The California Hospital Association volunteered to be the lead agency on the grant and the grant was funded. So in 1998, the task force turned into the Coalition for Compassionate Care.

The Coalition established a Steering Committee to provide guidance on implementation. We asked the various statewide trade associations representing health care providers—including physicians, hospitals, nursing homes, hospice, and others—to join the Steering Committee. We sought out the participation of key state agencies—including agencies with oversight of medicine, health care, and aging. We invited consumer advocates and representatives to participate. Individual folks who were passionate about improving care toward the EOL also joined us at the table.

The Steering Committee formed three workgroups, one to oversee each aspect of our original grant. The Steering Committee and the workgroups—public engagement, skilled nursing facilities, and professional education—met three times a year to provide input and advice on the Coalition's activities.

Over the years, the Coalition's relationship with the hospital association evolved. The Coalition started out as a project of the hospital association, which allowed us to focus on grant activities rather than day-to-day business operations. Over time, the Coalition took on more and more responsibility for fully supporting and funding itself. In 2010, the Coalition became separately incorporated.

The Coalition started out with an executive director at 20% time and a half-time administrative assistant. We have grown to a mix of six full-time and part-time staff. Much of our work has been accomplished through other organizations or individuals that we use as independent contractors to help us achieve certain objectives.

Originally, the Coalition was led by an executive committee, comprised of two cochairs of the organization and the chair of each of the workgroups. That evolved into an advisory board, which evolved into a governing board when the Coalition became separately incorporated.

Eventually, the steering committee and workgroup structure became stale. After 10 years, instead of hosting tri-annual steering committee meetings, we switched to a single, annual membership meeting and conference. We also traded standing workgroups for specific-purpose, time-limited advisory groups and task forces. We implemented a dues-paying membership structure.

The Coalition exists through philanthropic support, namely grants and donations. To date, most of our funding has been from grants. While we are eternally grateful for the grant funding we have received, the challenge with grant funding is that it limits an organization to activities that a grant funder believes is important. Just because we see a need, just because our members ask us to do something, doesn't mean we can secure the resources to do work on that issue.

Throughout the Coalition's existence, our hallmark has been collaboration. For people who want to make bigger changes than they can do on their own, the Coalition is the way to make that happen.

PRIMARY FOCUS ON ADVANCE CARE PLANNING

The Coalition has had two primary areas of focus—ACP and palliative care. Between those two, the majority of the Coalition's activities have focused on ACP. The reason is that no one profession or health care institution has taken responsibility for ACP. Physicians find themselves interpreting advance directives (ADs), but often have no role in completing them. Hospitals have an obligation to ask about ADs, but no responsibility to encourage their completion. Attorneys, emergency responders, and others have a piece of ACP, but not the whole picture.

In addition, often the time between execution and implementation of an AD is multiple years. Thus, the provider who helps a patient complete an AD is not the one who reaps the benefit of it. Moreover, while medical knowledge is helpful to ACP, quality planning also requires consideration of the patient's psychological, emotional, social, and spiritual values and beliefs. This causes many health care providers to view ACP as "taking too much time." For all these reasons, ACP was ripe for being the focus of a collaborative approach.

PHILOSOPHICAL UNDERPINNINGS

Coalitions can be very powerful. At the same time, they are very fragile. A successful coalition requires two things: (a) everyone needs to feel that they are heard and (b) they need to see progress. So it's a combination of process and outcome. Both process and outcome are needed; otherwise, you risk losing participants because they don't feel ownership of the coalition's efforts or they lose interest in an effort that appears to be going nowhere.

Ownership is particularly important. This is where the magic happens. When all participants feel that they own the efforts, outcomes, and successes of the coalition, they look for opportunities to promote the coalition and further its efforts. This is when synergy starts to happen. Connections are made. Impacts are bigger and further reaching.

When it comes to ACP, we firmly believe that it is a process that happens over time, not a one-time event. Conversation is the foundation. Really good conversations—among loved ones and between patients and their health care providers—can prevent the majority of controversies and challenges. For healthy people, naming the person you want to speak for you and discussing your goals and values with them is a critical step. This can be documented in an AD. For people with advancing illness, frailty, or chronic conditions, discussing what medical treatment you want based on your diagnosis and prognosis is beneficial. This can be documented in a Physician Orders for Life-Sustaining Treatment (POLST) form.

The traditional approach to education, that is, lecture, has been shown to have limited impact in creating change. The Coalition strives to incorporate adult learning principles into all of our educational efforts, including interactive exercises, real-life case examples, and personalized application. Being clear on the goal of the educational effort can be helpful. Sometimes, the goal is to impart a particular attitude, transfer knowledge, develop skills, establish behaviors, or bring about institutional change.

In the following section, I focus on the Coalition's work that has been most fundamental to our impact on ACP practices in the state of California.

PUBLIC ENGAGEMENT

From the beginning, public engagement was a core part of our work because it was required by our grant. Given the size of California, we needed a strategy that enabled us to reach groups of people throughout the state. Working one-on-one with individual consumers was not realistic.

We structured our public engagement work based on the following assumptions:

- ACP can begin in non–health care settings.
- Interactive small group discussion can be an effective format for stimulating reflection and discussion about EOL issues.
- Organizations and community members can be equipped, through a variety of tools, to plan and implement ACP activities on a largely volunteer basis consistent with their time, resources, and interests.
- With common tools and activities to link them, multiple organizations can form effective, locally based coalitions to bring attention to EOL issues.

Thus, we decided to focus on promoting ACP activities in community settings, rather than medical or individual settings. We targeted settings where people were already naturally gathering, such as churches, senior centers, and assisted living facilities.

We used a number of tools to encourage and assist consumers in engaging in ACP, including:

- A booklet to assist consumers in talking with their loved ones about their treatment wishes.
- A series of articles on EOL issues that could be published in local newsletters or church bulletins.
- An AD fact sheet.

Several of these materials were culturally and/or linguistically translated into Spanish or Chinese.

An important component of our work was development of a discussion guide for lay leaders, *Talking It Over*. The guide provides a program and exercises for three sessions to give people ideas for thinking and talking about their wishes at EOL. Some people were comfortable using the discussion guide after reading it. Others felt they needed training before they would feel confident in leading a discussion. So we developed a companion training to compliment the guide. The guide was translated into Spanish and Tagalog.

As we did this work, we started connecting with a number of local community-based coalitions with similar missions. We soon realized that these local coalitions would benefit from networking with each other. We invited local coalition leaders to join our public engagement workgroup. These meetings allowed local coalitions to share information about their activities, what worked, and any lessons learned. Those coalitions that were in driving distance or had travel support attended in person. Others attended by conference call. The Bill Moyers series *On Our Own Terms* prompted the creation of many local coalitions after its broadcast in 2000. At the height of activity, 23 local coalitions existed in California. Today, about half a dozen of those local coalitions continue to exist.

After our original grant ended, we were unable to secure significant funding for public engagement activities. Due to our reliance on grants, our focus moved away from continued formal public engagement.

NURSING HOMES

Since the Coalition grew out of the original task force that focused on nursing homes, working to improve EOL care in this setting has been a core part of our work. One of the Coalition's first acts was to publish the *ECHO (Extreme Care, Humane Options) Recommendations*. This document, created at a time when palliative care was still in its infancy, brought together the basic precepts of palliative care and applied them to the nursing home setting. It focused primarily on the ethical principles of ACP and medical decision making regarding life-sustaining treatment, which was cutting edge at the time. Bringing these principles together in one place resulted in the "light bulb going on" for many nursing home leaders. The document was groundbreaking in that it was the first set of guidelines in the nation that were specific to EOL care in nursing homes.

The ECHO Recommendations were field tested with a handful of facilities before being finalized. Field testing consisted of a small team of a physician, nurse, and attorney who trained facility staff on the principles in the Recommendations. This field testing gleaned valuable information about how to convey the principles in a way that nursing home staff would understand. These lessons were incorporated into the final document.

To encourage adoption of the *ECHO Recommendations*, the three associations representing nursing homes participated in creation of the document, as did the California Department of Health Services (DHS). Nursing homes are a highly regulated industry and DHS is the agency in our state that licenses and surveys these facilities. Nursing homes are hesitant to adopt new practices—even if they will result in better care—unless DHS "blesses" the new practice. With the *ECHO Recommendations,* DHS went so far as to write an "All Facilities Letter," which was sent to every nursing home in the state, encouraging them to adopt the principles in the *ECHO Recommendations.*

Different people learn in different ways. Some can read the written word and know how to incorporate it into their daily practices. Others may benefit from hearing the information presented, participating in small group discussion about the information, or engaging in exercises that apply the information to hypothetical or real-world situations.

For this reason, once the *ECHO Recommendations* were finalized, the Coalition created a training based on the Recommendations. We wanted the Recommendations to be adopted by entire organizations, not just individual staff, so we required that participants attend with a group of three or more staff from different disciplines from the same facility. Nearly 300 professionals from 109 nursing facilities participated in the training. We built time into the workshop for each team to create an action plan that they would follow once they were back at their facility to implement what they had learned at the training.

In 2009, the Coalition revisited the ECHO Recommendations and decided it was time to update them. We convened another task force with representatives of the same key organizations to make revisions. Upon review, the task force felt that the field of palliative care—and the knowledge and care practices in nursing homes—had progressed enough that new (rather than revised) recommendations were warranted. From this, the *CARE Recommendations* (*Compassion and Respect at the End of Life*) were created.

Many nursing homes have recently started to embrace "culture change," the common name given to the national movement for the transformation of older adult services, based on person-directed values and practices where the voices of elders and those working with them are considered and respected. Core person-directed values are choice, dignity, respect, self-determination, and purposeful living. The *Care Recommendations* incorporate these principles.

The *CARE Recommendations* guide nursing homes in increasing their capacity to provide compassionate, quality EOL care that is consistent with residents' wishes. The recommendations contain tools and resources that support the development of the attitudes, knowledge, and skills nursing homes need to provide the best possible EOL care for residents. The guide is comprised of three steps: (a) ACP, (b) clinical practices, and (c) other considerations, including grief, bereavement, spirituality, and cultural issues. The *Care Recommendations* handbook detailing how to approach each of these important areas is available at www.coalitionccc.org

In addition to *ECHO* and the *CARE Recommendations*, the Coalition has engaged in a number of projects aimed at improving EOL practices in nursing homes. Through these efforts, we have identified the following challenges when trying to change ACP practices in this setting:

- Turnover is high among staff and administration alike.
- Nursing homes have limited resources and time to devote to changing practices. Physicians have limited presence in nursing homes.

- Support of the administrator and, if appropriate, corporate office is key.
- Nursing homes tend to be highly risk adverse. They have strong culture of "we've always done it this way." Change, however, often requires moving out of one's comfort zone.
- In California, the staff is ethnically quite diverse. For many staff, English is a second language and they have limited English proficiency. Many grew up in cultures that don't have the same concept of ACP.
- ACP is seen as a task. Often, it's seen as a task to be completed upon admission.

We've found that the following approaches help support changes in ACP practices in nursing homes:

- Offer ACP as a solution to a problem about which they are concerned. Be clear on "what's in it for them."
- Get the blessing of the state agency that surveys nursing homes.
- Make it simple.
- Provide ready-to-use tools for implementing the change.
- Keep following up. You have to reinforce the change over and over and over. Ongoing education is important.
- Celebrate the facility's willingness to change. Celebrate staff's accomplishments.
- Be patient.

The bottom line is that to have a broad impact on nursing home practices, collaboration is required. Bringing together key stakeholders who know and can influence the industry is key.

PHYSICIAN ORDERS FOR LIFE-SUSTAINING TREATMENT

Our work with POLST perhaps best exemplifies the value of a coalition. Successful establishment of POLST in a state requires working collaboratively with a wide range of stakeholders on both a statewide and local level. We've been so successful that sometimes people equate the Coalition with POLST in our state.

POLST is a physician order that gives patients more control over their EOL care. Produced on a distinctive bright pink form and signed by both the physician and patient, POLST specifies the types of medical treatment that a patient wishes to receive toward the EOL. It encourages communication between providers and patients, enables patients to make more informed decisions, and clearly communicates these decisions to providers. As a result, POLST can prevent unwanted or medically ineffective treatment, reduce patient and family suffering, and help ensure that patients' wishes are honored.

For years, the Coalition had heard about POLST. Several times, CCCC leaders and members discussed whether to bring it to California. Each time the decision was not to do so. We knew that establishing proper usage of POLST would take more than just putting POLST into law or encouraging use of the form. We knew that it would take education—lots of education. That, in turn, would require committed resources sustained over time.

In 2007, three local communities in California expressed interest in using POLST in their local area. Because the Coalition believed that it was important to have statewide standards and consistency for POLST to work in our state, the Coalition made a commitment to establish POLST in California.

The Coalition approached the California Health Care Foundation (CHCF) with a grant proposal to establish POLST in our state. CHCF approved the grant, which provided start-up funds for the Coalition to lead statewide efforts, as well as funds to support efforts in eight communities.

The National Hospice and Palliative Care Organization (NHPCO) had announced a one-day workshop on POLST to be held three months after CHCF committed to funding POLST activity. So the Coalition and CHCF quickly developed a call for proposals for local community leaders and organizations that wanted to be one of the eight initial POLST coalitions. In November 2007, a group of about 20 people from California attended the NHPCO POLST workshop. This provided a strong informational foundation for our POLST work, as well as created a common identity among our initial POLST leaders.

Early on in our efforts to spread word about POLST in our state, we learned:

- POLST is only as good as the conversation on which it is based. The role of POLST is to document the conversation.
- POLST compliments an AD. ADs fill another, just as critical, need.
- POLST helps systematize solicitation, documentation, and transfer of patient wishes. By doing so, it highlights weaknesses in our health system. This may be disconcerting to some and appear that POLST is causing problems. In reality, POLST provides us a service by highlighting where we need to focus our efforts to improve our system.

The Coalition established a Task Force to oversee all statewide aspects of POLST, including public policy, content of the form, communication and messaging, standardized education, quality improvement, and evaluation of our efforts. The California Task Force is comprised of the following:

1. Twenty organizations that represent providers impacted by POLST, such as the medical association, hospital association, nursing home associations, and organizations representing emergency responders;

2. Eight state agencies that oversee those providers, including the Medical Board, Department of Public Health, and Emergency Services Authority;

3. Five organizations representing the consumer perspective, such as AARP and California Advocates for Nursing Home Reform; and

4. Three EOL coalitions.

We continue to add Task Force members as additional organizations and agencies are identified.

One of the strengths of POLST is that it applies across care settings. At the same time, one of the challenges of POLST is that it applies across care settings. The way that health care providers in one part of the health care continuum view and react to POLST can be very different from providers in another part. For example, emergency responders have limited training, have to act in a split second, and are trained to follow protocols. Physicians, on the other hand, have extensive education and exercise a lot of clinical judgment. This can impact how different Task Force members, representing different parts of the health care continuum, view various issues related to POLST. Thus, it's critical to have the perspective of all interested parties represented on the Task Force.

Because California is such a large state, we believed that it would be helpful to establish POLST in state law. We wanted to make it clear that POLST was "legal" and to provide an incentive to providers to honor POLST forms by providing immunity for doing so. We decided to take the legislative route.

To minimize potential opposition, we amended California's existing do not resuscitate (DNR) statute, rather than creating a brand new statute. We did our work behind the scenes, by addressing concerns raised by various constituencies and educating legislative staff on the bill. As a result, California Assembly Bill (AB) 3000 went through both houses of our legislature with unanimous support. AB 3000 was signed into law in 2008 and went into effect on January 1, 2009.

To facilitate uniform adoption of POLST in our state, we developed standardized messaging to explain what POLST is, who would benefit from POLST, how it operates, and how it relates to ADs. We use the message platform throughout all our materials.

In addition, we developed a standardized 2-day, train-the-trainer curriculum on POLST. The curriculum emphasizes the importance of the POLST conversation and involves extensive role play and skill building in having the conversation. As POLST can be used with children, the Coalition collaborated with the Children's Hospice and Palliative Care Coalition to create a 1-day curriculum on POLST in the pediatric population. Providing education on POLST, particularly the POLST conversation, is important for maintaining quality POLST form completion.

To further emphasize the importance of the POLST conversation, we developed a video on POLST conversations. The video is comprised of eight vignettes between real physicians and actor patients that highlight different aspects of the POLST conversation. None of the conversations in the vignettes are perfect. Rather, the vignettes provide rich learning opportunities for both what works and what doesn't work in the POLST conversation.

The Coalition also created numerous materials to support POLST implementation, including a brochure on POLST for providers; a brochure written at sixth- to eighth-grade reading level for consumers; model policies and procedures on POLST for hospitals, nursing homes, and hospices; a quick reference guide on POLST in nursing homes; and frequently asked questions for consumers.

In our early days, the question arose whether we should pilot a single form in the state or, in attempt to identify the best version, pilot multiple versions in different communities. The national POLST leadership wisely urged us to have a single version for the entire state even during our pilot phase. Once multiple versions are introduced, people might become wedded to their version.

Next, we needed to decide on the content of the form. To keep our efforts focused on implementation, we decided to begin with the Oregon form, which had benefited from years of collective wisdom about what works and doesn't work. This eliminated our need to have extensive discussion about every detail on the form. We chose not to include a section on antibiotics, however, because research showed that this section had little impact on the care patients received.

We followed the advice of national POLST leaders, so 2 years into implementation we solicited suggested changes to the form. The thinking is that updating the form periodically based on actual usage in the field serves as a mechanism to maintain POLST quality.

In response to our call for suggested changes, we received more than 300 comments. To process these suggestions, the POLST Task Force created a committee that developed a process for sorting through, evaluating, and deciding on which suggestions to adopt. We found that many of the suggested changes actually reflected a breakdown in education rather than a weakness in the form. As a result, the committee set the standard that any suggested change would need to provide a substantial benefit in order to be adopted.

The committee reviewed the suggestions and developed a subset that they moved forward to the full POLST Task Force for input. The committee then met again to consider the feedback from Task Force members and developed a recommended revised form. The revised form went to the full Task Force for approval.

Given our state's diverse population, the California POLST form has been translated into Armenian, Chinese, Farsi, Hmong, Korean, Pashto, Russian, Spanish, Tagalog, Vietnamese, and Braille. The translated form helps facilitate communication between providers and patients. Since English is the language of emergency responders, the signed form must be in English.

The Importance of Local Leadership

One of the hallmarks of California's POLST work is the recognition that successful establishment of POLST requires two strategies—one for impacting care on a statewide basis and one for impacting care at the bedside. Extensive statewide efforts don't guarantee that anything will change in the way care is actually provided. To make that impact, it takes local leadership.

In California, we used local coalitions to make that happen. We're now up to 27 local POLST coalitions. These coalitions, headed up by local champions for POLST, convene other leaders from across the continuum of care, pilot interventions, conduct education with groups of people and one on one, and assist in collecting data regarding POLST usage in their community. They are led by a wide variety of organizations, including local medical societies, hospitals, medical groups, educational and bioethics consortia, local coalitions already working on EOL issues, and others. As POLST is a physician order, local coalitions are expected to work with a physician who will champion POLST in the local community.

To keep the local coalitions connected to the statewide work as well as each other, we host monthly conference calls and annual in-person gatherings. The monthly conference calls are with the POLST physician champions and provide a forum for discussing clinical issues related to POLST, making sure that our efforts are always grounded in good clinical practices. POLST trainers—those who've attended our standardized train-the-trainer seminar—are supported on an ongoing basis through quarterly conference calls and webinars.

Effective implementation of POLST requires collaboration. California's success with POLST is a direct reflection of the extensive collaboration that has occurred on both a statewide and local level.

CULTURAL DIVERSITY

In California, an ethnic majority does not exist. At least 59 languages are spoken in the state's public schools, 27% of Californians are foreign born, and people of color make up 60% of California's population. California has more foreign-born, limited-English proficient residents that any other state in the union.

Thus throughout the Coalition's existence, finding a way to address the impact of cultural diversity upon ACP has been a priority. We've had several projects related to diversity, including translation of materials, supporting an outreach worker to the Latino community, and helping create the Chinese American Coalition for Compassionate Care.

Our work we believe to have the most potential to broadly impact ACP is our educational curriculum on EOL from a multi-cultural perspective. To develop the curriculum, we convened an advisory group made up of experts on cultural diversity, EOL care, and POLST education.

Soon after the group met, it was clear that the idea of anyone being "competent" in the cultural richness that comprises California seems questionable. Thus, we took the approach of addressing diversity from a multicultural perspective. We adopted the belief that culture involves more than ethnicity. To the contrary, culture is shaped by numerous factors, including socioeconomic status, birth order, geography, religion, family history, education level, professional training, personal experiences, and much more. As a result, a person is expert only in his/her individual, personal culture.

We identified several models to reflect our view of culture. One is the use of an iceberg to illustrate that certain aspects of culture are easily seen by others, whereas other just-as-important aspects are "below the surface" and out of sight. As a result, health care providers need to "become a student of the patient" to understand the patient's perspective.

Another model is to view culture as a "pair of glasses" or a lens through which we interpret our lives, including how we understand treatment options, medical decision making, pain and suffering, interactions with health care providers, dynamics with loved ones, death and the afterlife, and more. Our views of illness and medical care are seen through the "lens" of our personal culture.

Health care providers also need to be aware that they have their own unique culture—the culture of health care. Health care has its own language and communication style, its own way of viewing relationships, and its own concept of time. Within health care, each health care profession has its own sub-culture. The culture of physicians is different from the culture of nurses, which is different from the culture of social workers, chaplains, aids, and others. Furthermore, palliative and EOL care has its own subculture.

As a result of this effort, the Coalition created *Building Bridges*, a 4-hour curriculum that is highly interactive and involves self-reflection. To personalize this training, participants in the workshop are asked to draw their own cultural maps—a visualization of their lives and culture. Participants are also asked to describe the prominent "cultural" features of their work environment and how EOL care is viewed within that environment. The workshop also includes discussions of acculturation versus assimilation, challenging cross-cultural experiences and eliciting a patient's explanatory model. The training closes with a case study and role play during which participants take on different roles and discuss the conversation about goals of care in the context of culture.

The goal of this training is to transform the way attendees think about themselves, and the patients and families they serve. We've received feedback from attendees that confirm the *Building Bridges* curriculum has achieved this objective, such as:

■ I realized that one of my "negative" patients was not actually non-compliant. Rather, I was simply imposing my values on him.
■ For the first time, I see that culture, race, and nationality are not the same thing. The workshop made me change the way I've been thinking about culture my whole life.
■ I had never thought of becoming a student of my patients.

The Coalition's success in this area is a direct result of our collaboration with a range of people from a variety of backgrounds. Through that process we listened and learned. We became students of our collaborators.

DEVELOPMENTAL DISABILITIES

In 2005, staff from the California Department of Developmental Services, which oversees services and supports for persons with developmental disabilities, contacted the Coalition. They were concerned that another state agency, the California Department of Public Health, was requiring that terminally ill individuals living in "intermediate care facilities for the mentally retarded" (ICF-MR) move to a nursing home in order to receive hospice care. The thinking was that terminally ill persons required more nursing support than ICF-MRs provide. The result was that these individuals were forced to leave the place they called home and spend their last days in an unfamiliar place.

This is not an uncommon scenario. Regulatory agencies play an important role in making sure a minimum standard of care is provided in licensed settings. Regulatory staff often carry out their duties in a void without knowledge or appreciation of the unintended consequences of their interpretation of state law. The Coalition helped open a dialogue between the two agencies and eventually the state's position changed.

This experience helped us realize that persons with developmental disabilities were living longer and aging, much like the general population.

Many of these individuals were now outliving their parents, the people who had traditionally spoken for them.

Believing there was more we could do to improve care for seriously ill persons with developmental disabilities, the Coalition talked to our contacts at the state agencies to find out who needed to be at the table and then invited them to be part of a workgroup.

Some workgroup members warned that this was a "hot topic" and that it would be difficult to make progress. Others thanked us for convening the workgroup. During a particularly robust discussion at one of the meetings, one attendee who had a developmental disability simply asked us, "Why can't we have this information?" In that moment, it became clear that it didn't matter what the "professionals" or those who were in positions of power thought. The matter was that we had people in our midst who wanted information. It's a basic human right that people be provided the means to be as engaged as possible in the process of making decisions about their medical care.

Through discussion, we identified the issues related to EOL for this population and possible projects that might move things forward. One of the ideas was developing materials to help enable people with developmental disabilities to engage in ACP. A few years later, we obtained the resources to follow up on this idea.

The first thing we did was convene three focus groups of people who had developmental disabilities in different parts of the state. Each focus group met three times. Through the guidance of these focus groups, we crafted *Thinking Ahead,* an easy-to-use workbook in plain language, using symbols and pictures that enables people to make and document their wishes regarding health care treatment and related issues. A companion DVD features vignettes that illustrate the purpose and use of the materials, enabling people with limited reading comprehension to use and understand them. *Thinking Ahead* also features interviews with three individuals with developmental disabilities talking about real life experiences they've had that would have gone smoother if their loved one had completed an AD.

We have found that whenever we address the needs of a "special" population, it benefits all of us. Through this work, we have come to believe that many more patients would have "capacity" if health care providers communicated in a way that more people could understand. Responsibility for making the conversation understandable is on the health care provider. This shift in thinking will benefit all patients.

As with many of our projects, this one required us to collaborate with a new set of stakeholders. We needed to become familiar with the issues, dynamics, and politics that surround this community. By taking a collaborative approach, we were able to take a "hot topic" and create a situation that benefits all stakeholders.

FUTURE

The Coalition has had tremendous success collaborating with individual physicians, nurses, and others who are champions for ACP. Now, with health care reform in law, we have a new opportunity to connect with those charged with managing the operations of large health systems. Our society is realizing that we need to obtain better value for our health care dollar and ACP is a way to honor patient preferences. This is an exciting time to be a collaborator.

REFERENCES

Lynn, J., Arkes, H. R., Stevens, M., Cohn, F., Koenig, B., Fox, E. et al. (2000). Rethinking fundamental assumptions: SUPPORT's implications for future reform. Study to Understand Prognoses and Preferences and Risks of Treatment. *Journal of the American Geriatrics Society, 48* (5 Suppl.), S214–S221.

Lynn, J., De Vries, K. O., Arkes, H. R., Stevens, M., Cohn, F., Murphy, P., . . . Tsevat, J. (2000). Ineffectiveness of the SUPPORT intervention: Review of explanations. *Journal of the American Geriatrics Society, 48* (5 Suppl), S206–S213.

The SUPPORT Principal Investigators. (1995). A controlled trial to improve care for seriously ill hospitalized patients: The study to understand prognoses and preferences for outcomes and risks of treatments (SUPPORT). *Journal of the American Medical Association, 274,* 1591–1598.

CHAPTER 18

Passion, Persistence, and Pennies

Cari Borenko Hoffmann

Since 2003, Fraser Healthy Authority (FHA) in British Columbia, Canada, has championed the development, implementation, and dissemination of its advance care planning (ACP) work. Given the scarcity of dedicated resources, the program has benefited from the passion and persistence of not only colleagues within the health authority but patients and families to influence and spread the ACP initiative locally, provincially, and nationally.

The program, committed to system-level change and standardized education, has developed user-friendly, culturally sensitive tools and resources that have been adapted by health and community organizations across Canada, the United States, and New Zealand.

This vision led to a national symposium and other initiatives that support a pan-Canadian approach to ACP implementation and the development of a Canadian research agenda. Program leaders in FHA have been invited to a variety of speaking engagements at provincial, national, and international conferences. FHA has also been able to influence legislation, policy, and uptake related to ACP within British Columbia.

Fraser Health is one of five health authorities in British Columbia (see Figure 18.1). We serve over 1.6 million people with 12 acute care hospitals operating over 2,000 beds, 7,760 residential care beds, and a comprehensive home health program that provides 630 home nursing visits daily. FHA has 26,000 staff and 2,500 physicians. Our communities consist of large Asian, Indo-Canadian, Filipino, Korean, and First Nation people.

Discussions began in 2003 among Palliative Care providers and the Executive Team of the Fraser Health Authority regarding the need to develop resources and systems for advance directives (ADs) and ACP. These

FIGURE 18.1 Map of British Columbia and Fraser Health Authority.

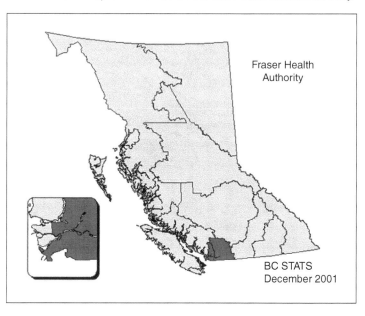

discussions were initiated in large part because many substitute decision makers (agents or proxies) struggle with end-of-life (EOL) medical decisions when the wishes of their loved ones are seemingly unknown. These types of situations profoundly affect not only families but health care providers. Media coverage, often sensationalized, added to the need to develop a program that would support families and health care providers to engage in ACP conversations prior to a medical crisis and before a state of patient incapacity.

Initially, the Palliative Care Program provided six months of funding for a nursing Project Leader to develop ACP tools. In large part due to time constrictions, our initial program ideas consisted of the promotion of physician-directed orders. The initial model was a tick-like box "form" on which the patient indicated acceptable and unacceptable mental and physical conditions. Clinicians in our health authority strongly opposed this type of care planning and rejected the proposed model. Physicians and other clinicians advocated and stated unequivocally that patients and families would want and benefit from a program that focused on conversations, not checkboxes.

As a result of this and other clinician feedback, we began to research successful ACP programs both nationally and internationally. We recognized that Respecting Choices® in Wisconsin (http://respectingchoices. org) was not only a best practice program but unique, as it used an integrated systems approach, and aligned with our philosophy of the delivery of patient-centered care, not only at the EOL but throughout the trajectory of a patient's journey of care.

Our expertise with ACP has grown significantly since 2003 and continues to be an area of learning and adaptation to an increasingly complex health care environment. The implementation of ACP within our health care system has touched cultural and community boundaries unlike any other program area we have worked within. Two successful components that continue to be relevant to the success of our program include physician support and dedicated regional implementation leadership.

Our ACP program has evolved uniquely and has been characterized by the following:

- Passion: We have embraced and involved health care professionals and public members who are passionate about the need for promoting living well, dying well, and conversations to improve EOL care within our health care systems, homes and communities.
- Persistence: As individuals and program leaders, we have been persistent in our efforts to move ACP forward within our health authority, British Columbia, and Canada. Simply put, we just never gave up.
- Pennies: Our program has funding for one full-time equivalent permanent employee. We quickly learned one person really can make a difference.

This chapter describes our journey based within the building blocks (Figure 18.2) published initially in the *Implementation Guide to Advance Care Planning in Canada: A Study of Two Health Authorities* (2008) and the subsequent publication, *Advance Care Planning in Canada: National Framework* (2012).

ENGAGEMENT

A Steering Committee was formed in 2004 to provide guidance to the program and a conscious decision was made to include community members as well as health care professionals. Membership consisted of a librarian; a hospice organization representative; leaders from the Punjabi and Chinese communities; the executive director for a volunteer center; a retired ombudsman; physicians specializing in palliative care, geriatrics, and renal diseases; a clinical nurse specialist; a social worker; and a spiritual care practitioner.

In 2007, Calgary Health and Fraser Health partnered and sponsored the first Canadian Inaugural National Symposium on ACP. This event brought together leaders and supporters of ACP across Canada. Health Canada, our national organization, provided opening remarks and supported our endeavors to move ACP forward in a sustainable and systematic way. The goal of this symposium was to share experiences and promote national collaboration. The Canadian Hospice Palliative Care Association also supported this event and has become the central repository of ACP resources

FIGURE 18.2 Canadian National Framework for Advance Care Planning.

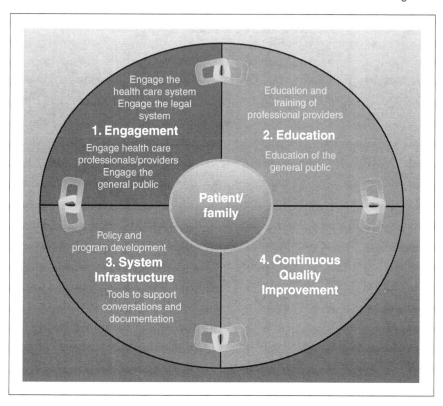

in Canada (Canadian Hospice Palliative Care Association, 2012). Together, as a national group, we have written a variety of consensus and framework documents, collaborated on a national approach to ACP, and developed a Canadian research agenda. A number of national sub-committees have formed, such as the National Community of Practice ACP Educators, with the goal to share materials and learn collectively.

Within FHA, we have been fortunate to have forward-thinking leaders in our Hospice Palliative Care Program. As a result of leader ingenuity, we have a well–coordinated and integrated Hospice Palliative Care Consultation Team in each of our 12 communities. Team members have been integral in "spreading the word" of ACP to their colleagues in acute and community settings. They act as mentors and assist in the sustainability of ACP.

Public presentations have been an important part of supporting, promoting, and sustaining ACP in communities. The Project Implementation Coordinator, hired in 2006, accepts invitations to do presentations and presents at least monthly. Marketing of presentations is by word of mouth. Presentations are by invitation from particular organizations and have included churches, disease-specific support groups, and retired groups. Presentations are 1 hour in length and generally include a 30-minute presentation that includes stories and then a question-and-answer period. PowerPoints and DVDs are not generally used unless there are more than 30 people in attendance. Written ACP materials such as brochures and booklets are distributed widely. The Project Implementation Coordinator presented to a "Walking Group" in a local mall as well as over a cup of tea in the kitchen of a seniors co-op housing apartment complex.

An Ipsos-Reid poll in March 2012 indicates that 86% of Canadians have not heard of ACP, less than half have had a discussion with family about medical treatments they would want for themselves in the future, 9% have spoken with a health care professional, 80% do not have a written plan, and 46% have a designated substitute decision maker (Ipsos-Reid Poll, 2011). While these results are daunting and perhaps discouraging, the respondents from the communities of Fraser Health are significantly more likely to have heard of ACP, and are more likely to have discussed their wishes with family, friends, or a health care professional as compared to the respondents from the rest of Canada (www.advancecareplanning.ca/news-room/ national-ipsos-reid-poll-indicates-majority-of-canadians-haven't-talked-about-their-wishes-for-care.aspx). We feel this is due to the standardized and regularly offered education of health care professionals as well as regular information sessions held in community settings.

Summary of Engagement

- One engagement action can lead to national advances.
- Public presentations are important; present where people gather.

SYSTEM INFRASTRUCTURE

Since 2005, with the support, wisdom, and guidance from the ACP Steering Committee, we began to develop a variety of tools and resources that proved to be foundational to the success of our program. These resources were developed over the course of several years and with one-time money.

Resource Development

In 2005, work began on the first iteration of the Fraser Health My Voice Workbook. This workbook was modeled after Respecting Choices. It was finalized in 2006 and has been pivotal to our program. It has often been said that the Fraser Health My Voice Workbook was developed "by the public for the public."

The last page of our workbook, "Expressing Your Wishes," is referred to as the "heart page," and it is suggested individuals complete this first before other engagement in the ACP process. People are asked to reflect on and write about the following:

- When I think about death, I worry about the following possible situations: For example, "I worry I will struggle to breathe," or "I worry that I will be alone."
- If I am nearing my death, I want (and/or do not want) the following: For example, "I want soft music playing," or "I want someone to hold my hand," or "I want my minister or priest to perform the necessary religious rituals."
- When I am nearing my death and cannot communicate I would like my family and friends to know and remember these things: For example, "I love you" or "I forgive you."

This workbook is complemented by two brochures: *Making Informed Choices about CPR* and *Information Booklet on Advance Care Planning*. These publications as well as the workbook were translated and are available in English, Punjabi, and Chinese.

Educational DVDs were also produced at this time. These are also available in the above-noted languages. The DVDs have been utilized in patient education sessions, community presentations, as well as for health care professional learning sessions. These DVDs are available in all of the libraries in British Columbia, all libraries in our health authority, as well as on the Internet. Clinicians have also utilized these DVDs in one-to-one sessions with patients and families, some of whom are struggling with engaging in the ACP process.

Posters are also available in seven languages. These have proven effective when placed in physician offices as well as public areas in hospitals and clinics. Posters have basic information about ACP, contact information, and a suggestion to speak with your physician. An ACP e-mail address and toll-free telephone number for the public is available and included on all printed resources. All resources have been made available on our Fraser Health website (www.fraserhealth.ca/your_care/advance-care-planning/), which has been an effective dissemination strategy for the community/public.

The My Voice Workbook as well as the brochures have been adapted in various countries. Fraser Health has shared their resources and has formal letters of agreement with health organizations throughout Canada, the United States, New Zealand, and Singapore.

Policy and Medical Orders

In 2006, a regional CPR and do not resuscitate (DNR) policy came into effect for acute care settings. The policy included some elements of ACP. Building our ACP program, including policy, has been incremental in nature. The ACP elements that were included in the CPR/DNR Policy were the implementation of the Greensleeve, Greensleeve processes, and ACP Record. A Greensleeve is a green page protector that is kept at the front of binder charts and holds ACP materials. The ACP Record is a communication tool that all health care professionals can document on and provide a quick look at where people are in the ACP process. The early introduction of both the Greensleeve and ACP Record proved pivotal in the coming years.

An audit of the policy, DNR form, and Greensleeve processes in our 12 acute care sites from December 2009–April 2012 provided the following data:

- 62% of patient charts had Greensleeves.
- 45% of patients had a DNR.
- Of those patients with a DNR:
  - 80% wanted medical treatment but no Critical Care Interventions.
  - 10% wanted Critical Care Interventions.
  - 8% wanted comfort measures.
  - 2% had specific instructions not captured on our form.
- 83% of physicians had spoken with someone prior to completing the DNR.
  - 41% had documented the conversations.

Additional audit information that assisted in the further development of policy and implementation strategies included the following:

- The ACP Record form was not being consistently used in acute settings; however, social workers and physicians often noted conversations in their respective chart sections.
- The DNR form provided a place to document refusals only, not wishes.
- Greensleeves did not house ACP documents, but held only DNRs.
- Many patients in acute settings had multiple acute admissions and multiple programs involved in their care, which added to the complexity of care planning and illustrated the need to improve communication among providers.

Building on the CPR/DNR Policy, in 2010, the Executive Team approved the *Making the MOST of Conversations: Medical Orders for Scope of Treatment* (MOST) initiative (http://www.fraserhealth.ca/professionals/advance-care-planning/). A variety of clinicians had, throughout the years, identified the need to standardize resuscitation status and medical intervention policy and language in all sectors of care, particularly residential and acute care. A physician focus group was convened in 2007 to begin the initial thoughts surrounding this policy and form.

Throughout 2010 and 2011, focus groups were held with over 200 clinicians to begin revisions and changes from the current CPR/DNR to the MOST policy and form. Key learnings from these focus groups included the following:

■ General awareness in all groups of the concept of ACP and need for conversations. Wide variation on what people considered as ACP, for some it was specifically a DNR discussion, for others understanding was full scope;
■ Consensus that there are many layers of education and information required within the health authority; for example, promoters, supporters and responders. Most groups supported ACP to become part of all assessments and admissions processes.

Key challenges identified included:

■ Time and resources for conversations
■ Patients' lack of information regarding diagnosis, prognosis, and information about illnesses and/or interventions
■ Health care professionals' lack of legal understanding, most notably substitute consent
■ Transfer of information between health care professionals and programs has been fragmented

Summary of System Infrastructure

■ ACP is first and foremost about the messages we hold in our hearts.
■ Develop resources and materials as finances prevail.
■ Public input is invaluable and resources should be user-friendly and in plain language.
■ Incremental policy development builds upon implementation experience.

EDUCATION

In 2004, the Health Authority Executive Team approved and supported a team of health care professionals to attend education with Respecting Choices in Wisconsin. The foundational building of our program is owed in large part to this program and the founders of Respecting Choices for sharing wisdom, knowledge, challenges, and pragmatic suggestions.

Following the visit to Wisconsin, the FHA Executive Team and Advance Care Planning Steering Committee supported bringing Respecting Choices Faculty to the health authority to train both Facilitators and Instructors. As a result, in 2005, 60 facilitators and 16 instructors completed the Respecting Choices course.

Education for health care professionals as well as the public has been an important aspect of our program. In 2006, we developed education specific and applicable to Fraser Health policies and procedures as well as provincial law. This included a 30-minute online learning module (www. fraserhealth.ca/professionals/advance-care-planning/) with the following learning objectives:

- Define ACP.
- State and explain who can legally make an ACP.
- State and explain three reasons why it is important to have an ACP.
- State and explain who should be included in ACP discussions.
- State and explain when health care providers, family, or friends would apply someone's ACP.
- State and explain when it would be appropriate to begin having ACP discussions with people.

The module is complimented by 6 hours of classroom learning. Role playing is an integral part of learning. Although sessions are structured, scenarios and case studies are revised based on disciplines and programs in attendance. All health care professionals are supported and encouraged to attend this educational session. Sessions are interdisciplinary and include a multitude of programs such as renal, intensive care, medical/acute care, residential care, and community/clinic. This has proven to be successful as participants are able to learn from one another, begin to understand the complexity of all program areas, and see the need for effective communication between health care professionals. Sessions are limited to 21 participants and include the following objectives:

- Describe the basic concepts of ACP.
- Initiate an ACP conversation.
- Describe the fundamental legal aspects of ACP.
- Describe the challenges and opportunities involved with creating a personal ACP.
- Discuss the importance of developing and maintaining organizational systems and practices for ACP.

These initial education sessions are open to all health care professionals. Unit clerks in hospital settings as well as office managers in home health programs are welcome to attend. Although they will not be engaging in ACP conversations with clients, it is imperative they are aware of ACP—what it is and why it is important, as well the system processes. These health care providers are an important part of our health care systems, are often the first point of contact for patients and families, and can provide written materials as well as contact information. They often attend for personal reasons, and this supports, enhances, and facilitates sustainability in community. Organizations such as the Catholic Healthcare Association, Parkinson's Society, and Lymphoma and Leukemia Society have also attended and further enhance our philosophy that ACP is a shared responsibility. Health care professionals from other Canadian provinces have also attended the sessions and completed the online learning modules.

In 2008, a second online module and classroom session was developed in response to a growing need to further the learning of health care professionals. The online learning objectives include:

- Define and explain the use of listening, questioning, exploring, and reflecting back while initiating and following up on ACP discussions.
- Describe the importance of facilitating ACP conversations throughout the continuum of care and in what settings these conversations should take place.
- Describe the elements of documenting ACPs and how to use the My Voice Workbook with clients.
- Identify and effectively manage potential for conflict within ACP conversations.
- Describe ACP policies and processes.

This module is also complimented by 6-hour classroom learning sessions. These classroom sessions are for clinicians who engage in ACP conversations routinely in their practice. Learning objectives include the following:

- Describe the basic concepts of ACP, including who, why, and when individuals should have ACP conversations.
- Define and explain the use of listening, questioning, exploring, and reflection while initiating and following up on ACP discussions.
- Describe the importance of facilitating ACP conversations throughout the continuum of care and in what settings these conversations should take place.
- Initiate an ACP conversation with a client and client's substitute decision maker.
- Describe the elements of documenting ACP: how to use the My Voice Workbook with clients, and how to use the ACP Record.
- Describe how to identify and manage potential for conflict within ACP conversations.
- Describe ACP policies and processes.

In December 2008, a survey was completed by students who had attended the Level One 6-hour education session. Students stated that following ACP education, they included individuals who they had not previously included in ACP conversations. In fact, there was an 11.2% increase in conversations with those with chronic illness and a 20.8% increase with healthy adults. Students noted that when clients and families engage in ACP, it helps with decisional conflict as well communication within the family and health care team. Most notably, when ACP took place, students stated client wishes were "always" honored.

Examples of specific program involvement include the Emergency Program where all directors, managers, and nurse supervisors complete the 30-minute online module. Following this, all nursing staff have been mandated to do the same. This will ensure that all Emergency Program staff have a common understanding of what ACP is and be better able and comfortable to support ACP with clients and families in this setting. As well, one of our surgical units supported all clinicians to attend the education. As a result, this unit distributes ACP materials to all adult patients when discharged and they organized a display of all ACP resources and materials.

Summary of Education

- Be responsive to clinicians' educational needs.
- Development and objectives of education must take into consideration the culture and history of your organization.
- Review what ACP is throughout sessions.
- Include legalities (state/provincial law) as well as organizational policies in sessions.
- Welcome community organizations and members to attend sessions.
- Sessions should be inclusive for all disciplines and all programs—community, hospital, and clinic settings.

CONTINUOUS QUALITY IMPROVEMENT

In 2004 and 2005, pilots and partnerships with both the Renal and Residential Care programs were initiated and both continue to be ACP leaders in our health authority. In the Renal Program, a nurse was hired 1 day per week to engage in ACP conversations with patients and families. Included in a renal pilot were 35 patients who had been on dialysis an average of 31 months and were on average 64 years of age. ACP conversations took place over time and averaged 2 hours in length. The pilot concluded that with this type of intervention:

- 86% of patients had an ACP on their chart,
- 100% of patient wishes were honored; patients and families stated they felt relief and gratitude following engaging in ACP.

While this was certainly successful, in retrospect, the hiring of a specific person hindered embedding ACP into all clinicians' practice. Additionally, this funding was not continued and, as a result, sustainability was not achieved. Funding for an EOL and ACP Coordinator for the Renal Program was secured for 2 years. This person does not engage in ACP conversations directly with patients but, rather, coordinates implementation among the teams and regional program.

From 2006 to 2007, the FHA embarked on a pilot program to implement ACP in a single community to further gain experience prior to implementing across the health authority. The goals were to implement in all health sectors including acute, residential, and community care programs and to promote it in the public sector by placing information and materials in areas such as libraries and community centers. From our experience, implementing in a single community across all sectors and care delivery settings is more successful than implementing in single program areas such as a hospital or renal care center. Insights from this pilot showed the public is interested and eager to engage in ACP as illustrated by the number of community presentations requested. Physicians were open to engage in ACP with patients, particularly those with shortened life expectancy, and health records departments were willing to file documents. The pilot also provided the following information, which assisted the growth of the program: More physician offices needed to be engaged, communication between hospital and home health needed to be enhanced, and community information/education was vital.

Summary of Continuous Quality Improvement

- Successes are measured one unit/program, sometimes one clinician, at a time.
- Patient competence/capacity was a barrier and, as such, residential care was a difficult place to begin ACP.
- Work together as a team to respond to ACP roles and responsibilities.
- Support programs (e.g., our Renal Program) have grown and adapted into successful examples and provide opportunities to share with other programs.
- Never give up on learning and adapting; pace change; set small, achievable goals.

OVERCOMING CHALLENGES

Whose Role Is It Anyway?

One of the challenges faced includes the long-standing myth that ACP is a role exclusively for physicians. Other successful ACP programs have implemented a facilitator role where this person's job is to accept referrals and engage in ACP conversations with patients and families. Due to lack of resources, we have not been able to fund a role such as this. As a result, the FHA promotes and supports an interdisciplinary approach to ACP conversations. While it has been a challenge to delineate the roles of nurses, social workers, spiritual health practitioners, respiratory therapists, and other allied health professionals, the development of our five Core Elements of ACP conversations have assisted these professionals to work out who is doing what with a particular individual. (For more information, see www.fraserhealth. ca/professionals/advance-care-planning/) These elements are:

1. S.P.E.A.K. to adults about ACP.
2. Learn about and understand the adult and what is important to him/ her. Involve substitute decision makers.
3. Clarify understanding and provide medical information about disease progression, prognosis, and treatment options.
4. Ensure interdisciplinary involvement and utilize available resources/ options for care.
5. Define goals of care; document and create a plan (including potential complications).

Some programs do not employ allied health professionals, such as social workers; therefore, nurses' scope of practice may include Core Element 2 as well as 3.

How Is Information and Education Provided to Almost 30,000 Staff?

As previously mentioned, FHA has 26,000 staff and 2,500 physicians. Educating and providing information to them has been one of our most significant challenges and one that has been extremely difficult to resolve. One method of communication, the development of online learning modules, has assisted with the challenge of educating large numbers of staff. We also place news items in e-newsletters and have an internal website where we host information.

ACP education sessions prepare students to become mentors and leaders in their programs and settings. This by far has been the most successful communication strategy. Following education, students are supported by the Project Implementation Coordinator, particularly when individual patient and family situations, as well as implementation issues, arise.

As part of the MOST initiative, Program and Implementation Leads have been identified in all 15 adult program areas and are supported by the ACP Project Implementation Coordinator as well as Clinical Nurse Specialist from the End of Life Program.

Who Has the Time?

We have heard many times through the years that clinicians do not have time to engage in ACP conversations. As part of our ACP education, role playing is an integral part. This is certainly due in part to practice engaging in ACP conversations, and to illustrating how much ACP can be accomplished in a focused 20-minute discussion. Noting and highlighting this during the education sessions has been eye opening for people. We do, in fact, have the time.

In addition, ACP is a shared responsibility. For example: social workers' or nurses' roles are to learn about and understand the adult and what is important to them (Core Element 2); physicians or nurse practitioners' roles are to speak to patients and families about their diagnosis, prognosis, and treatment options (Core Element 3). All clinicians are involved in ensuring interdisciplinary involvement (Core Element 4) and defining goals of care, documenting, and creating a care plan (Core Element 5). The ACP Record Form has been instrumental in illustrating this concept and clinicians feel confident in filling out "Next Steps" for colleagues to follow up and continue the conversation.

How Do You Reach the Physician Group and Move From a Curative Medical Model of Care?

The medical model prevails in health care. We continue to be challenged with changing the culture of "treatments and cure," to openly discussing the risks and benefits of treatment options with individuals, and grounding decisions in quality of life and personal goals and wishes. From our experience, individuals will often choose pain and symptom treatments that provide improved quality of life. Certainly the goal of ACP is not to promote less medical interventions, but to promote decisions based on fully informed and accurate medical information.

The education of and information sharing with physicians has also been a challenge. We have developed physician-specific education modules for ACP that includes pre-work, a 4-hour classroom session, completion of a 20-minute online module, and a follow-up 3-hour classroom session. Classroom session objectives include:

1. What is ACP and how we can be more effective as physicians in initiating these conversations and in overcoming barriers?
2. What are the legal issues and applicable provincial legislations related to ADs and the role of substitute decision makers?
3. What are the skills needed for effective ACP conversations and to practice them?

4. How do we recognize and resolve potential conflict situations?
5. Review of the Medical Orders for Scope of Treatment (MOST) form and policy.

SUMMARY

Our personal experiences with illness, disease, death, and dying within our families and communities shape how we engage in ACP with the people we support and care for in health care, regardless of our culture or our discipline.

Building a successful ACP program in any organization requires passion, persistence, and pennies. The ACP journey requires patience and paced change initiatives. Change needs to be coupled with a sense of knowing (a) the system readiness, (b) clinician readiness, and (c) community readiness. The path is not linear, but the path is an adventure!

REFERENCES

Canadian Hospice Palliative Care Association. (January, 2012). *Advance care planning in Canada: National framework.* Retrieved from http://www.advancecareplanning.ca/media/40158/acp%20framework%202012%20eng.pdf

Ipsos-Reid Poll. (March, 2011). Retrieved from http://www.advancecareplanning.ca/news-room/national-ipsos-reid-poll-indicates-majority-of-canadians-haven't-talked-about-their-wishes-for-care.aspx

Systems Level Change: Charting a New Path for Dying, Death, and End-of-Life Care

Introduction

Leah Rogne

This final section presents big-picture thinking from leading scholars of end-of-life (EOL) care about what is at stake and what it will take for us to transform how we deal with dying, death, and care. Writers, including a bioethicist/anthropologist, a political theorist, a sociologist, and a British National Health Service physician and leader in health care quality improvement, draw on their disciplinary knowledge and orientations to outline the historical, social, and ideological challenges we face and to call for large-scale initiatives that could fundamentally shift our approach to death and care as health care professionals, as citizens, and as communities.

These leading-edge ideas reflect what appears to be a heightening energy around the need to confront—indeed, embrace—the enormity of the concept and reality of death in our health care system and in our society. It is emblematic of this new energy that Pulitzer prize-winning columnist Ellen Goodman has taken on as her retirement project, The Conversation Project, a cooperative effort including Goodman, the Institute for Healthcare Improvement, and other leading thinkers on health care and EOL (http://theconversationproject.org). Along with high-profile initiatives such as Goodman's, we see more and more health care professionals speaking out about the need to deal with issues of EOL care, and more and more local and state advance care planning (ACP) initiatives springing up throughout the country. (See Chapter 22 in this volume for links to some of these initiatives.)

Chapters in this part are intended to inform, inspire, provoke, and challenge. In their chapter, Chapple and Pettus raise the bold question of whether the nation's survival depends on a new EOL conversation. They identify rescue as the dominant ideology and central paradigm guiding health care in the United States and point to tragic consequences that follow from the rescue paradigm, including a failure to recognize the importance of and reimburse adequately for prevention, rehabilitation, long-term care, mental health, or public health. Chapple and Pettus discuss the ways in which medical interventions are automatically applied—almost as a reflex—with an expectation of universal technological triumph over death. The authors point out that economic engines—the businesses of biomedical technology—fuel automatic application of complex biomedical interventions and that these businesses are a powerful driving force that benefits from, and perpetuates, rescue ideology. The authors convincingly argue instead for classical citizen virtues of civic friendship, honesty, and courage—virtues they identify as embodied in palliative care and ACP, and a positive counterpoint to ideology of rescue. Complexity and chaos theory are presented as more appropriate conceptualizations for EOL care, an approach that can encompass the uncertainty and surprises that can accompany dying and death.

In Chapter 20, British National Health Service physician and health care quality improvement champion Dr. Ben Lobo describes how organizations, health care systems, and societies perceive the value of providing high-quality service to people who are dying, and the opportunities to achieve the "Triple Aim" of improved health care outcomes and a positive experience at an affordable cost. He describes how quality improvement techniques may also help to achieve wider aspects of improving access and equity to services in a timely and effective way. At a patient level, the key to this is the need to make proactive case management for individuals and ACP the common approach. In the face of spiraling health care costs and higher expectations of patients and their families, Dr. Lobo discusses the challenge of engaging with patients and professionals to improve systems to identify and treat patients who will gain measureable benefit, prevent harm by not treating those who won't, and deliver a good and natural death. He discusses the role of effective leaders and great teams in health care improvement related to EOL care, and points to key elements important to implementing large-scale change in how we deal with dying and death. Finally, he asks leaders (public, professional, and political) how they will pass the "Moral Test" (Berwick, 2011) by doing the right thing, including challenging entrenched financial and other conflicting interests that stand in the way of positive change that can provide the opportunity for patients to have a good death.

Finally, in Chapter 21 sociologist Allan Kellehear makes a passionate and compelling case for a public health approach to dealing with dying, death, loss, and care, arguing that no campaign to encourage ACP can succeed without a community-wide approach that normalizes death and dying and reduces societal fear of death. Kellehear urges for development of a comprehensive grassroots community development-focused public health plan that identifies discussing and planning for death, dying, loss, and care as a fundamental component of national policy. Sharing examples of community approaches undertaken in various countries to demystify and de-stigmatize conversations about dying, death, loss, and care, Kellehear outlines how such initiatives can address barriers to appropriate ACP and community-based EOL care, and go "straight to the heart" of what it truly means to commit ourselves as a society to human well-being in living and dying.

CHAPTER 19

Does the Nation's Survival Depend on a New End-of-Life Conversation?

Helen Stanton Chapple
Katherine Irene Pettus

Rescue medicine is a staple of U.S. health care. As a defensive strategy for individuals, advance care planning (ACP) has arisen partly in reaction to the primacy of a rescue ideology in our health care system. The impetus to snatch life from death's very jaws is tied to prominent themes in American ideology such as self-reliance and overcoming adversity. The relentless medical pursuit of rescue from death reflects this ideology. As overall health policy, however, rescue medicine is ruinous to the nation's future. The classical citizen virtues of civic friendship, honesty, and courage are embodied in the modern ethics and practice of hospice and palliative care. A meta-ethic of palliative care provides a positive counterpoint to the ideology of rescue and sets up the coordinates for a new national EOL conversation, including ACP. Rescue recedes as a central goal within the worldview of chaos theory, which comprehends turmoil and progress, living and dying, overcoming and succumbing. In this chapter, we describe the dynamics of a health care delivery system that reflects the classic virtues of citizenship.

THE MAJOR KEY: RESCUE AS NATIONAL IDEOLOGY

Since the invention and proliferation of CPR in the 1960s, rescue has become the central paradigm of health care in the United States. More dollars go toward acute care than to prevention, rehabilitation, long-term care, mental

293

health, or public health combined (U.S. Department of Health and Human Services Public Health Service, 1994). Why have rescue and stabilization come to dominate health care delivery in the United States? To understand why overcoming imminent peril resonates so strongly throughout the health care system, it is instructive to consider how well rescue embodies the dominant U.S. ideology. It is also helpful to ask what the general public wants to be rescued *from*, and therefore, how the mainstream culture views death and dying.

Respiratory or cardiac collapse is a dramatic event, signaling imminent death. But with the application of speed, intensity, and complex technology, it is potentially reversible—in some cases, under the right conditions. The juxtaposition of imminent death with its potential reversal through tools of human design is irresistible to the American imaginary. Rescue embodies many of the themes of the dominant U.S. ideology, what we are calling the "major key" emphasized in media messaging. Other values built into American citizenship, which seem to command less media attention, form a "minor key."

The United States was founded on a shared ideology rather than a shared history. That circumstance serves as a source of ongoing insecurity for its citizens regarding the stability of its foundations and the viability of its future (Cavell, 1976). As a result, many people in the United States cling tenaciously to nationalizing narratives as a stronghold against perceived threats (Nichols & Mathewes, 2008). Themes of triumph, heroism, and overcoming adversity through determination and innovation run deep. Never give up, never say die. Drama and display are also important in the United States (Nye, 2001), making technological innovations in health care settings especially salient, particularly if they can delay death. When individualism, entitlement, and choice are paired with the idea of equal opportunity for all, they become legitimized as national aspirations (Bauman, 1992). Francis Hsu (1972) has summed up American psychology as self-reliance, noting its corollary, the abhorrence of dependence. Yet there is a tension here, because many Americans think of themselves as altruistic, always ready to extend a hand to those in legitimate need.

Rescue from calamity fits with this ideology of heroism and triumph, especially if it involves technology and drama. Body trauma television programs capitalize on the appealing combination of a high stakes threat, intensity, urgency, and valiant intervention. Rescue is individualized, customized care made available to anyone, as long as she or he is in extremis. As rescue is understood as being universally available, privileged access to health care can exist in an egalitarian society. In fact, rescue may be the one part of health care in the United States that the system attempts to guarantee to everyone. (The problem is that those who have inadequate insurance must collapse and have the collapse be witnessed before they will become eligible to have "everything done.") Excellence in the intensity and complexity of rescue medicine implies overall excellence in U.S. health care delivery. It is clear that this display of fervor, intricacy, and speed is perceived as the gold standard of medical care, the apex of medicine as it is understood and delivered in America. The most cultural value accrues to conquering the highest perceived threat. In the United States, that threat is death.

Minimizing the Dying in Death

Partly because of rescue's prominent role in the U.S. health care system, death seems distant from everyday life, bolstered by the "mythology" of CPR (Codagan, 2010; Timmermans, 1999). Many people believe that death comes only after an unforeseeably bad accident, or only after all contingencies are exhausted (Callahan, 2003). Media reporting of dramatic medical breakthroughs make them seem both routine and far-reaching. One could easily believe that because medical technology for rescue is both limitless and unknowable, scientific advances seem unending, and every contingency will be explored, one's death will be postponed for so long that it may never come at all.

Under such circumstances it seems neither necessary nor worthwhile to prepare for death, much less for dying. The concept of death rarely enters the national conversation. However, dying is even more troublesome than death, to be avoided even more strongly. Its proximity to nonbeing and inherent disorder are disturbing. Will it be painful? Many hope that death will come in sleep, unawares, so that they might avoid the dying part altogether. In the United States, dying must be properly contained so as to protect the living (Mellor & Shilling, 1993). Recognizable dying should certainly be removed from the public gaze.

Perhaps it is unsurprising, then, that clinicians are so reluctant to think of their patients as "dying." Seriously ill patients are assumed still to have a future available to them, making them eligible for the gold standard of medical care in the United States until the last possible minute. To be dying in the hospital, by contrast, is to have no future, to be a second-class citizen compared to those deemed still rescuable (Chapple, 2010). Clinicians automatically apply advanced interventions to serious illness when initial efforts fail to arrest it, unless or until something happens to obviate the strategy. This rescue trajectory is compelling for staff, patients, and families alike. It is difficult *not* to be swept up in the enthusiasm for treatments that promise to reverse this or that complication. Ironically, when death's arrival proves that the patient was in fact dying, these same patients are blamed for costing too much, even though the prevailing social contract ensures that the U.S. health care system will fight to the death to rescue every life. Opportunities for a more meaningful process are lost.

Calculating Value

Up to this point the weight of the national ideology falls on the side of attempting rescue from the threat of death rather than allowing death, even if hospice and/or palliative care are available as alternative modes of care. Market forces and reimbursement patterns reflect and reinforce the priority of overcoming adversity. The ideology that makes rescue so appealing also capitalizes the health care industry. Together they complicate any objective assessment of what constitutes value in health care delivery. This confusion manifests itself at the bedside of dying patients.

The business of the biomedical project, which profits from providing goods and services for patient management, and the altruism of health care, which attends to patient well-being, coexist uncomfortably in a market system. The awkward symbiosis between the two animates the U.S. hospital, whose very survival may depend on its ability to produce more time alive for patients while reducing their length of stay. Rescue maps onto commerce when technological patient management is invoiced. Throughput and productivity ride piggyback on rescue's rapid response, speeding up and quantifying every patient encounter for reimbursement.

Hospitals juggle their competing priorities, working to keep the business end from contaminating their altruistic public image. On one side of the equation are the countable items and services, to which price tags can be affixed: technological interventions, drugs, procedures, and vital sign monitoring. Interestingly, the very multiplicity of interventions confers legitimacy on a patient whose inherent dignity seems to command such investment. But they also bring alienation—so many specialized objects and actions attached to her body make her appear foreign to those who love her. Meanwhile, the priceless aspects of care are much less measurable, such as the compassion, trust, and relationship that grow from interactions between staff and patients and the education and training that permeate the hospital day. The immeasurable value of life itself forms the subtext of the acute care enterprise, not to mention the value of the particular lives that may be at stake. With such contrary forces at work, how is value to be understood?

Other industrialized countries have settled these questions with less confusion, lower costs, and better results. The burden of authenticating the social contract falls not on a commitment to rescue, but more straightforwardly on solidarity. This value is not unknown to mainstream U.S. ideology, but when self-reliance is driving the bus, social consciousness takes a back seat. Nations whose citizens have ready access to health care have demonstrated that it is less expensive and more effective to provide broad basic care than to fix problems after they have become severe, as shown in Figure 19.1.

FIGURE 19.1 Why Does the U.S. Spend More Than Other Countries?

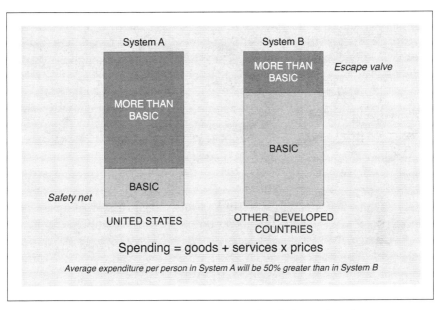

SOURCE: Engelhard, 2005, used by permission; adapted from Fuchs, 1993, p. 62.

Health Policy and End of Life (EOL) in the United States

Employer-based health insurance, the foundation of patient coverage in the United States, has been in place since World War II. Strong efforts at health care reform have modified but not dislodged this system, even though it is acknowledged to be inefficient and exclusionary. The struggle for reform has not accounted for the baseline ideological values that have combined capitalism and rescue in a self-reinforcing institutional framework. The progressivists' assumption that it is only a matter of time before all causes of death are eliminated (Callahan, 2003) continues to drive investment, derailing any serious challenge for a more holistic approach to patient care that would reinforce palliative care and symptom control. Meanwhile, public health initiatives that promote a broad understanding of prevention and wellness rarely address EOL care and actual dying situations.

The portion of gross domestic product consumed by health care costs in the United States has grown from 7.2% in 1970 to 17.9% in 2010 (The Henry J. Kaiser Family Foundation, 2012a). It consumes an ever-greater portion of the GDP, especially compared to other industrialized countries, whose per capita health care costs are a fraction of those in the United States (The Henry J. Kaiser Family Foundation, 2012a). As costs rise, the beneficiaries reap the benefits. But as costs rise, less and less money is available to spend on other national priorities, such as education and physical infrastructure. As these costs have been accelerating in the face of stagnant national income, the sustainability of the health care system is in question (Health Care Marketplace Project, 2006). As government programs strive to shift from a fee-for-service system to a value-based system with health care reform (Centers for Medicare and Medicaid Services, 2009; Smith, 2010), neither the hidden connection between fee for service and technological salvation nor the need to ground the transition in something more positive than the imminent death of capitalism is addressed.

The polarized U.S. political climate, a longstanding fear of "big government," and mistrust of the medical system that dovetails with a lack of universal health care have together made rational political deliberation about EOL and/or health policy virtually impossible at the community, state, or federal levels. Underneath the conflict simmers the fear of death and a fear that reform would put the brakes on technological innovation. According to a Kaiser poll, 36% of the public in 2012 believed that the Affordable Care Act would "allow a government panel to make decisions about EOL care for people on Medicare" 3 years after the term "death panels" was debunked and a provision to reimburse physicians to engage in ACP was removed from the legislation (The Henry J. Kaiser Family Foundation, 2012b).

So far we have been discussing rescue as being underpinned by ideology, and indeed it is. An ideology of self-reliance and overcoming adversity assumes a linear view of progress and time (see Figure 19.2).

A more comprehensive approach to health care delivery will require a more multi-dimensional worldview along with attention to the financial realities the current system has created.

In fact, the nation's economic survival depends on a new EOL care conversation. U.S. health policy must be grounded in palliative care principles, which hold that symptom control for the seriously ill and dying must be universally available. This conversation is justified by focusing attention on "minor key" aspects of a view of human society that does not promote conquering death as a legitimate "end" of health care policy.

Reforming Ideology, Reforming Worldview, Reforming Health Care

Just as U.S. hospitals weave industry together with life and death drama, combining speed and technology with throughput and saving lives, the U.S. health care system combines major themes of ideology with the nation's underlying fear of non-survival (Cavell, 1976). Here the news of medical breakthroughs that seem to hold back death for individuals also reinforces national pride and legitimacy for the United States as a nation.

This particular ideology of progress is based on a mechanistic, linear worldview that hearkens back to Isaac Newton. The underlying assumption

FIGURE 19.2 Traditional Linear Understanding of U.S. Health Care.

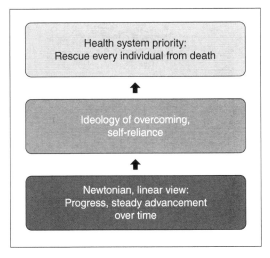

is that a continuous investment of energy and treasure in the medical project can extend the line of continuous innovation and advancement forever. Such an understanding maps closely to the interest in expanding rescue and life support technology to avoid personal finitude. Unfortunately, a strategy of progress cannot erase the anxiety of a nation founded on ideology, since it cannot guarantee its future existence. Furthermore, chaotic events inevitably interrupt the assumed linear progress. Getting back on track restores credibility. Anything that encroaches upon the U.S. ability to lengthen its lifeline, therefore, must be rejected. Perhaps the salience of the concept of "death panels" expressed the anxiety that slowing technological progress in any way would shorten the lives of both individuals and the nation itself.

In fact, as Albert Jonsen and Daniel Callahan warn, the project of continuous rescue is itself ruinous to the nation (Callahan, 2003; Jonsen, 1986). Prolonging an unqualified pursuit of more time alive is untenable for both individuals and for national economies. A belief that honest striving will make future events break largely in favor of the United States, that no abyss yawns ahead, is bravado. No one nation can hope to escape the effects of global warming, pandemic flu, economic collapse, natural disasters, and/or other yet unknowable forms of chaos. The U.S. faith that unlimited growth will enable the nation to prevail over such adversity interferes with realistic preparations for adverse events and could actually accelerate their arrival. The negative externalities of market transactions, which seem irrelevant when the deals are struck, can be expected to backfire, as the 2008 economic collapse showed (Chomsky, 2012). Not only is the view of progress as a linear advancement untenable, it is also deeply flawed. It does not account for the actual complexities of real-world phenomena, nor does it allow for the inevitability of chaos.

Taking Comfort in Complexity

There is good news, however. Now that computers analyze enormous sets of data, it is possible to appropriate more accurate depictions of reality that can incorporate chaos and complexity. Order can be created even without the luxury of predictability (Chinnis & White, 1999). In this more comprehensive view of the way things work, interconnectivity, creativity, and relationships become keys to thriving. Complex adaptive systems display openness, nonlinearity, self-organization, emergence, and the diffusion of local action to global effects (Anderson, Crabtree, Steele, & McDaniel, 2005; Malone & Tanner, 2008). Building social capital offers the resources to creatively manage bad times and the resilience to move beyond them (Campbell, 2006). Complexity science enables a revised view of reality as indicated below.

Those who have been working in the field of thanatology and EOL have long known that chaos is a common experience for patients and families when dying and death eradicate the illusion of linear progress. The events of serious illness and the reactions to those events are often complex and unpredictable, notwithstanding even comprehensive efforts toward ACP. Acute illness brings multiple attempts to rescue, diagnose, and treat with a momentum that has a life of its own, and chronic illness brings exacerbations that take one by surprise. The hoped-for orderly trajectory seems not to play out in reality. At these moments self-reliance fails. Advocates for hospice and palliative care are familiar with strategies of interdependence and resilience. Linking arms, connecting with spirituality, and riding out

FIGURE 19.3 Complexity Science Offers an Alternative View of U.S. Health Care.

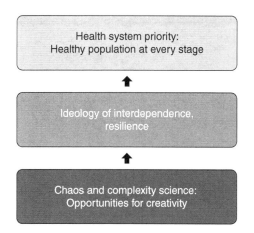

the storm with supports in place are more likely to bring everyone safely to the other side than fighting the good fight.

It is not necessary to abandon technology and its hope of progress, but in view of a chaotic reality, humans are compelled to find a broader base for creative management. Complexity science and palliative care both recognize human interdependence, and both exploit untapped resources in what is small and close at hand. These approaches challenge the reductionist emphasis on rescue in favor of more abundant perspectives demonstrating that chaos itself generates resourceful solutions. Those who are comfortable with dying and death understand the creativity engendered by chaos.

Using chaos theory and complexity science rather than progressivism to ground a national worldview provides an opportunity to bring underappreciated American values into the spotlight. Rescuing an individual from collapse demonstrates one portion of a social contract, the tacit agreement between a people and its government with regard to protection from untimely death. Emergency services (911) and the surprisingly unsafe health care "safety net" (Becker, 2004) are supposed to make rescue universally available, whereas public access to other areas of health care in the United States is less straightforward. William F. May (May, 2011) argues that the contractual understanding of the role of government in the United States is inadequate. It does not reflect the intentions of the founding fathers, who envisioned a wider role for government than that of being a party to the social contract. May claims that the founders saw government as a necessary refuge from the storms of less civilized influences. This view of government as a covenant with the people, rather than a contract, allows a more nuanced role in keeping with the needs of a pluralistic society.

THE MINOR KEY: PALLIATIVE CARE, THE VIRTUES OF CLASSICAL CITIZENSHIP, AND A NEW END-OF-LIFE CONVERSATION

Courage, friendship, honesty (truth-telling), and justice, also known as "virtues" in political theory discourse, were core values of classical citizenship. The virtues are integrally related to the concept—developed by Aristotle, St. Augustine, Thomas Aquinas, and the 20th century French Catholic philosophers—of the idea of the common good. We argue that the virtues are expressed in the praxis of palliative care, which contributes to the common good.

Palliative Care

Palliative care (from the Latin word *palliare*, meaning to cloak) is a specialized area of health care that focuses on relieving the suffering of patients and their families experiencing advanced illness. Dr. Balfour Mount coined the term in the mid-1970s. Palliative care in Great Britain grew out of a religious tradition and concerns about social solidarity, while the American palliative care movement grew out of legal and secular concerns, assertion of patients' rights, and debate over physician-assisted suicide (Fins, 2005, p. 14). Unlike hospice care, which it supports, palliative care is appropriate for patients in all disease stages. Most notably, it does not aim to *cure* illness: palliative care meets illness on its own terms and aims to relieve the suffering—physical, emotional, spiritual, and existential—that characterizes and accompanies both serious illness and the dying process. Ideally, palliative care is practiced by a multidisciplinary team: physician, nurse, pharmacist, psychosocial professional, chaplain, and volunteer. The patient or "unit of care" in the palliative care approach includes relevant family members and caregivers. Indeed, the long-term physical, mental, and spiritual health of family members and caregivers depends on seeing that their loved ones' suffering and symptoms are relieved, that opportunities to create meaning are made available, and that wishes to die at home or in hospice, rather than in a hospital or institution, are granted whenever possible. The discipline of palliative care also attends, crucially, to health care providers themselves, addressing burnout, conflict resolution, bereavement, and improving communication skills (Halifax, 2011). "This is the first discipline [to include] health care providers in its scope of attention" (Jazieh, 2012). In contrast with the biomedical model, where the operative unit is a binary (patient–physician) palliative care is paradigmatically practiced in, by, for, and *as* a community.

Palliative Care and the Virtues

Truth-telling or "parrhēsia" (Foucault, 2011) was a classical political virtue that can be loosely compared to the modern right to free speech, which is central to democratic citizenship. Establishing, revisiting, and revising patients' and families' goals of care through inclusive consultation, sensitive truth-telling, and ACP is also central to palliative care. In that it is conditioned by an ethic of truth-telling, palliative care both expresses and generates another of the virtues, known as "civic friendship" in the classical sense of *philia*, a "loving bond...involving altruism, reciprocity, and mutual recognition" (Konstan, 1997, p. 69). Friendship and honesty were considered core political virtues in the classical world, and are internally related to the common good: "Where there is justice, friendship is possible. And where there is friendship, there is the pursuit of the common good" (Smith 1995, p. 167).

According to Aristotle (1985, 212–213; *Nichomachean Ethics*, Bk.Viii, 9:35 1156b), "complete friendship is the friendship of good people similar in virtue; for they wish goods in the same way to each other insofar as they are good, and they are good in themselves. Those who wish goods to their friend for the friend's own sake are friends most of all; for they have this attitude because of the friend himself." This is closely related to the Buddhist concept of the spiritual friend (King, 1991, p. 119). The "goods" the palliative care team wishes for the patient and family (and ultimately, of course for themselves)—relief from physical, emotional, spiritual, or psychosocial pain—are "produced" in the community of friendship generated by the praxis of palliative care. The virtues condition the "energetic tone" of the family, the community, and even the polity as a whole when policies supporting palliative care ensure that it is fully integrated into the health care delivery system.

The core political virtue of civic friendship is classically twinned with the virtue of courage (*tharséō*). The courage of the soldier (the paradigmatic classical citizen) is the willingness to face death in battle, knowing he has the support and trust of the community he loves. The community, his group of comrades, is the wind at the soldier's back. The modern citizen/patient/community of the seriously ill has this same wind at its back when that citizen's fellows, her health care services, and her elected representatives treat her well-being, and that of her family, as their primary concern. The foundation of political courage, its molecular structure, is love and charity (*caritas*): love of country (*patria*), family, clan, and virtue (Viroli, 1995). That love can also be extended to suffering humanity, to our fellow inhabitants of the planet. These virtues are all immanent to the original institution of citizenship, which can be mapped in *praxis* onto international legal and biomedical regimes (Fins, 2005, p. xvi). The virtues we have identified are a synergistic source of authentic collective power for a terminally ill person and her caregivers: "communication confers communion and creates community" (Ward, 2000, p. 111). The Veterans Administration incorporates the virtues that have always been immanent to the soldier–citizen–polity continuum into its palliative care program for terminally ill soldiers through its Home-Based Primary Care and inpatient programs.

The Centrality of Truth Telling or Parrhēsia

The ethical premise of palliative care—which begins ideally at diagnosis and continues through bereavement services for caregivers—is that relief of suffering, and meaning-making, depends on increasingly transparent communication among all parties (friends) about the progress of the illness and the goals of care. These goals often change as the illness evolves. In the absence of intentionally honest speech among those joined in this particular community of friendship over time, the initiation and delivery of good palliative care is impossible. Clearly, truth-telling is also central to effective ACP, which ideally heads off the ideology of rescue medicine "at the pass" by prioritizing conversation about patients' wishes concerning futile treatment and how they wish to spend their last days.

Communication is a most important catalyst for the selection of palliation. Indeed, poor communication renders all other medical care ineffective. Without effective communication, palliative care will remain an unstated option. At worst, it can be one that is discounted. This might be through a careless phrase like, "Well, we could just palliate." ...Considered this way, communication—not opioid analgesia—becomes the central catalyst to effective palliative care. (Fins, 2005, p. 70)

As in palliative care, "healing" does not refer to "cure." Healing can take place during the last weeks, days, months, or even moments of a person's life. Once the palliative care needs of seriously ill patients and their families are met and suffering is brought under a modicum of control, patients and their families can experience a quality of life and an intensity of relationship—by means of truth-telling in multiple domains—that may have been previously unavailable to them during their productive, pre-illness lives. (See Byock, 2012; Callanan & Kelley, 1993; Grassman, 2009; Levine, 1984; Singh, 1999 to name only a few books that "redeem" dying from the narrative of failure and despair in the presence of good palliative care.) Relieved of the burden of intense pain and able, perhaps, to communicate coherently with family and caregivers, people can live more joyfully and meaningfully together, even when (or even because) they know their time together is limited.

Ira Byock, a passionate American campaigner for improved EOL services, calls palliative care "ardently life-affirming," adding, "If you are committed to affirming life, you have to affirm all of life, including that part we call dying" (Catholic News Service, 2011). Even more radically, we submit that the suffering and dying body cared for by a community of friends grounds a source of authentic power, and that the deathbed can be reinscribed in the national narrative as a site of connection and transcendence rather than of trauma, failure, and despair.

Palliative care and ACP both demand and exemplify the virtues of courage, friendship, and truth-telling for honing in on goals of care as conditions change for the patient. This practice occurs in what political theorists call the "private (non-public) sphere." Practiced systematically in the "public sphere," though, "truth-telling" becomes the ethical foundation of democratic citizenship and can, ideally, be a healing and regenerative political force. In this sense, truth-telling is aligned with John Dewey's theory of inquiry, in which truth claims are openly submitted for testing by a community of inquirers to clarify, justify, refine, and/or refute proposed truths (Bernstein, 1967).

The debate about what "truth" means can be endless. In this context, it is used in the sense of the Fourth Buddhist precept: to practice honest speech. The Fourth Precept has also been rendered as the "abstain from falsehood" or "practice [of] truthfulness." Zen teacher Norman Fischer (2003) says the Fourth Precept is I vow "not to lie but to be truthful" (p. 150). Palliative care practitioners value the virtue of truth-telling highly because they practice authenticity in close proximity to death, which calls forth (in some practitioners at least) the other core political virtue: courage, or fearlessness. It is the *sine qua non* of palliative care practice not to try to cheat death, but to meet it respectfully—to honor it as a teacher—to benefit the friend/patient traveling toward it.

We can extrapolate from the individual to the society in the following way: The healing, rather than curing, of a polity that has been distorted by inappropriate and aggressive diversions of resources into individual rescue medicine to the detriment of public health and the common good, must begin with honesty—ethical speech directed toward truth-telling— about the goals of care appropriate to U.S. society in the 21st century. The praxis of palliative care, truth-telling, and ACP situated in the private sphere—the microcosm of community that includes the patient, family, and palliative care team—must be reflected in the macrocosm, which includes the larger community, the state, and the country. In other words, Americans interested in redefining and expanding the national EOL conversation must adopt a "meta-ethic" of palliative care in terms of the values of the health system as a whole, not just in EOL care and ACP. This meta-ethic would by definition be inclusive, interactive, dynamic, creative, and—yes—probably chaotic, at least in the beginning. Individuals and communities must avail themselves of the political virtues of courage and civic friendship, which we have argued are available in the original institution of citizenship (Pettus, in press), if they are to begin the healing conversations that will serve the common good.

REFERENCES

Anderson, R., Crabtree, B. F., Steele, D. J., & McDaniel, R. R. (2005). Case study research: The view from complexity science. *Quality Health Research, 15*(5), 669–685.

Aristotle (1985). *Nichomachean Ethics* (translated, with an Introduction by Peter Irwin) Indianapolis/Cambridge: Hackett.

Bauman, Z. (1992). *Mortality, immortality, and other life strategies*. Cambridge, UK: Polity Press.

Becker, G. (2004). Deadly inequality in the health care "safety net": Uninsured ethnic minorities struggle to live with life-threatening illnesses. *Medical Anthropology Quarterly, 18*(2), 258–275.

Bernstein, R. J. (1967). Dewey, John. In P. Edwards (Ed.), *Encyclopedia of philosophy, volume 2* (pp. 383). New York, NY: MacMillan.

Byock, I. R. (2012). *The best care possible: A physician's quest to transform care through the end of life*. New York, NY: Penguin.

Callahan, D. (2003). *What price better health? Hazards of the research imperative*. Berkeley, CA: University of California Press.

Callanan, M., & Kelley, P. (1993). *Final gifts: Understanding the special awareness, needs, and communications of the dying.* New York, NY: Bantam.

Campbell, J. M. (2006). Renewing social capital: The role of civil dialogue. In S. Schuman (Ed.), *Creating a culture of collaboration: The international facilitators handbook* (pp. 41–55). San Francisco, CA: Jossey-Bass/The International Association of Facilitation.

Catholic News Service. (2011). *Palliative care expert sees essential role for Catholic health care.* Retrieved May 12, 2012, from http://www.catholicnews.com/data/briefs/cns/20110812.htm

Cavell, S. (1976). *The avoidance of love: A reading of King Lear. Must we mean what we say? A book of essays* (pp. 267–356). Cambridge, UK: Cambridge University Press.

Centers for Medicare and Medicaid Services. (2009). *Roadmap for implementing value-driven health care in the traditional medicare fee for service program.* Retrieved September 17, 2012, from http://www.cms.gov/Medicare/Quality-Initiatives-Patient-Assessment-Instruments/QualityInitiativesGenInfo/downloads/VBPRoadmap_OEA_1–16_508.pdf

Chapple, H. S. (2010). *No place for dying: Hospitals and the ideology of rescue.* Walnut Creek, CA: Left Coast Press.

Chinnis, A., & White, K. R. (1999). Challenging the dominant logic of emergency departments: Guidelines from chaos theory. *The Journal of Emergency Medicine, 17*(6), 1049–1054.

Chomsky, N. (2012). In Ashbrook T. (Ed.), *Noam Chomsky: On point with Tom Ashbrook.* Washington, DC: National Public Radio.

Codagan, M. P. (2010). CPR decision-making and older adults. *Journal of Gerontological Nursing, 36*(12), 10–15.

Engelhard, C. L. (2005). *Why does the U.S. spend more than other countries?* Unpublished manuscript.

Fins, J. J. (2005). *A palliative ethic of care: Clinical wisdom at life's end.* Sudbury, MA: Jones and Bartlett.

Fischer, N. (2003). *Taking our place: the Buddhist guide to truly growing up.* New York, NY: Harper Collins.

Foucault, M. (2011). *The courage of the truth: (lectures at the college de France, 1983–84)* (G. Burchell Trans.). Eastbourne, UK: Palgrave MacMillan.

Fuchs, V. R. (1993). *The future of health policy.* Cambridge, MA: Harvard University Press.

Grassman, D. L. (2009). *Peace at last: Stories of hope and healing for veterans and their families.* St. Petersburg, FL: Vandamere Press.

Halifax, J. (2011). The precious necessity of compassion. *Journal of Pain and Symptom Management, 41*(1), 146–153.

Health Care Marketplace Project. (2006). *Snapshots: Health care costs.* Retrieved September 17, 2012, from http://www.kff.org/insurance/snapshot/chcm050206oth2.cfm

The Henry J. Kaiser Family Foundation. (2012a). *Health care costs: A primer; key information on health care costs and their impact.* Retrieved September 17, 2012, from http://www.kff.org/insurance/upload/7670–03.pdf

The Henry J. Kaiser Family Foundation. (2012b). *Kaiser health tracking poll: Public opinion on health care issues.* Retrieved 06/22, 2012, from http://www.kff.org/kaiserpolls/upload/8285-F.pdf

Hsu, F. L. K. (1972). American core value and national character. In F. L. K. Hsu (Ed.), *Psychological anthropology* (pp. 241–262). Cambridge, MA: Schenkman.

Jazieh, A. R. (2012). What is palliative care? Towards better understanding of a core health care discipline. *Journal of Palliative Care & Medicine, 2011*, 1:1, available at http://dx.doi.org/10.4172/jpcm.1000e102.

Jonsen, A. R. (1986). Bentham in a box: Technology assessment and health care allocation. *Law, Medicine & Health Care, 14,* 172–174.

King, S. B. (1991). *Buddha nature.* Albany, NY: State University of NY Press.

Konstan, D. (1997). *Friendship in the classical world.* Cambridge, UK: Cambridge University Press.

Levine, S. (1984). *Meetings at the edge: Dialogues with the grieving and the dying, the healing and the healed.* New York, NY: Anchor.

Malone, D., & Tanner, M. (Producers), & Malone, D., & Tanner, M. (Directors). (2008, 14 October 2008). *High anxieties: The mathematics of chaos.* [Video/DVD] London: BBC Worldwide; Films on Demand. Retrieved from http://digital.films.com/PortalPlaylists.aspx?aid=3864&xtid=40397

May, W. F. (2011). *Testing the national covenant: American fears and appetites.* Baltimore, MD: Georgetown University Press.

Mellor, P. A., & Shilling, C. (1993). Modernity, self-identity and the sequestration of death. *Sociology, 27*(3), 411–432.

Nichols, C. M., & Mathewes, C. (2008). Introduction: Prophecies of godlessness. In C. Mathewes, & C. McKnight Nichols (Eds.), *Prophesies of godlessness: Predictions of American godlessness from Puritanism to the present day* (pp. 3–20). New York, NY: Oxford University Press.

Nye, D. E. (2001). Technology and cultural difference. In D. Carter (Ed.), *American exceptionalism revisited* (pp. 94–111). Amsterdam, the Netherlands: Aarthus University Press.

Pettus, K. I. (in press). *Palliative care and political theory: Honoring and healing the body politic.* Albany, NY: State University of New York.

Singh, K. D. (1999). *The grace in dying: How we are transformed spiritually as we die.* New York, NY: Harper Collins.

Smith, A. (2010). Moving from a medicare fee-for-service system to a pay-for-performance system. *Health Lawyers Weekly, 8*(19), 1–3.

Smith, M. A. (1995). *Human dignity and the common good in the Aristotlean-Thomist tradition.* Lewiston, NY: Edwin Mellon Press.

Timmermans, S. (1999). *Sudden death and myth of CPR.* Philadelphia, PA: Temple University Press.

U.S. Department of Health and Human Services Public Health Service. (1994). *For a healthy nation: Returns on investment in public health*. Washington, DC: U.S. Government Printing Office.

Viroli, M. (1995). *For love of country*. New York, NY: Oxford University Press.

Ward, G. (2000). Radical orthodoxy and/as cultural politics. In L. Hemming (Ed.), *Radical Orthodoxy? A catholic enquiry* (pp. 97–111). Aldershot: Ashgate.

CHAPTER 20

Inspiring Improvement and Leading Change in End-of-Life Care

Ben Lobo

Death is life's greatest change agent.

After Steve Jobs

This chapter reflects on how leaders and great teams can and must rise to the challenge of improving health care systems and provide high-quality services to people who are dying. This challenge presents opportunities for leaders to achieve the "Triple Aim™" (Institute for Healthcare Improvement [IHI], 2012) of improved health of a population, improved experience of care, and a decreased cost per capita affordable cost.

This chapter describes how quality improvement (QI) techniques may also help to achieve wider aspects of improving access and equity to services in a timely and effective way. This approach to drive up quality and provide value will help us address the demographic change of people living longer and dying with long-term health conditions and social deprivation. In part, the key to address this need is to make proactive case management for individuals and advance care planning (ACP) the common approach and to have simple but standardized measurement and align financial incentives from the payer. To provide guidance to practitioners who want to advance the cause of best practice in ACP and end-of-life (EOL) care, I discuss the role of effective leaders and great teams in health care improvement, review key elements of QI initiatives applied to EOL care, point to key elements important to implementing large-scale change (LSC), and present the "Moral Test" put to health care planners by health care improvement leader Donald Berwick (Berwick, 2011).

LEADERSHIP AND GREAT TEAMS

Effective Leadership

I am privileged to share my personal experience of leadership as a corporate director and as a senior clinician dedicated to improving EOL care through ACP. Rising to the leadership and QI challenge in general has taught me much about people (myself as well as those I affected), the change process, and local and national politics. Leadership in austere times is tough, and my approach to survive and thrive is built on simple principles, no Ivy League MBA required. My leadership and QI learning journey has highlighted the importance of defining and communicating a simple and clear vision, and a realistic ambition with tangible stretch built into specific objectives.

Taking people with you is fundamental to positive change. It can only be achieved by sharing and understanding the common values and culture that make us human. I have learned how to use my behaviors to *accentuate* the positive and to get people to be hungry to *acquire* new knowledge and skills and be the *architects* of future services. It helps me to connect to people by explaining how I am, and most of us are, driven by vocation, and the fundamental and intense desire to do the best for patients and their families. I have learned to understand my own and other people's ideas, concerns and expectations, as well as in some circumstance real fears, and turn this into positive energy for front line change.

I recognize that because I, like other leaders, am under intense pressure to deliver on the bottom line with quality and cost improvements, I have to be careful not to unfairly push and exceed the team's ability to respond. Sustainable change is built upon a strong foundation, the team, the coalition, and the collaborative network. This is of paramount importance to teams dealing with high pressure and stressful roles in diagnosing (or acknowledging) for the first time a person is dying and needs support through ACP.

Mastering resilience and managing adversity are essential in maintaining growth and delivering on the bottom line in a time of organizational and system turmoil. Leaders of organizations must understand that to deliver success there must be synergy between frontline staff and the board members built by and maintained with openness and transparency. Every member, whether doctor, nurse, or assistant, must work at the top of his or her license. What does this mean in practice? I suggest it is about getting the basics right, being professional, using years of knowledge and experience to open conversations at the right time, understanding and sharing information with the patient and their families, and not being frightened to tell some they are dying. A different approach is needed, away from hopes of cure and aggressive treatment and its concomitant harm.

The paraphrased quotation that opens this chapter is from Steve Jobs, the cofounder of Apple Inc. It has many both positive and potentially negative meanings, but to me, in the context of improving EOL care, getting quality right has been a foundation stone in my positive approach to my personal and professional life. There are no second chances and the moral stakes are high.

I learned the essence of medical ethics and morality as a child listening to the stories of my father, a pediatrician, and how he had the successes and challenges of looking after critically ill children. I have learned as a doctor that despite, and as a consequence of, medical advances, the greatest need now is to be good at controlling symptoms and offering a positive patient experience as people live longer and become frailer. Steve Jobs died in 2011 at the age of 56 of pancreatic cancer. Even this business leader and icon of the 21st century with the benefit of huge wealth, influence, and cutting edge medical treatment could not beat nature. He will be remembered not because of how he died but how he lived a life where he challenged traditional belief; pushed for perfection in the quality of his products; and achieved, as some believed, the impossible.

The question is not whether we will die, it is about how we will live.

Joan Borysenko

Great Teams

Leaders who build great teams not only push for perfection in the products; they only tolerate "A" team players. Jobs was famously impatient, petulant, and tough with the people around him (Pentland, 2012). Everyone finds his or her leadership style; Jobs clearly had his own, and his style is not necessarily advocated explicitly by me. The principle is simple: to aspire to be the best, you must get together the most effective team. The best leadership teams in history not only have a great leader but have committed players who are usually highly talented leaders in their own right. Great teams and their constituents all contribute high energy; they communicate effectively because they are engaged. This ability to be engaged, use effective communication, and channel intrinsic energy allows robust and fast exploration of opportunities and threats and conversion to action with rapid improvement and sustained improvement.

At this point, I would like to ask the reader to rise to my first challenge. Rather than give an obvious example of an international leader or champion of palliative EOL care, I would ask the reader to think of a person or professional who does this day in day out in his or her own community. Think why they do this and how they succeed. In my experience, these leaders have drive, motivated by ethical and altruistic reason to deliver care to people, because they know it will make that positive difference, often without accolade. This primary drive to help is often aligned with their spiritual energy and connection to people, the patient, their family, and the team(s) around them. Whether born into a vocation or grown into, the difference these dedicated people make is huge, by reducing fear, ameliorating pain and distress, and giving realistic hope when hope and spirit had been taken.

> *Leadership is not about making clever decisions and doing bigger deals. It is about helping release the positive energy that exists naturally within people.*
>
> Henry Mintzberg

When Great Teams Are Not Enough

In today's fast-moving ultracompetitive global business environment, you can't rely on stable teams to get the work done (to deliver exceptional results). Instead you need "teaming," which is flexible teamwork where you gather experts from different divisions and disciplines into temporary groups to tackle unexpected problems or emerging opportunities. To "team" well, employees and organizations must embrace principles of project management and team leadership. Those who master teaming will reap benefits. Teaming allows individuals to acquire knowledge, skills, and networks, and accelerates the delivery of current offerings while responding to new challenges (Edmondson, 2012). This is in clinical terms the basis of multidisciplinary and interagency working. The team knows that in some cases they must think and act differently, often with a pressing time scale for completion. Dying often finds its own schedule, waiting for neither man nor priest. Therefore, it is essential to start earlier, getting the right team together and approach for the job, actively seeking and listening to preferences and making decisions. Starting with the end in sight helps to give that focus and produce the right outcome. In health care "business" terms I have often seen teams become ineffectual and unable to respond to new or different challenges or increase productivity at scale because they become static or concrete in their thinking. All "A" teams, including clinical "A" teams, need new player acquisitions and sometimes a bench of talented specialists or special teams to bring onto the field—a new team for a new play. In simple clinical terms, for example, bringing in a professional with specialist palliative care skills to a team focused on renal replacement to support the transition from dialysis to EOL care, when the dialysis ceases to be an effective or tolerated treatment.

QUALITY IMPROVEMENT AND LEADING LARGE-SCALE CHANGE

The global economic instability and the demographic time bomb have delivered an imperative to all cultures and nations. In these austere times with ever changing national politics, government policy and cut backs, and health care delivery systems changes, there has never been a greater need for clinical and managerial leadership. This has put pressure on health systems to reduce expensive emergency admissions to hospitals, especially of people whose real "presenting complaint" might be recorded as dying but without support or ACP.

In my own experience I continuously try to turn the pressure of ever-higher demand and expectations of the public, payers, regulators, and media into opportunities for quality and performance improvement.

Intensive care and cancer treatment are two excellent examples where QI delivered through LSC should have great financial return and positive impact on the quality of clinical care by reducing harm of necessary and unnecessary treatment. Cancer treatment especially has been driven by research to find what works to cure or control disease. Unfortunately, there is a great limitation of this research science, as it does not often tell people (patients and professionals) when to stop because the treatment has become ineffective and when to switch focus to palliation and EOL care. How many patients admitted as an emergency to intensive care with respiratory failure from end-stage chronic obstructive pulmonary disease will survive and be discharged home?

Quality Improvement in End-of-Life Care

The reality of the current performance in health care and EOL care is far from the "Six Aims of Institute of Medicine" (Committee of Quality of Life in Health Care, 2001), with wide variance from quality standards with inconsistent or no measures in some specific areas. A significant step forward was taken in 2011 with the launch of the English National Institute of Health and Clinical Excellence End-of-Life Quality Standards (National Institute of Health and Clinical Excellence, 2011).

The following statistics from the National EOL Intelligence Network for England have been quoted in national strategy. These facts help to demonstrate the scale of challenge.

Currently in the United Kingdom, around 1% of the population around (approximately 600,000 people) die each year (National End of Life Care Intelligence Network, 2009); 66% are aged over 75; and the majority follow a period of chronic progressive illness. The place of death is 58% hospitals, 18% home, 17% care homes (nursing homes), 4% hospices, and 3% elsewhere. If the long-term trend in home death proportions observed over the last 5 years continues, less than 10% will die at home by 2030. When the public are surveyed, 60% say they would like to die at home. Institutional deaths would increase by over 20% and at an increasing age, with the percentage of deaths amongst those aged 85 and over rising from 32% in 2004 to 44% in 2030. The total monetary and quality cost of institutional deaths is expected to rise.

Projections from critical/intensive care experts support the concerns about the emerging clinical crisis and population change. This will mean that either there is an increase in resources to meet this need by increasing traditional capacity models, and/or a different way is required to manage this demand. Multiple independent and dependent factors are involved, such as clinical advances that can prolong life or slow death, ethical decisions about resource allocation combined with economic constraint and market recession, and socio-political factors.

Every reader will have his or her own opinion about which hero first established and embedded QI in health care, whether it be British nurse practice trailblazer Florence Nightingale (Stanley & Sherratt, 2010); early 20th century U.S. hospital reformer Ernest Amory Codman, who pioneered the concept of outcomes management (Codman, 1916); or more modern leaders such as Donald Berwick (2011), founder and former chief executive officer (CEO) of the IHI and champion of evidence-based practice, currently senior fellow at the Center of American Progress.

What is clear is that QI became a science driven by large-scale commercial production in the post-World War II era. Quality Measurement and Production Performance Management has been a powerful tool to supplement the medical model of evidence-based medicine, which tends to be defined and driven through research methodology. It is this same positive and disciplined mentality that is required to meet the huge health and socioeconomic need for changing the way we approach death and improve systems to deliver better the tsunami of EOL care that the statistics predict. Of course, we would never want to make dying a soulless production line; on the contrary, QI can help deliver both savings and improved personalized care.

The Institute of Medicine Principles and Advance Care Planning

Between the health care we have and the care we could have lies not just a gap, but a chasm.

Institute of Medicine, "Crossing the Quality Chasm"

The Institute of Medicine (IOM) is an independent, nonprofit organization in the United States that provides unbiased and authoritative advice to decision makers and the public (see www.iom.edu). Established in 1970, the IOM is the health arm of the National Academy of Sciences, which was chartered under President Abraham Lincoln in 1863.

The IOM claims to ask and answer the nation's most pressing questions about health and health care. The report from the committee on the Quality of Health Care in America made an urgent call for fundamental change to close the quality gap, recommending a redesign of the American health care system, and providing overarching principles for specific direction for policymakers, health care leaders, clinicians, regulators, purchasers, and others.

"To Err Is Human": Building a Safer Health System

"To Err Is Human" (Institute of Medicine, 1999) was a groundbreaking report that brought into sharp reality the harm that health care can cause patients. It stated:

> Health care in the United States is not as safe as it should be and can be. At least 44,000 people, and perhaps as many as 98,000 people, die in hospitals each year as a result of medical errors that could have been prevented, according to estimates from two major studies. Even using the lower estimate, preventable medical errors in hospitals exceed attributable deaths to such feared threats as motor-vehicle wrecks, breast cancer, and AIDS.

It is important to include this report, as it highlights the scale of harm in health care when professionals thought they were delivering good care.

"The Quality Chasm"

"Crossing the Quality Chasm" is a subsequent IOM report (Institute of Medicine, 2001) that describes broader quality issues and defines six aims of quality care: care should be safe, effective, patient centered, timely, efficient, and equitable. This report also presents 10 rules for care delivery redesign.

Table 20.1 summarizes the IOM quality aims and rules for care delivery redesign from the Quality Chasm. These aims and rules are generic and apply to ACP and EOL care. Looking back at these proposed rules, it is timely to review them in the context of ACP and EOL care to highlight the importance of items **2** and **3** (care is effective and is customized according to the needs of the patient, with the patient as the source of control); **4** (knowledge is shared in a timely fashion and information flows freely); **8** (needs are anticipated); and **10** (cooperation among clinicians is a priority).

Improvement Science

Some readers will be familiar with the work of august institutions that promote and support the implementation of improvement science. Research and its methodology are distinct from improvement science. Research is often orientated around summative evaluation and is designed to answer very specific

TABLE 20.1
Crossing the Quality Chasm: A New Health System for the 21st Century
March 1, 2001 Consensus Report IOM

IOM QUALITY AIMS	10 RULES FOR CARE DELIVERY REDESIGN
1. Safe	1. Care is based on continuous healing relationships.
2. Effective	2. Care is customized according to patient needs and values.
3. Patient-centered	3. The patient is the source of control.
4. Timely	4. Knowledge is shared and information flows freely.
5. Efficient	5. Decision making is evidence-based.
6. Equitable	6. Safety is a system property.
	7. Transparency is necessary.
	8. Needs are anticipated.
	9. Waste is continuously decreased.
	10. Cooperation among clinicians is a priority.

IOM, Institute of Medicine.

questions, "Does the treatment work?" QI is orientated to learning how to apply the knowledge in effective systems and often uses formative evaluation. QI also incorporates cultural/social and behavioral factors. Again, these techniques can be used to improve ACP and EOL care. These people or community factors are even more relevant to get people and professionals to treat patients with respect and allow or facilitate communication and engagement in change programs that deliver better ACP and EOL care.

Improvement and the Institute for Healthcare Improvement

The IHI is an international organization based in Cambridge, Massachusetts, that promotes QI science. It builds motivation and will for change, identifies and test new models of care in a partnership approach, and ensures the broadest adoption of best practices and effective innovations. The aims of the IHI are to inspire and train the current and future workforce to be skilled agents of change. Improving EOL care is a priority for the IHI. It is important to discuss their work from both the United States and international perspective.

Figure 20.1 shows the IHI core strategies for driving improvement. This simple figure has been included for those readers preparing for or engaged in leading change to deliver ACP to gain or maintain focus.

The IHI has its own method of working. Figure 20.2 shows how the IHI executes aims that grow from the will to change with defined ideas. These are then described in an aim, which is developed, and tested before disseminating successful programs at large scale.

FIGURE 20.1 Core Strategies for Driving Improvement.

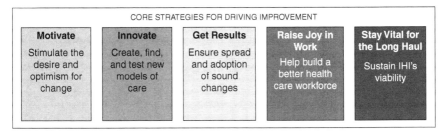

IHI, Institute for Healthcare Improvement.

FIGURE 20.2 The IHI Method of Executing Aims.

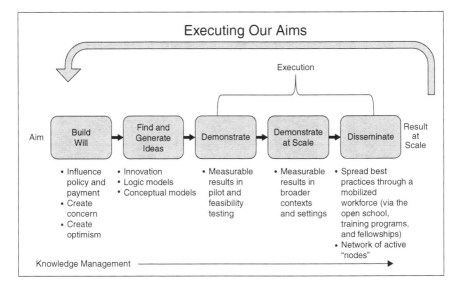

IHI, Institute for Healthcare Improvement.

The IHI describes many of its approaches by building on the prototype (the microlevel—testing out new ideas with small and trusted teams most likely to succeed), then taking to a pilot phase (the meso or organizational level) before large- and rapid-scale implementation (the macro or whole system change through collaborative networks). The system requires the ongoing degree of belief to build in system change reinforced by getting results, hitting the step-wise improvement gains.

The "end of life" is more, much more, than health care, as dying is a predestined human condition and is a social phenomenon within cultural boundaries. Determinants in health care show that there is much to gain from addressing nonmedical factors considered in a social and cultural context. Providing EOL health and social care is highly complex, varies in different societies, and is challenging to change. However, this is not an excuse but a clarion call to people and professionals to get organized and be disciplined about QI and change. In part, this chapter begins to advocate the de-medicalization of dying and the normalization of the inevitable. Despite the will and motivation of patients and their families, significant sections of society have limited choice because of social exclusion as a result of, for example, poverty, illiteracy, war, and famine.

Driver diagrams are promoted by the IHI to help the QI process. They can organize what factors or drivers are important and how they are related. Figure 20.3 is the Driver Diagram created by the IHI for the appropriate utilization of resources for EOL care. This process helps people engaged in QI understand better the limits and opportunities for change in systems or pathways of management.

FIGURE 20.3 IHI Driver Diagram for Appropriate Utilization of Resources at the End of Life.

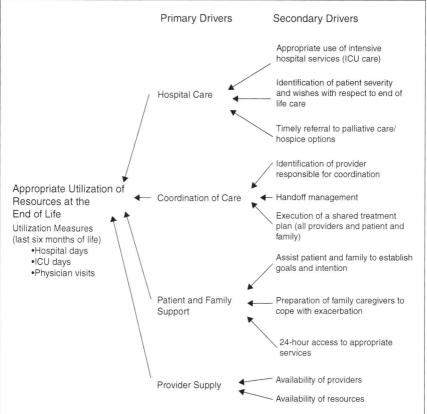

ICU, intensive care unit; IHI, Institute for Healthcare Improvement.

Making Quality Improvement Easier

Leaders need to talk to the front line of care and talk to patients, carers, and staff. They need to understand what future success might look and feel like, then work systematically through their current reality of what goes well and what needs to change. Do the systems they operate work the rubric of: "Who, What, Where, When, How, and With What?" What reliability levels does the service need to operate? Most services don't look at pathways this way. Sometimes people strive for 100% or perfection every time. In non-critical systems, 100% is extremely difficult to achieve and to achieve at an affordable cost when a "reasonable" level of reliability (say 95%) would have been acceptable. In some circumstances positive change and greater reliability requires less complexity rather than more, reducing steps, handovers of care, multiple providers, and repetitive processes. A paradigm shift needs to take place to identify and share what the patient- and family-centered priorities are so that effort and limited resources are focused on key outcomes. This "keep it simple" approach for ACP is vital, as any extra and unwarranted complexity can unnecessarily make a crisis out of a drama. Case or care managers play a vital part in ACP because of the positive impact of care coordination.

Process design must make hard work easier, building in less dependence or necessity on vigilance, removing pointless steps, and stopping futile interventions that can lead to harm. Knowing where QI opportunities relate to the key functions and care delivery will help us get EOL care services right, and the quality outcomes will follow. Classic examples of positive change have been through the improvements delivered by case management, coordination of care providers, unified communication and documentation systems, and effective, efficient clinical navigation. This does not currently happen routinely and at large scale in most health and social care systems. When it does happen and care is planned and coordinated, it dramatically reduces the risks that previously drove the litigation-fearing health care behaviors. This means when treatment is futile, it is stopped and a natural death is allowed to happen, hopefully away from a potentially harmful, and costly, and intensive medical environment in a hospital. A natural death is currently more likely to happen in the United Kingdom in health social care facilities where palliative care is routine and in large care homes (nursing homes) with well-trained staff. It is possible by extrapolation to anticipate that ACP may improve outcomes for community-dwelling older people (Conroy, 2011). The figures included in this section from the IHI and their approach help keep the method simple and increase the chances of achieving QI and LSC.

Figure 20.4 summarizes the model for improvement, which is entirely appropriate to consider in ACP and EOL care. To help implement the model, the three questions noted in the figure must be asked and then answered so

FIGURE 20.4 Model for Improvement.

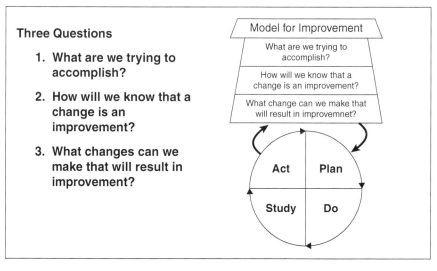

Three Questions

1. What are we trying to accomplish?

2. How will we know that a change is an improvement?

3. What changes can we make that will result in improvement?

Model for Improvement

What are we trying to accomplish?

How will we know that a change is an improvement?

What change can we make that will result in improvemnet?

Act   Plan

Study   Do

SOURCE: *The Improvement Guide*, Langley et al., p. 24.

that specific improvement aims with realistic gains can be achieved for each change or Plan Do Study Act (PDSA) cycle.

Making Quality Improvement Difficult

Change should be from the bottom up or, better described, from where the care is given. Change must be supported by committed leadership and management technique.

Don't make change difficult or, worse still, irrelevant by ignoring the patient and family. Make use of Experience-Based Design techniques with the patient and family as collaborators to initiate ACP programs and drive improvement. The case and method for change can then be properly understood. Not getting the basics right and not achieving clear communication of the benefits to patients and staff multiplies fear, and failures can occur. Usual public fears of change include the fear of the nihilistic cost-cutting exercise; or worse, still as part of a program of euthanasia; and in the extreme, linked to eugenics aimed against the poor, the disabled, the frail, and the elder.

Failure or Success?

Sometimes, despite starting out with the best of intentions, some organizations initiate programs with a "top-down" approach by imposing onto their staff and systems a process in which staff don't believe and on which they can never realistically deliver. Imposing a process without support never works and leads to alienation and disengagement. Not paying close attention to the change process and failing to show discipline make achieving meaningful results unlikely. The lack of accountability and commitment without the guiding force of a champion and senior leadership sponsorship is again a critical failure in project management. The terminal phase of a project comes when there is an irrecoverable loss of trust when people see the approach of failure and start blaming others.

Generating success requires us to consider and use the Seven Leadership Leverage Points for Organization-Level Improvements (Reinertsen, Bisognano, & Pugh, 2008). Start by setting specific system-level aims with less but more meaningful measures monitored by the organization's board of directors. Build an executable strategy to achieve the aims. Channel attention to system-level aims and measures. Get patients and their families on your team. Engage key players often overlooked or not used effectively, such as the Chief Financial Officer, as persons in that position should be interested in what positive results the resources will bring. Engage the front line in achieving the aims, and make them own and be proud of positive change. Build improvement capacity and capability.

I have observed the worst-case scenario even in EOL care initiatives where a regional attempt to design a standardized and uniformly recognized do not attempt cardio pulmonary resuscitation form (DNARCPR in the United Kingdom or DNR in the United States), a great idea, was hijacked by political masters and given to those who are not able to perform QI. This resulted in the failure of this vital initiative when success was required. It added to complexity, with a chance of increasing patient safety risks. It has a wider future impact, as it has now made it so much harder for QI for DNARCPR or related EOL decision-making initiatives at a later date, as well as adding to the general negative sense of de-motivation, loss of will and hope, and disengagement.

IMPLEMENTING LARGE-SCALE CHANGE

The enormity of the English challenge is not too dissimilar to many other populations where needs cannot be met by resources within traditional systems. This challenge requires QI techniques to deliver LSC. In the United Kingdom and some other countries, the individual has high expectations often for free or subsidized health and social care.

There has been significant investment in the U.K. health care system and in palliative and EOL care in the last decade. The evidence of the return on this investment is small in terms of how we currently measure quality and performance. One good example is the relative small reduction in hospital deaths, approximately 2% to 3% over three years in England. Dying at home is preferred by many patients and is a national marker of higher-quality experience if planned and supported well. In order to change this national statistic and, more importantly, health outcomes, we must challenge whether national strategy is achievable, and appreciate that there is a need for the fundamental process and evidence base of delivering LSC and delivering it at pace if in England we are to meet our challenge. While we are making change to improve the quality of EOL care and strengthening ACP, we must ensure that the majority of patients that still die in hospitals must also have improved care. While change brings a rebalance about the mechanism and place of death, we must have a commitment that no matter how and where we find people entering into this state, we look after them and those close to them with dignity, compassion, and respect.

A working definition of LSC is the emergent process of moving a large collection of individuals, groups, and organizations toward a vision of a fundamentally new future state by means of high-leverage key themes, distributed leadership, massive and active engagement of stakeholders, and mutually reinforcing changes in multiple systems and processes, leading to such deep changes in attitudes, beliefs, and behaviors that sustainability becomes largely inherent (Fraser, 2012). LSC has significant pervasiveness to effect whole pathway and system change, depth of thinking causing cognitive and behavioral change to create a paradigm shift, and size impacting on many people.

To fuel such LSC leaders must understand and fuel organizational energy. Organizational energy can be described as the extent to which the leaders of an organization or system are able to put things in motion (change, core initiatives, innovations, etc.) that mobilize the intellectual, emotional, and behavioral potential of the people in the system to pursue its goals. Bruch and Vogel (2011) wrote about how great leaders boost their organization's positive energy and ignite high performance. Bruch and Vogel also describe how to minimize inertia and resignation or complacency (low-energy states) and corrosive (high-negative) energy states.

According to Bruch and Vogel (2011), sustaining LSC requires a proactive approach to managing energy levels, staying focused on altruistic outcomes, and forcefully cut corrosion to help build energized leaders, their teams, and organization. The four energies are intellectual, physical, emotional, and spiritual. The last two energies are often underestimated in unleashing energy but are fundamental in engagement strategies of involving people in and delivering results from change. Emotional and Spiritual energy bring human connection and enhance relationships, and add to the sense of hope and optimism often so important to promote but easily lost in EOL care. The best leaders use this to engage and motivate through simple stories told well. The well-known speech by Martin Luther King, Jr., in 1963 made on the steps of the Lincoln Memorial catalyzed not only the 200,000 civil rights supporters present but a generation for change with his "I have a dream" theme, because he mobilized people by tapping into their emotional and spiritual energy. Let us all have a shared dream that by working together we can drive positive change to deliver better EOL care through ACP.

All organizations, according to Bruch and Vogel (2011), must create an unleashed managed high positive energy by:

- Mobilizing: escaping the complacency trap
- Rebuilding: escaping the corrosion trap
- Focusing: escaping the acceleration trap (where elements run away from plan)
- Sustaining: for the long haul

In the United Kingdom, we are proud of our National Health Services (NHS), which, despite all its failings, still performs well in systematic reviews on quality and cost effectiveness (Schoen et al., 2011). Aneurin Bevan, founder of the NHS said, "Society becomes more wholesome, more serene, and spiritually healthier, if it knows that its citizens have at the back of their consciousness the knowledge that not only themselves, but all their fellows, have access, when ill, to the best that medical skill can provide" (Bevan, 1952, p. 79).

Delivering Higher System Performance

What do we need to change to deliver higher system performance to enable high-quality EOL care?

We are presented with a challenge of engaging with dying patients, families, and professionals to improve systems to identify and treat patients who will gain measureable and, hopefully, longer-lasting benefit. We also need to prevent harm, including not treating those who won't gain treatment benefit, but still deliver good care and allow a natural death. The system must reduce fears of discrimination and lack of patient safety by using transparent decision making and clinical audit to account for all outcomes as part of good governance.

The Conversation Project

This is a contemporaneous example of a wider public engagement strategy in the United States. It is an example of how important an awareness and information-sharing campaign can be in influencing other more specific LSC projects. The Conversation Project, launched in August 2012 by award-winning U.S. journalist Ellen Goodman, seeks to encourage people to have conversations about their preferences for EOL care with people who are close to them. The Conversation Project was launched in collaboration with the IHI, which has also started an initiative called "Conversation Ready" to help health systems and providers gain the skills necessary to elicit patients' and families' EOL preferences, document them, and carry them out. The consequences of this project might include more direct involvement with people/patients in the future planning and design of services that will be needed to meet these objectives. The majority of Americans still die in acute hospital care, sometimes receiving inappropriate, expensive, and potentially harmful treatments such as intensive care or chemotherapy fuelled by fear of litigation and payment systems. Readers are directed to the project website for further information: www.theconversationproject. org. For more about "Conversation Ready," see www.ihi.org/offerings/ Initiatives/ConversationProject/Pages/ConversationReady.aspx.

The Leadership Challenge

If ACP is considered a good and moral thing, how can we get it implemented on a large scale? Having considered many theories and reflected on experiences, the following summary on leadership challenges helps us to consider in this context of how we get started and lead change.

Kabcenell and Conway (2011) describe the key role that executives play in initiatives to honor preferences of patients with advanced illness. There are many programs in the United States that engage in and promote ACP from the early conversation to decisions in the last stages of life, including in sectors of high-cost and high-harm environments such as ICUs. What Kabcenell and Conway describe includes engaging the workforce in new programs of care and new ways of thinking. It is now the expectation certainly in the United Kingdom that clinical leaders in responsible roles in organizations should take charge, lead change, and be accountable. Analysis of the national NHS End-of-Life Care Programme initiatives demonstrates that key clinical leaders are identified and supported by academic, managerial, and administrative staff. Further reflection on these NHS programs unfortunately shows less strength in improvement science, LSC, business skills, or entrepreneurial spirit.

Six Leadership Actions From Kabcenell and Conway

1. *Know Your Organization's Current Performance*

   "Understanding the realities of current practice in your organization concerning advanced illness is essential to charting a course forward. Do staff reliably elicit and respect patient preferences?"

2. *Set Bold and Measurable Aims*

   "Governance and executive leadership should set a bold aim to always honor a patient's preferences at the end of life, providing no more care than desired and no less. Communicate this aim clearly to all staff members and explain why it is important, not only for patients and families but also for the organization."

3. *Prepare People for Success*

"With the expectation set, leaders need to position their staff (including all physicians) to be knowledgeable, competent, and compassionate about the preferences of patients with advanced illness. Palliative care education should be tailored to match the different needs of various types of practitioners (e.g., primary care staff, oncology staff, ICU staff, etc.)."

4. *Establish Systems to Support Effective Care Delivery*

"Training, while important, is insufficient to support respectful practices 100% of the time. Patients, families, and staff need a system they can rely on to reinforce what has been learned."

5. *Create Measures and Accountability*

"Establish specific measures for palliative care programs, and have your organization's leadership team and the board review the data for these measures periodically. While structure and process measures, such as 'access to a palliative care program,' and 'percentage of patients dying at home or in hospice' or 'number of palliative care consults,' are all important, leaders should also track and report patient and family experience outcome measures, including the number of times a patient's state preferences for EOL care are known and carried out correctly."

6. *Remove External Barriers*

"Barriers to effective, respectful care for patients with advanced illness include reimbursement systems that don't cover hospice or palliative care and the absence of systems that enable clinicians to seamlessly address the palliative care needs of patients also receiving curative therapy. As health care executives experiment with provider–payment systems, and other reforms, they should seek to identify mechanisms that support advanced illness planning (ACP) and care delivery. Efforts to improve care transitions and continuity of care across settings can have a huge impact as long as the associated financial requirements are met and incentives are aligned" (pp. 74–76).

Identifying Patients With Particular Needs: The Gold Standards Framework

Some particular patient needs are disease specific. One of the major barriers to the delivery of good-quality EOL care is the fact that people who are approaching the end of their lives are not identified at an early enough stage. Consequently, they and their families are not provided with the support they need. This may lead to poor care provision, inappropriate hospital admissions, preventable suffering, or crisis events. This is a particular problem for patients with non-malignant diseases, frailty, and dementia, as the illness trajectories of such conditions are not as predictable as those of malignant disease.

The Gold Standards Framework (GSF) is a result of a grassroots initiative of primary care providers to improve palliative care in the United Kingdom (Gold Standards Framework, 2012). The GSF Prognostic Indicator Guide was developed by the GSF Central Team to assist generalist clinicians with early identification of people approaching the end stages of their disease process. The guidance provides useful prompts or "triggers" to health care professionals, making them aware that supportive measures for EOL care should be initiated promptly.

Triggers include multiple comorbidity, frailty, and excess mortality: Muscle weakness, bone fragility associated with falls and fractures, malnutrition, delirium, and frailty exacerbated by the risks of recurrent and possibly inappropriate admission to acute hospital services can accelerate death though a range of avoidable physical and psychological harms.

Expert clinicians, especially case managers (often advance practice nurses) and geriatricians, are aware of the inherent risks the older and or frail patient faces. Timely and accurate assessment as part of proactive management or ACP linked with objective critical decision making delivers a higher chance of securing the right outcomes. Individual tools and intervention might have limited impact. Health care decisions that are subject to direct or indirect bias of financial incentives might lead to skewed and unfavorable outcomes too, such as the exclusion of intensive care for an elder where there might have gained benefit because of age discrimination.

Universal Positive Change

U.K.-based systems of integration of health and care delivery systems give some hope for more universal positive change over and above either disease-specific and small-scale initiatives. The basic ingredients remain the same: keep the patient (and family) at the center of what we do and provide good clinical care, a multidisciplinary focus, anticipatory treatment and care decisions, coordination of services, and access to specialist advice and support for the patient and frontline staff.

Informed treatment and care decisions in anticipation of future predicted events can lead to the formulation of legally binding advance directives (ADs) (e.g., advance decisions to refuse treatments). Statutes enshrine the legal principles of autonomy and self-determination of people with mental capacity, even if the decisions they make may seem unwise to others. Advance decision making is not new. The expected benefits of these decisions have had uncertain impact in the United States. In England, the statute is still markedly underutilized and enacted when judged against the expected need of the 1% per year dying. The overarching principles of ACP include ADs that compel health care workers to follow their legally binding decisions. ACP systems must include the structured approach to set patient priorities, including ADs and preferences of where and how to die if we are ever to achieve the IHI's Triple Aim of (a) improving the patient experience of care (including quality and satisfaction); (b) improving the health of populations; and (c) reducing the per capita cost of health care.

The Triple Aim

According to the IHI (2012), Triple Aim "is a framework developed by the IHI that describes an approach to optimizing health system performance. It is IHI's belief that new designs must be developed to simultaneously pursue three dimensions, called the 'Triple Aim'." The Triple Aim is portrayed in Figure 20.5.

The Triple Aim of ACP could be to demonstrate (a) improved health outcomes for patients at the end of their lives in a defined community (including improved clinical decision making with safer and better access to services with more professional/organizational accountability and transparency to the public); (b) enhanced patient experience (the right care at the right time and

FIGURE 20.5 Institute for Healthcare Improvement Triple Aim.

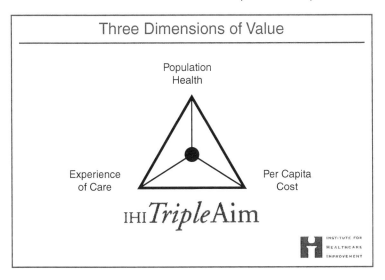

place, avoiding harm); and (c) reduced per capita cost of care supported by the financial alignment of payment systems to promote and deliver ACP.

Author and poet Maya Angelou described one of her perceptions on change as, "the need for change bulldozed a road through the center of my mind." The potential of the Triple Aim to support this case for universal change to improve treatment decisions at the EOL has had the same "bull-dozer" effect on me. The need for change delivered by ACP is to stop futile, expensive, and harmful treatments (e.g., chemotherapy, resuscitation, or intensive care) for people who might want and need a natural, good death in a place they prefer (often their home, avoiding hospitalization). ACP, when done well, has the ability to utilize resources in a different way, improve patient flows and access away from expensive and harmful treat-ment for those who will not gain benefit, supporting a demedicalized and less costly care and death out of hospital. Dignity and privacy for people at the end of their lives is much easier to achieve in a place other than the ER on a gurney. Where there is no AD and/or ACP, doctors sometimes resort to imposing DNARCPR orders too early and not treating the reversible presenting problem or too late, having pursued futile treatment and there-fore causing harm and adding cost. In the United Kingdom, DNARCPR orders are not often supported by proper best interests assessments and are implemented without true accountability. Real fear exists in the United Kingdom that there is excess mortality in Trusts/organizations driven by the bottom line. Patients with capacity have the statutory power to make their own legally binding AD, but the evidence tells us that the majority do not do this often. Doctors too often and too late impose do not attempt resuscitation (DNAR) orders, and in the worst-case scenarios discriminate against the frail and vulnerable.

The Physicians/Medical Orders for Life-Sustaining Treatment (POLST or MOLST) programs in North America in part meet the chal-lenge of better decision making with more accountability. These programs are still yet to prove significant benefit at large scale. The application of improvement science to support a Triple Aim program has the potential to achieve this.

In the United Kingdom, there is no validated standard, audit, or other publicly accountable mechanism for decisions about life-sustaining treat-ment plans. There is no standardized provision for the communication and documentation of clinical decisions that travel with patients across all boundaries (ward to ward, hospital to hospital, county to county). National public inquiries including the Francis Report (2012) have identified signifi-cant concerns about the quality and safety of care, including excess and avoidable harm and mortality of older and vulnerable patients. They call for greater transparency and accountability. This should bring the reader back to the seminal IOM consensus reports on *To Err is Human* (see p. 315 of this chapter).

Kotter's Change Management Tools

Research by leadership guru Dr. John Kotter (Kotter International, 2012) has proven that 70% of all major change efforts in organizations fail. Failure occurs because organizations often do not take the holistic approach required to see the change through. Table 20.2 outlines the Eight-Step Process by Professor Kotter, which helps organizations to avoid failure and become adept at change. By improving their ability to change, organizations can increase their chances of success, both today and in the future. Without this ability to adapt continuously, organizations cannot thrive. It is important for the reader to consider these eight generic steps and relate them to the specific six leadership actions for EOL care set out on page 316 of this chapter.

TABLE 20.2
Eight-Step Process for Leading Change by Dr. John Kotter

1. Establishing a Sense of Urgency
   - Examine market and competitive realities
   - Identify and discuss crises, potential crises, or major opportunities
2. Creating the Guiding Coalition
   - Assemble a group with enough power to lead the change effort
   - Encourage the group to work as a team
3. Developing a Change Vision
   - Create a vision to help direct the change effort
   - Develop strategies for achieving that vision
4. Communicating the Vision for Buy-In
   - Use every vehicle possible to communicate the new vision and strategies
   - Teach new behaviors by the example of the Guiding Coalition
5. Empowering Broad-Based Action
   - Remove obstacles to change
   - Change systems or structures that seriously undermine the vision
   - Encourage the risk-taking and non-traditional ideas, activities, and actions
6. Generating Short-Term Wins
   - Plan for visible performance improvements
   - Create those improvements
   - Recognize and reward employees involved in the improvements
7. Never Letting Up
   - Use increased credibility to change systems, structures, and policies that don't fit the vision
   - Hire, promote, and develop employees who can implement the vision
   - Reinvigorate the process with new projects, themes, and change agents
8. Incorporating Changes Into the Culture
   - Articulate the connections between the new behaviors and organizational success
   - Develop the means to ensure leadership development and succession

CONCLUSION: THE MORAL TEST

This chapter has touched on many areas important in QI to promote and deliver better ACP and EOL care. It has been written by a U.K. health care leader who has had the benefit of time studying the U.S. health care system and the challenges it faces. U.S. clinical leaders tend to promote their optimism and positive belief that they can effect change in some states and health care organizations. This external optimism may well be real and unfettered, or perhaps we must remember the commercial pressure of competing for the patient dollar. It is at this last section of the chapter I would like to introduce the "Moral Test."

Dr. Donald Berwick, the founder and former CEO of the IHI and former Administrator of the Centers for Medicare & Medicaid Services in the United States, presented a keynote speech at the IHI National Forum conference in 2011. He presented his personal view about the approach to and resistance of change he has faced, as well as more public, professional, and political pressures. I have provided an edited excerpt from this address covering key aspects of EOL care. Readers are encouraged to go to the full text available online (Berwick, 2011).

> Cynicism diverts energy from the great moral test. It toys with deception, and deception destroys. Let me give you an example: the outrageous rhetoric about "death panels"—the claim, nonsense, fabricated out of nothing but fear and lies, that some plot is afoot to, literally, kill patients under the guise of end-of-life care. That is hogwash. The truth, of course, is that there are no "death panels" here, and there never have been. The *truth* is that, as our society has aged and as we have learned to care well for the chronically ill, many of us face years in the twilight of our lives when our health fades and our need for help grows and changes. Luckily, palliative care—care that brings comfort, company, and spiritual and emotional support to people with advanced illness and their families—has grown at its best into a fine art and a better science. The principle is simple: that we can and should offer people the very best of care at all stages of their lives, including the twilight. (Berwick, 2011, p. 9)

Berwick recommended five principles to guide efforts to transform our health care system:

1. Put the patient first. Every single deed—every single change—should protect, preserve, and enhance the well-being of the people who need us. That way—and only that way—will we know waste when we see it.

2. Among patients, put the poor and disadvantaged first—those in the beginning, the end, and the shadows of life. Let us meet the moral test.

3. Start at scale. There is no more time left for timidity. Pilots will not suffice. The time has come, to use Göran Henrik's scary phase, to do everything. In basketball, they call it "flooding the zone." It's time to flood the Triple Aim zone.

4. Return the money. This is the hardest principle of them all. Success will not be in our hands unless and until the parties burdened by health care costs feel that burden to be lighter.

5. Act locally. The moment has arrived for every state, community, organization, and profession to act. We need mobilization—nothing less (Berwick, 2011, pp. 22–23).

Clearly Berwick made this speech during the political turmoil of U.S. health care reform, as he was leaving his role as the Administrator of the Centers for Medicare and Medicaid Services. The negativism he was facing included reform to EOL care. His eloquent soliloquy emphasizes the last simple principle "that we can and should offer people the very best of care at all stages of their lives, including the twilight" (Berwick, 2011, p. 9).

Leadership and the Commitment to Change

As a clinical leader driven by my vocation to effect positive change, I use this question at key times to test myself or to help colleagues, "Do you have the commitment, competence, confidence, and clarity of purpose to deliver excellence reliably?" This, I find, is a good way to build will and motivation and be action focused.

Finally, this is my last personal reflection dedicated to all those converted to change management and improvement science: I don't pretend to have all the answers because I haven't finished learning yet. What I do know is that I have the confidence to lead a coalition of passionate believers with the tools of improvement science to make positive change. Most importantly I am not afraid to demand change and get people to do the right thing, do it better and do it for less, and give patients a good death.

REFERENCES

Berwick, D. (2011). The moral test. *Keynote presentation at IHI 23rd Annual National Forum on Quality Improvement in Health Care, December 7.* Retrieved from http://www.ihi.org/knowledge/Pages/Presentations/TheMoralTestBerwickForum2011Keynote.aspx

Bevan A. (1952). *In place of fear.* New York: Simon and Schuster.

Bruch, H. & Vogel, B. (2011). *Fully charged: How great leaders boost their organization's energy and ignite high performance.* Boston Massachusetts: Harvard Business Review Press, 2011 – ISBN 978–1–4221–2903–6.

Codman, E. A. (1916). *A study in hospital efficiency: the first five years*. Boston: Thomas Todd Co.

Committee of Quality of Life in Health Care. (2001). *Crossing the quality chasm: A new health system for the 21st century*. Retrieved from www.nap.edu/html/quality_chasm/reportbrief.pdf

Conroy, S. (2011). End-of-life decisions in acute hospitals. *Clinical Medicine, 11*(4), 364–365.

Edmondson, A. C. (2012). The importance of teaming. *Harvard Business Review* April 25: Foot, M. Aneurin Bevan Vol. 2 1945–1960 London Granada 1975.

Francis Report. (2012). *Robert Francis Inquiry report into Mid-Staffordshire NHS Foundation Trust*. Department of Health. Retrieved from http://www.dh.gov.uk/en/Publicationsandstatistics/Publications/PublicationsPolicyAndGuidance/DH_113018

Fraser, S. (2012). *Leading large scale change*. Retrieved from www.institute.nhs.uk/leading_large_scale_change_homepage.html

Gold Standards Framework. (2013). Gold Standards Framework. National Gold Standards Framework Centre. Retrieved from http://www.goldstandardsframework.org.uk/

Institute for Healthcare Improvement (IHI). (2012). *The IHI triple aim*. Retrieved from http://www.ihi.org/offerings/Initiatives/TripleAim/Pages/default.aspx

Institute of Medicine. (1999). *To err is human: Building a safer health system, November 1, 1999*. Consensus Report Institute of Medicine, Crossing the Quality Chasm. March 1, 2001 Consensus Report.

Kabcenell, A., & Conway, J. B. (2011). End-of-life care: 6 leadership actions. *Healthcare Executive, 26*(1), 74–76.

Kotter, J. (2012). *The 8-step process for leading change*. Kotter International. Retrieved from http://www.kotterinternational.com/our-principles/changesteps/changesteps

National Institute of Health and Clinical Excellence. (2011). *NICE publishes new end of life care quality standard*. Retrieved from http://www.nice.org.uk/guidance/qualitystandards/indevelopment/endoflifecare.jsp

National End of Life Care Intelligence Network. (2009). *End of life care profiles: place of death*. NEoLCIN. place_of death/atlas.html

Pentland, A. (2012). The new science of building great teams. *Harvard Business Review* March 20.

Reinertsen, J. L., Bisognano, M., & Pugh, M. D. (2008). *Seven leadership leverage points for organisational –level improvement in health care* (2nd ed.) IHI Innovation series White Paper.

Schoen, C., Osborn, R., Squires, D., Doty, M. M., Pierson, R., & Applebaum, S. New (2011, November 9). Survey of patients with complex care needs in 11 countries finds that care is often poorly coordinated. *Health Affairs* Web First.

Stanley, D. D., & Sherratt, A. A. (2010). Lamp light on leadership: Clinical leadership and Florence Nightingale. *Journal of Nursing Management, 18*(2), 155–121.

CHAPTER 21

Advance Care Planning as a Public Health Issue

Allan Kellehear

Advance care directives often ask too much of the people who should be making them. The usefulness of making advance care directives is commonly eroded by the widespread lack of understanding about death, dying, and health care in the wider community beyond health care services. In this chapter, I argue that no health care movement in favor of advance care directives can push this separate from an equal momentum around a public health approach to EOL care that promotes and supports death education in the community. In this way, community learning about death, dying, and care is as fundamental to EOL care planning as community learning about health, fitness, and well-being is to health care planning. Understanding this linkage between advocacy of the policy and its adoption and actual practice by communities is crucial to the success and sustainability of advance care planning. Acknowledgment of the linkage between death education and the empowerment of individuals and families to make *informed* plans for the EOL is crucial to any future campaign to promote advance care planning (ACP) as a sustainable, nonthreatening, and community-friendly practice.

WHAT DOES ADVANCE CARE PLANNING ASK OF US?

In basic terms, advance care directives are the formalizing of our plans for what treatments we wish to have—or not have—when we near death. They can be negative statements such as advanced wishes/expectations about

333

what treatments we will refuse to have (e.g., resuscitation, artificial ventilation, or artificial feeding), or they can be more positive preferences about
what we would like to experience or receive while near death (e.g., a preference to die at home if possible, or a preference for treatments to keep us
"comfortable" or pain free) (Seymour & Horne, 2011; Thomas, 2011). These
plans can be informal, that is, written literally as preferences to be shared
with one's family physician or residential care staff at a nursing home; or
they can be more formal, as they might be when completing a "living will";
and legal as when witnessed, notarized, and/or written with legal counsel
and support with provisions made for a lasting power of attorney. Either
way, such provisions help prepare health care staff, families, and individual
patients for future personal incapacity and/or dying.

To participate in the kinds of decisions, preferences, and planning
about anticipated medical and health services matters near one's death,
advance care planning requires certain basic social conditions and/or
knowledge from all of those who would participate in this process. Most
of the challenges to ACP are discussed earlier in this book but I will remind
readers of the broad outline of their technical and sociological features for
the purposes of providing a context for the role of public health activism
in this area.

First and foremost, there must be a personal and family *willingness to
discuss matters of death, dying, and EOL care*—a requirement that has associated with it a long- discussed series of cultural, religious, and social barriers. Academic and clinical commentators have long observed how difficult,
even taboo, the subject of death and dying has been to most Western societies, including the United States (DeSpelder & Strickland, 2009; Howarth,
2007). The obsession with medical rescue has made personal discussions
about death and dying, or hospice and palliative care, commonly associated in the public mind with medical failure, the loss of hope, and social
abandonment (DeSpelder & Strickland, 2009; Kaufman, 2005).

The second major requirement of ACP asks of all those who participate in its process an understanding of the possible health service and
medical treatments commonly associated with your own possible future.
These will differ widely depending on whether one is anticipating a dying
from cancer, motor neuron disease, AIDS, or multiple strokes in a nursing home. The medical crises associated with a catastrophic motor vehicle
accident, head injuries from falls or gunshot wounds, or from accidental
or intentional poisoning are often a mystery to most people, and there are
not always disease-related support associations available to help patients
or families navigate the different possible scenarios. The medical and sociological technicalities surrounding determination of brain death are also difficult, not to say inaccessible, to most people in the general community. Yet
a basic understanding of these is crucial in making plans for any advanced
care, particularly in medical circumstances of trauma. In general, there is a

woeful lack of public understanding about life-extending, life-saving, and palliative treatments and the differences and inter-related nature of all three (Mason, Sives, & Murray, 2011).

Third, the cyclical nature of dying in modern societies makes any ultimate determination of what to do when "dying" or "near death" uncertain and contingent (Kellehear, 2007). In a context of chronic, life-threatening, or life-limiting illness, how is one to determine when one should accept "dying" or not? When is the "right time" to "let go" for patients and or their families? Do the decisions one makes when in comparative health remain relevant when one is in severe pain, anxiety, or away from one's family home? People often change their minds about inheritance as they grow older, for example, or as relationships change and evolve through different friendships, marriages, and work circumstances. The same is true of what one would wish to happen in poor health when one remains in good health. Things change, sometimes by the month, in one's view of what one would *like to happen or not happen* in anticipation of a collapse of personal health and well-being. How is one to decide in circumstances that are regularly changing? (Seymour & Horne, 2011, p. 21). Some philosophers take this idea of the continuity of personal identity, experience, and decision making even further by asking: In what sense is the brain-dead person still the person who originally made the advance care directive? How are we to understand the continuity of "personhood" in the presence of subsequent severe neurological damage such as occurs in dementia or brain trauma? (Buchanan, 2007; George & Harlow, 2011). *a deeply personal determination...*

Finally, the push for advance care directives (promoting autonomy, planning, and choices) without general education about death and dying (knowing what the social, spiritual, or psychological alternatives and possibilities are) is like asking people to choose to eat better (autonomy, planning, and wise choices) when they don't understand what's in the daily food products they are buying (knowing what the alternatives are) (Watson, 2011). The public understanding of what being in a coma is like, or what dying from cancer is like in the final 24 hours, or what the final hours of dying from motor neuron disease is like is mostly slim to nothing (Kellehear, 2008).

The different challenges underlying ACP are both sociological (the reluctance to publicly and personally engage in discussions about death, dying, and care; diverse ethnic and religious understandings and preferences around individual autonomy and dignity; different understandings about personal identity and continuity) and technical (different treatment options and their differing purposes and consequences). *Both* sociological and technical forms of these challenges are public health challenges—not simply for health care institutions, but for everyone. Just as health care is not solely the responsibility of the unwell or ill but also the healthy and the well, so too, death, dying, and care are the responsibility of everyone, not simply those who are old or at risk of injury or life-threatening illnesses such as cancer or HIV. Just as "healthy communities" rely on community education to make decisions about diet, exercise, avoidance of harmful substances and circumstances, as well as the protective value of certain technologies (seat belts, bicycle helmets, condoms, etc.), so too a public health education approach to death, dying, and care places public discussion about ACP squarely in the domain of a broader death education context.

It is quite common to overlook death education as a public health concern, with many clinical and academic colleagues viewing this as a specialized form of raising awareness about grief and loss and of principle interest only among "thanatologists" or counselors. However, death education is more than "raising awareness" and it addresses wider topics than simply "grief and loss." The problem of mortality goes to the heart of living with all forms of life-threatening or life-limiting illness, living with grief, and long-term care for all these kinds of people. Death education in this way is a broad population health issue because few people are not untouched by cancer, serious accident and trauma, aging and dementia, suicide, or grief, and far greater numbers of people are also actively involved in their care as family, friends, coworkers, or neighbors. As a population health matter, death education as a form of health promotion has a number of important harm-reduction and prevention targets that are quite specific and relevant to engaging publics in their own EOL care decision making and planning.

THE PUBLIC HEALTH ROLES OF DEATH EDUCATION IN SUPPORTING ADVANCE CARE PLANNING

✗ *Normalizing death education*

Like all public health campaigns for weight loss, smoking cessation, or workplace safety, a public health approach to death, dying, loss, and care encourages a normalization of discussion and support for these matters in the wider community. As part of the push to normalize topics about mortality, health education and community engagement practices commonly target procrastination, apathy, stigma, and superstition around all matters that erode good health and well-being: in other words, they can and should target community barriers toward openness in matters to do with death if these experiences erode good health and well-being. People living with life-threatening or life-limiting illness should not be precluded from efforts toward keeping them healthy or restoring well-being any more than we currently do for people living with disabilities.

Current community engagement practices in death education are designed to minimize or reduce fear and anxiety around death, dying, loss, and care and can limit its negative social, psychological, and spiritual

Treating death awareness much as health awareness has been handled

outcomes. For ACP, this can provide a broader and more "usual" context for discussions about EOL care. The "shocking," "morbid," or "distasteful" dimension of discussing matters to do with death and loss for many people can be eroded by placing these discussions in a broader and more widely accepted context. In this way, the specific topic of advanced care planning is given a "healthy" context. The discussion is couched in terms of future well-being.

This achievement is created by building on, consolidating, and linking personal experiences of death, dying, loss, and care with wider community experiences of these verities to strengthen the support capacity of both. This is commonly called "capacity building"—building a capacity for resilience and support that is sustainable because it relies on ordinary members of the community and not simply health services.

Furthermore, making death, dying, loss, and care a key part of the usual health promotion activities of any community provides a context to the more problem-focused image of death, dying, loss, and care. Just as "health" is now widely viewed as more than "avoidance of illness," so too death, dying, loss, and care might be viewed as more than "tragic problems" and their creative and positive confrontation viewed instead as part of building personal well-being and resilience. This will encourage the maximizing of personal and community sources of hope, as well as personal control and social support. At the same time, such health-promoting ideas about death, dying, loss, and care may help combat ignorance and superstition as they enhance informed choices.

Just as health education and community engagement programs mobilize and maximize family, community, and workplace supports and reorient them to what they can do to keep each other healthy, so too this kind of approach to death and loss can reorient a culture of denial toward a culture of acknowledgment and support for life's commonplace and universal losses. It may do so by fostering an openness toward personal troubles in the face of mortality and this, in turn, can encourage individuals, institutions, and communities to learn more about the technical complexities of living and dying in medical contexts. In all these public health roles, death education becomes a population health approach that builds on existing health education and community engagement strategies for health promotion for other health topics. Because the strategies are identical, the goals are also the same—to not only change social attitudes but also the behaviors and qualities of experiences at the EOL. Like all modern public health campaigns, the pursuit of death education programs in the community seeks to create social changes that promote healthy behaviors; reduce or prevent physical, social, and psychological harms; and maximize well-being and resilience in the face of death, dying, loss, and long-term care. I review some examples and briefly summarize some of their achievements below.

What a hopeful vision!

[Handwritten margin notes: "Changing the attitudes + avoidance of death + replacing it + processing it w/ actively acknowledging it." "Challenging Publics"]

A HEALTH PROMOTION AND COMMUNITY ENGAGEMENT CONTEXT FOR ADVANCE CARE PLANNING

Public health approaches to death, dying, loss, and EOL care—employing "new" public health ideas such as health promotion and community development—have been increasingly popular internationally (see Cohen & Deliens, 2012; Conway, 2011; Monroe & Oliviere, 2007; Sallnow, Kumar, & Kellehear, 2012). These approaches also have their advocates in the United States (see Rao, Anderson, & Smith, 2002; Rao et al., 2005). The social philosophy behind public health strategies is principally to "normalize" care in the contexts of death, dying, loss, and care for carers, and to build community capacity for resilience inside these experiences. By encouraging the major social institutions—schools, workplaces, churches/temples, or local media—to take some small responsibility for care in these areas, ordinary community members gain a greater capacity for understanding, caring, and resilience about death, dying, and loss while at the same time minimizing their own shock, trauma, or avoidance responses. *These contexts promote responsiveness, active compassion, openness, and resilience toward difficult but regularly occurring death-related events and experiences.*

In Australia (Kellehear & O'Connor, 2008) many "health-promoting" palliative care services have created partnerships with schools and workplaces to develop school- or workplace-based policies on death, dying, and loss. Such policies help create structured or formal responses to unexpected serious illness, death, or bereavement, and encourage whole systems such as schools or workplaces to react formally with support. Like policies for health and safety, policies for death, dying, loss, and care encourage everyone to publicly acknowledge the health and well-being of all workers or all students, teachers, and parents, and under the rubric of the policy, create a safe environment for support, resilience, and openness. It's okay to speak openly about serious illness, death, loss, and the difficulties of caring in these matters. Workplace and school policies publicly endorse and encourage care. *[Handwritten: A marked contrast to my work exp]*

In Japanese villages, shops in the main business district help share the burden of respite care for families living with dementia (100-Member Committee, 2012). Businesses have volunteered to provide and share short-term "minding" of ambulant people living with dementia with other businesses, temples, or public associations to relieve families and share this responsibility with existing health and social care providers. This public recognition and sharing of respite care is also part of other programs on "wandering-senior safety networks"—a network of neighbors and businesses who take it upon themselves to look out for wandering seniors who appear lost.

Other dementia-friendly programs bring young people at school in close relationship with people living with dementia by including people living with dementia in their sports day organization and management, or by encouraging seniors with dementia to provide street safety patrols for the purposes of watching over children traveling to and from schools. These kinds of programs allow *all* people to gain greater insight and understanding of dementia and the complexities of care. These community programs break down the common isolation of not only seniors living with dementia but also the families that care for them. Talk about dementia and dementia care becomes ordinary, routine, and open, and stigma and embarrassment are minimized or banished all together.

Towns in India partner with local palliative care services to share and participate in EOL care (Kumar, 2012). Housewives, lawyers, university teachers, taxi drivers, builders, school children, or police volunteer their time to a "neighborhood network" that provides transport services and needed medical supplies to patients and their families. People from all walks of life commit a certain amount of their time to a "time bank" for the neighborhood network—sometimes just a couple of hours per week, up to several days per week, depending on occupation and personal preferences. In these ways, living with dying and living with loss evolves to become a shared and public experience. The isolation of private grief, the burden of complex care, the difficulties of arranging transport to services, or even the high costs of needed drugs, is shared by these communities of "neighbors." Death, dying, loss, and care become everyone's responsibility.

In the Republic of Ireland and the United Kingdom, local palliative care services have developed "compassionate communities" to raise awareness and encourage participation in matters to do with death, dying, loss, and care (Conway, 2012; Kellehear, 2005). Just as "healthy cities/communities" encourage multisector community support for health and well-being by endorsing or engaging in healthy activities for a community, so too "compassionate community" programs encourage people to participate in support experiments and projects around death, dying, loss, and care—from public ceremonies around memorialization, to "trivial pursuit" game nights at pubs where most of the questions and answers relate to "death & dying," to book clubs that encourage reading of first-person accounts of serious illness or loss. Other examples include libraries that place helpful suggestions on the back of their regularly printed, free bookmarks on how to support friends and families living with loss; art or short-story writing competitions about living with a life-threatening or life-limiting illness, living with loss, or living as long-term carer; and arranging and promoting annual "open days" at local funeral businesses or hospices.

All these above examples employ mainstream health promotion, health education, and community development theory and interventions for the promotion of health and well-being for those living with life-threatening or life-limiting illness and bereavement, as well as all those who care for them. Care for everyone touched by serious illness or loss becomes shared. Awareness of the fragility of life becomes a regular and "normal" remembered experience. Discussions about will-making or advanced care directives in this wider context become a non-threatening topic of conversation that is both meaningful and relevant for the volunteer work, school experience, or workplace policy in which they are currently involved and engaged. Topics such as advance care planning become topics of concern that are included seamlessly into other—and now related—community activities that have a similar role and purpose.

These broad experiences—coming as they do from key social institutions in their community—act as "early interventions" in the service of prevention and harm reduction strategies that alter and reshape the social and cultural environment to promote a greater awareness and participation context. This altered context in turn promotes a more open, relaxed, less threatening, and more receptive context for discussion and activities for topics such as advance care planning.

HOW PUBLIC HEALTH CONTEXTS ADDRESS CHALLENGES AND BARRIERS TO ADVANCE CARE PLANNING

A broad-based health promotion and community development focus on death, dying, loss, and care is able to address the different challenges and barriers to ACP by providing a sustained and sustainable interest in preparing for personal trouble and grief. A concerted health promotion approach to death, dying, loss, and care, one that involves a long-term partnership between health services and key community institutions, has demonstrated a capability in breaking the taboo on the topic of death. By making concerns about serious illness, loss, or long-term care the subject of community policies in schools and workplaces, by interesting the local media in stories of personal and community resilience, and by encouraging the reduction of personal isolation during illness and care, ACP simply starts to make "common" sense. Such a context robs superstitions and fears about death of their common surprise, shock, or "morbid" appearance, allowing these topics to be assimilated into routine community and personal discussions of health and wellness. ⟨Normalizing conversations + support for each other around death⟩

Second, a community interested in addressing the support needs of people living with serious illness, loss, or long-term care will inevitably and invariably learn more about what these experiences entail. At the same time, they will be able to compare and contrast their own personal and cultural experiences of illness and care with those of others. They will gain comparative social and ethical perspective and a deeper understanding of social, religious, and cultural diversity in the face of mortality.

Third, at the same time as these communities become familiar with other people's experiences of illness and loss, they will also learn more about the technical aspects of those experiences. Less confined to one-off learning experiences associated with themselves and their wider family, their own families will learn of the diseases and treatment regimes that effect other families and their struggles with illness, medical crises and decision making, or home care.

With an ever-widening potential to learn about the verities of death and dying, there will come a "naturally occurring" demand for more information about life-threatening or life-limiting illness beyond the usual life-saving information most people seek. The complexities about the determination of death, the economic arguments for and against indefinite treatments, and the vested interests and social needs behind vacating intensive care beds or of organ transplant campaigns might be discussed more openly and be subject to greater media attention and public debate.

A community interested in increasing supports for people living with serious illness, loss, and long-term care will learn or demand to learn the major EOL scenarios and care choices available for themselves and their families. The differences between intensive care dying, hospice dying, home care dying, or nursing home dying will be important to know, as well as what treatments to expect in those contexts. However, this interest and demand for more information and learning will not be a one-way street. Health services and their individual practitioners might also expect similar learning at their end of the health promotion and community development partnership.

Partnering with schools, workplaces, public media, recreation clubs, or church and temple groups will also provide health care professionals insights and awareness of the plurality and diversity of EOL care preferences and related concepts of autonomy and dignity that exist within their own health service catchment area. For many professionals, this might mean learning first hand that many preferences are *not* the result of superstitions or fears but rather different (and legitimate) outcomes of clear and autonomous decision making from different religious, cultural, or social beliefs. This is a realization that might lead to the further realization that ACP, for example, is for a limited few (however large the actual numbers) or that such planning may need to target groups and families rather than individuals.

For other health care professionals and services, community partnerships may raise awareness of the very significant challenges in informing publics of the different clinical purposes of the same or similar medical, pharmacological, or nursing interventions at the EOL. Such public education challenges bring with them not only challenges of explaining the complex in accessible ways but also the challenges of language/jargon translation and understanding the diversity of public audience education levels and ethical values systems. Effective public education campaigns in smoking cessation or healthy dietary promotion have also usually required non–health service allies such as local media services and service clubs. If the local health service does not have existing links or networks in these kinds of information and social systems, this too will become an apparent need during any community partnership that places death, dying, loss, and care at the center of its service approach.

Finally, community partnerships in health promotion as outlined above can also be valuable and important to closing the gap between health services and the general public expectations and information about what to expect at the EOL. The more this gap is reduced between health services and the general public during times of health and well-being, the greater the chances of better communication, cooperation, and support for the work of health services during times of serious illness and crisis. At the same time, this helps reduce misunderstanding, ignorant and hostile responses, and poor attention to each other's needs (patients, families, and health care staff) during times of formal care and aftercare.

Overall, providing a broad health promotion and community development context for ACP ensures not only cooperation and willing interest, but most importantly, sustainable and genuine community buy-in. This provides a firmer basis for both commitment and informed choice, making ACP a true partnership with health care services rather than a policy imposition by what might otherwise be negatively viewed as a self-interested health care culture. What must American public health interests do in order to mentor these kinds of directions in their health services?

THE CHALLENGE OF FACING DEATH FOR AMERICAN PUBLIC HEALTH

The Ottawa Charter for Health Promotion (1986) has been adopted and promoted by the World Health Organization for over 25 years now. Its charter of principles is as relevant and important today as ever: To build public policies that support health; to create supportive environments; to strengthen community actions for their own health; to help people to develop their own personal health-promoting skills; to reorient health services from solely focusing on cures and encourage them to help with prevention, harm reduction, and early intervention. Prevention is always better than cure.

Furthermore, health promotion is everyone's responsibility—not simply hospitals and health services. The promotion of health is a community task not simply for the ill, but also the well who will eventually become ill or vulnerable. Any health promotion activity must be participatory—not imposed by health services. For communities to "own" and "take responsibility" for their own health, health services must work *with* and *not on* their communities. Education is important, but that education must be a result of a felt-need by communities and not simply a result of health services preaching to patients and families.

All these principles of health promotion apply to death, dying, loss, and long-term care. We now need to build public policies that support health and well-being at the EOL. Supportive environments need to be created—not simply hospice and nursing homes—but also inside schools and workplaces too—wherever people grow old, experience serious illness or loss, or wherever people who care for those latter people are to be found. In these matters, community actions need strengthening and personal skills enhancement. Above all, health services that now view death and dying as someone else's responsibility (e.g., viewing mainly hospices or residential aged care services as the services who take this type of lead) need to reorient themselves to understand the important role they too can play to promote well-being at the EOL. Prevention is always better than cure, and for matters of death and loss this means addressing these concerns and verities *before* they arise.

For U.S. public health, this means that there must be formal national recognition by the American Public Health Association (APHA), from all their clinical and academic membership, that U.S. public health has an important and unique role to play in matters to do with death, dying, loss, and care. Alongside other recognized public health priorities such as the national reduction of drug and alcohol use, obesity, accident and injury, and environmental hazards must come a recognition of the role public health can play in reducing the morbidities and mortalities associated with living with life-threatening or life-limiting illness, loss, and long-term care. The traditional public health concern with health inequalities should also encompass how this problem continues to manifest at the EOL. Death should not continue to be viewed as a failure of public health. We should continue to wage our war on illness, disability, and unnecessary deaths but only in the context of a broader human acceptance of the inevitability of death and the universality of loss in every human and animal life cycle. Eventually, all living things die.

There should be formal recognition, better national identification, and greater public education efforts about the morbidities (e.g., stigma, loss, depression, social rejection) and mortalities (e.g., suicide) associated with living with a life-threatening/limiting illness, loss and grief, and long-term care. This information should be part of the development of national policies that recognize that these troubles *are* amenable to prevention and harm-reduction strategies. We do *not* have to leave these matters to health professions and services alone. There is much useful work we can do as communities and as communities in partnership with our health care services. Early interventions for social and health difficulties, including those associated with the EOL, are possible and necessary. ACP will be a natural outcome of these kinds of community concerns, policies, and actions.

There should be recognition that the commonly observed procrastination, antipathy, and outright fear that often underlie poor or absent ACP is rooted in a broader, deeper cultural malaise and anxiety around death and loss. This is a public health matter that goes straight to the heart—not only to the human confrontation with mortality—but also human well-being and the sociological basis of human caring itself. To promote and encourage communities to participate in ACP without a broader conversation about mortality is no less than missing the forest for the trees—a narrow and decontextualized approach to health care always doomed to partial success at best. The task of promoting ACP, and the freedoms and opportunities that such planning can offer to all those who participate, cannot be enjoyed and understood separate from the related freedoms and opportunities that will ultimately come from liberating ourselves from our longstanding, traditional fear of death itself.

REFERENCES

Buchanan, A. (2007). Advance directives and the personal identity problem. In M. P. Batten, L. P. Francis, & B. M. Landesman (Eds.), *Death, dying and the ending of life* (Vol. 1, pp. 173–198). Aldershot, UK: Ashgate.

Cohen, J., & Deliens, L. (Eds.) (2012). *A public health perspective on end of life care*. Oxford, UK: Oxford University Press.

Conway, S. (Ed.). (2011). *Governing death and loss: Empowerment, involvement, and participation*. Oxford, UK: Oxford University Press.

Conway, S. (2012). Public health developments in palliative care services in the UK. In L. Sallnow, S. Kumar, & A. Kellehear (Eds.), *International perspectives on public health and palliative care* (pp. 85–97). Oxford, UK: Routledge.

DeSpelder, L., & Strickland, A. (2009). *The last dance: Encountering death and dying* (8th ed.). New York, NY: McGraw-Hill.

George, R., & Harlow, T. (2011). Advance care planning: Politically correct, but ethically sound? In K. Thomas & B. Lobo (Eds.), *Advance care planning in end of life care* (pp. 55–69). Oxford, UK: Oxford University Press.

Howarth, G. (2007). *Death and dying: A sociological introduction*. Cambridge, UK: Polity.

Kaufman, S. R. (2005). *And a time to die: How American hospitals shape the end of life*. Chicago, IL: University of Chicago Press.

Kellehear, A. (2005). *Compassionate cities: Public health and end-of-life care*. Oxford, UK: Routledge.

Kellehear, A. (2007). *A social history of dying*. Cambridge, UK: Cambridge University Press.

Kellehear, A. (2008). Dying as a social relationship: A sociological review of debates on the determination of death. *Social Science & Medicine, 66*(7), 1533–1544.

Kellehear, A., & O'Connor, D. (2008). Health-promoting palliative care: A practice example. *Critical Public Health, 18*(1), 111–115.

Kumar, S. (2012). Public health approaches to palliative care: the Neighborhood Network in Kerala. In L. Sallnow, S. Kumar, & A. Kellehear (Eds.), *International perspectives on public health and palliative care* (pp. 98–109). Oxford, UK: Routledge.

Mason, B., Sives, D., & Murray, S. A. (2011). Advance care planning in the community. In K. Thomas & B. Lobo (Eds.), *Advance care planning in end of life care* (pp. 148–157). Oxford, UK: Oxford University Press.

Monroe, B., & Oliviere, D. (Eds.). (2007). *Resilience in palliative care: Achievement in adversity*. Oxford, UK: Oxford University Press.

100-Member Committee. (2012). The campaign to build a dementia-friendly community. In L. Sallnow, S. Kumar, & A. Kellehear (Eds.), *International perspectives on public health and palliative care* (pp. 123–138). Oxford, UK: Routledge.

Ottawa Charter for Health Promotion (1986). Retrieved from http://www.who.int/healthpromotion/conferences/previous/ottawa/en/

Rao, J. K., Alongi, J., Anderson, L. A., Jenkins, L., Stokes, G. A., & Kane, M. (2005). Development of public health priorities for end of life initiatives. *American Journal of Preventive Medicine, 29*(5), 453–460.

Rao, J. K., Anderson, L. A., & Smith, S. M. (2002). End of life is a public health issue. *American Journal of Preventive Medicine, 23*(3), 215–220.

Sallnow, L., Kumar, S., & Kellehear, A. (Eds.) (2012). *International perspectives on public health and palliative care*. Oxford, UK: Routledge.

Seymour, J., & Horne, G. (2011). Advance care planning for end of life: An overview. In K. Thomas & B. Lobo (Eds.), *Advance care planning in end of life care* (pp. 16–27). Oxford, UK: Oxford University Press.

Thomas, K. (2011). Overview and introduction to advance care planning. In K. Thomas & B. Lobo (Eds.), *Advance care planning in end of life care* (pp. 3–15). Oxford, UK: Oxford University Press.

Watson, M. (2011). Spiritual aspects of advance care planning. In K. Thomas & B. Lobo (Eds.), *Advance care planning in end of life care* (pp. 45–54). Oxford, UK: Oxford University Press.

PART V

Selected Resources on Advance Care Planning and End-of-Life Care

Leah Rogne
Susana Lauraine McCune

This chapter includes selected resources on advance care planning (ACP) and end-of-life (EOL) care, including selected state and national initiatives, professional associations, books, and journals, as well as items of general interest. It is not intended to be inclusive but rather to point to a growing array of resources currently available on EOL decision making and care. Readers should be aware that web links are subject to change.

NATIONAL INITIATIVES

Aging With Dignity

Resources, action, and advocacy to promote better care at EOL. Promotes "Five Wishes," a popular guide to communicating about EOL care and preparing advance directives (ADs). Documents translated into 24 languages. Includes Voicing My Choice: A Planning Guide for Adolescents and Young Adults, a guide to help young persons living with serious illness communicate their preferences.

www.agingwithdignity.org

American Bar Association

Consumer's and Lawyer's Tool Kits on ACP, emphasizing conversations with clients. Includes a Proxy Quiz to assess the agent's knowledge of the principal's wishes.
www.americanbar.org/groups/law_aging/resources/health_care_decision_making.html

Americans for Better Care of the Dying

Dedicated to improving EOL care, including building momentum for reform, exploring new models and systems for delivering care, and shaping public policy through evidence-based understanding.
abcd-caring.org

Caring Connections

A program of the National Hospice and Palliative Care Organization (NHPCO); national consumer and community engagement initiative to improve care at the EOL. Has provided more than 1.3 million ADs to individuals free of charge since 2004. Links to download ADs for each state.
www.caringinfo.org/i4a/pages/index.cfm?pageid=1

Caring Conversations (Center for Practical Bioethics)

Provides a booklet and other resources designed to help guide individuals and families through the process of ACP.
www.practicalbioethics.org/resources/caring-conversations.html

Center to Advance Palliative Care (Robert Wood Johnson Foundation)

Palliative care tools, education, resources, and training for health care professionals.
www.capc.org

Centers for Disease Control and Prevention

Information on ACP; online course for professionals.
www.cdc.gov/Features/AdvancedCarePlanning

Coalition to Transform Advanced Care

Promoting best practices in care for advanced illness. Education for the public and professionals, creating policy change.
advancedcarecoalition.org

Compassion and Choices

Provides education and advocacy to change attitudes, practices, and policies to assure patients' rights and provide choices related to EOL. Chapters throughout the United States.

www.compassionandchoices.org

Consider the Conversation

One-hour video produced by Rainbow Hospice Foundation (Jefferson, Wisconsin) that promotes communication about EOL choices. Links and resources, including podcasts on conversations about EOL.

www.considertheconversation.org

The Conversation Project

Collaboration including columnist Ellen Goodman, the Institute for Healthcare Improvement, and other leaders to encourage conversations about dying, death, and EOL care. Provides a "Starter Kit" to facilitate conversation and features real-life stories of persons dealing with death and dying.

theconversationproject.org

Conversation Ready

Initiative of the Institute for Healthcare Improvement to give health systems and providers the skills to communicate with patients and families about EOL preferences and to document and carry out their wishes.

www.ihi.org/offerings/Initiatives/ConversationProject/Pages
/ConversationReady.aspx

Dying Well

Website for Dr. Ira Byock, author and palliative care physician. Includes free "Assessment and Outcome Measure for Palliative Care," which helps assess quality of life for persons experiencing life-threatening illness.

www.dyingwell.org

Education in Palliative and End-of-Life Care

Develops curricula and training products, including distance learning, in palliative and EOL care.

www.epec.net

End-of-Life Nursing Education Consortium (ELNEC), American Association of Colleges of Nursing

National education initiative to improve palliative care. The project provides undergraduate and graduate nursing faculty; continuing education providers; staff development educators; specialty nurses in pediatrics, oncology, critical care, and geriatrics; and other nurses with training in palliative care so they can teach this essential information to nursing students and practicing nurses.
www.aacn.nche.edu/elnec

Five Wishes Online

Step-by-step guide for completing an AD using popular "Five Wishes" model; initiative of Aging with Dignity.
fivewishesonline.agingwithdignity.org

Hospice Foundation of America

Discussion and explanation of ACP and documents.
www.hospicefoundation.org/advancecare

International Palliative Care Initiative (Open Society Foundations)

List of International Palliative Care Initiative Grants.
www.opensocietyfoundations.org/about/programs/public-health-program/grantees/international-palliative-care-initiative-grants-0

Institute of Medicine

Has convened Committee on Transforming End-of-Life Care to examine the current state of EOL care with respect to delivery of medical care and social support; patient–family–provider communication of values and preferences; ACP; health care cost, financing, and reimbursement; and education of health professionals, patients, and their loved ones.
www.iom.edu/Activities/Aging/TransformingEndOfLife.aspx

Life and Death Matters

Teaching resources, online newsletter, and online training and courses in hospice and palliative care.
www.lifeanddeathmatters.ca

Making Your Wishes Known (American Geriatrics Society)

Provides guidelines for legal and ethical decision making, including ACP.
www.healthinaging.org/making-your-wishes-known

MediCaring Project

Working to improve the health care system for people living with serious and chronic conditions. Includes Action Guides for care transitions.
medicaring.org

Project on Death in America (Open Society Foundations)

Report on Project on Death in America, 2001–2003.
www.opensocietyfoundations.org/reports/project-death-america-january-2001-december-2003-report-activities

Talk Early Talk Often

Website of Rev. Dale Susan Edmonds on dealing with aging parents, including talking about EOL decision making.
www.talk-early-talk-often.com

Your Life Your Choices (Veterans Affairs Health Services Research and Development Service)

Comprehensive booklet and planning guide for future medical decisions.
www.innovations.ahrq.gov/content.aspx?id=795

STATE OR REGIONAL INITIATIVES

British Columbia (Canada)

Fraser Health
Coaching on how to start a conversation with family, videos, and resources for ACP.
www.fraserhealth.ca/your_care/advance-care-planning

California

Center for Healthcare Decisions
Provides educational materials, trainings, and policy recommendations to help to implement new EOL policies and practices.
chcd.org/what-endoflife.htm

Coalition for Compassionate Care of California
A statewide partnership of regional and statewide organizations, state agencies, and individuals.
coalitionccc.org

Coda Alliance
Community education to empower the public and help foster conversations about what it means to "live well" at the EOL; provides assistance with ACP and offers "Go Wish Cards" for facilitating conversations.
  www.codaalliance.org/home.html

Colorado

Colorado Advance Directives Consortium
Information organization of professionals in health care, senior services, law, and ethics dedicated to improving the tools and processes for health care decision making in Colorado.
  www.coloradoadvancedirectives.com

Hospice and Palliative Care of Western Colorado
ACP initiative with forms and links.
  www.hospicewco.com/i4a/pages/index.cfm?pageid=3633

Life Quality Institute
Advancing palliative care through education. Provides forms and educational presentations on ACP.
  www.lifequalityinstitute.org

Connecticut

Connecticut Coalition to Improve End-of-Life Care
Working to improve the care of people who are dying and their families, and to ensure that every individual has information about and access to compassionate, quality EOL care. Provides booklet *Beginning the Conversation about Death, Dying and End-of-Life Care in Connecticut.*
  www.ctendoflifecare.org/index.html

Delaware

Delaware Decisions
Devoted to educating the community about ACP.
  delawaredecisions.org/index.htm

Hospice and Palliative Care Network of Delaware
Working to improve access to quality EOL care by identifying barriers and working to overcome them. Provides slide show "As You Wish" on ACP.
  www.hpcnd.org

Florida

Department of Elder Affairs — State of Florida
Information on EOL initiatives and resources in Florida.
elderaffairs.state.fl.us/doea/hospice_eol.php

Center for Hospice, Palliative Care and End-of-Life Studies
University of South Florida initiative to optimize care and systems of care for patients and families faced with non-curable diseases by generating new knowledge through interdisciplinary research, educating health and human service professionals, and influencing public policy to support quality EOL care.
health.usf.edu/medicine/eolcenter/index.htm#

Project Grace
Partnership of physicians, elder care providers, and concerned citizens of Florida dedicated to changing the death-defying, technology-driven approach to EOL care to a holistic, compassionate one that respects human dignity and the individual's best interests and personal wishes. Provides community and corporate presentations on ACP, booklets, links, and a resource library.
www.projectgrace.org

Georgia

Georgia Health Decisions' CRITICAL Conditions Planning Guide
Provides The CRITICAL Conditions[SM] Planning Guide, emphasizing conversation and documentation of wishes for EOL care.
georgiahealthdecisions.org/critical1.html

Georgia Hospice and Palliative Care Organization
Information, education, and advocacy. Links for ACP.
www.ghpco.org

Hawaii

End-of-Life Care for Hawaii's Ohana
Group-targeted messages and individually tailored support on EOL planning for family caregivers of elders receiving long-term care services. Downloadable booklets on various aspects of ACP. Initiative of the University of Hawaii Center on Aging.
www.hawaii.edu/aging/endoflife_hiohana.html

Kokua Mau: Hawaii's Hospice and Palliative Care Organization
Organization includes individual and organizational champions and supporters from hospitals, education, consumers, insurance, long term care
and hospices; provides resources and links on ACP, including POLST.
   kokuamau.org

Idaho

Idaho End-of-Life Coalition
Resources about compassionate care for people as they complete life,
including resources on ACP.
   www.idahoendoflifecoalition.wildapricot.org

Intermountain Healthcare
ACP conversation guide and planning booklet.
   intermountainhealthcare.org/health-resources/hospitalstay/Pages/
   advanceplanning.aspx

Illinois

Chicago End-of-Life Coalition
Links and resources; speakers bureau on EOL care, including ACP.
   www.cecc.info/end-of-life-care

Iowa

Honoring Your Wishes (Iowa City Hospice)
Provides free consultations with ACP facilitators who help individuals
explore options and prepare written plans.
   iowacityhospice.org/advance-care-planning/honoring-your-wishes

Indiana

Indiana Hospice and Palliative Care Organization
Provides ACP booklet emphasizing conversation.
   www.ihpco.org/consumer/welcome-ihpcoorg-families

Louisiana

LaPOST: A Health Care Quality Forum Initiative
Initiative of the Louisiana Health Care Quality Forum to empower consumers and health care professionals with easy-to-access, simple-to-understand
information and resources to make educated decisions about EOL care;

emphasis on LaPOST, a Louisiana version of POLST (Physicians Orders for Life-Sustaining Treatment).
lhcqf.org/lapost-home

Maine

Maine Hospice Council and Center for End-of-Life Care
Promoting excellence in EOL care; promotes POLST as well as EOL planning in prison.
www.mainehospicecouncil.org

MaineHealth Palliative Care Initiative
Promoting education and support for health care professionals to conduct conversations with patients and their families to help them make medical decisions about the care they wish to receive.
www.mainehealth.org/mh_body.cfm?id=5754

Massachusetts

Better Ending
Nonprofit community coalition in Central Massachusetts working to help individuals and their families plan for EOL and receive community support. Provides planning guide and "Personal Wishes" form.
www.betterending.org

Michigan

End-of-Life Care Committee
Organized to disseminate information about and engage in educational initiatives to promote knowledge about ADs and other planning processes associated with EOL decision making.
www.cahealthalliance.org/end-of-life_care_committee.php

MI Seniors: Michigan Office of Services to the Aging
ACP booklet.
www.michigan.gov/osa/1,4635,7-234----,00.html

Minnesota

Honoring Choices (Twin Cities Medical Society)
Designed to inspire and support community-based conversations regarding EOL care planning. Includes a toolkit of video, text, and web links to support these conversations.
www.honoringchoices.org

Mayo Health Systems-Mankato
Resources for ACP, emphasizing how to have conversations with physicians, family, and friends; includes volunteer "ambassadors" who give consultation to patients and families on ACP.
  mayoclinichealthsystem.org/locations/mankato/for-patients/
  advance-care-planning/have-conversations

Missouri

Missouri End-of-Life Coalition
Education and empowerment for policy makers and dying persons and their families. Includes "Life Choices" workshop on ACP and other resources.
  www.mo-endoflife.org

Montana

Montana Department of Justice: End-of-Life Registry and
Advance Health Care Directives
Stores advance health care directives in a secure computer database and makes these documents available to health care providers; links to toolkits on ACP.
  doj.mt.gov/consumer/end-of-life-registry

Nevada

Nevada Center for Ethics and Health Policy (University of Nevada, Reno)
Resources and links on ACP, including discussion guide for group discussions on EOL care.
  www.unr.edu/ncehp/AdvanceCarePlanning.html

New Hampshire

New Hampshire Healthcare Decisions Coalition
Information to assist persons making EOL care decisions; planning guide, educational video, and booklet on ACP in the workplace.
  www.healthynh.com/advance-directives-healthcare-decision-coalition-home.html

New Hampshire Hospice and Palliative Care Organization
Links and conversation guides on ACP.
  www.nhhpco.org/advance.htm

New Mexico

Being With Dying
Initiative of the Upaya Institute in Santa Fe. Trainings for physicians, nurses, psychologists, social workers, hospice workers, and clergy to enhance competencies in EOL care and introduce innovative approaches in psychosocial, ethical, and spiritual aspects of care.
 www.upaya.org/bwd

New York

Compassion and Support at End of Life (Rochester)
Collaboration to increase acceptance of ADs in the community; emphasis on Medical Orders for Life-Sustaining Treatment (MOLST).
 www.compassionandsupport.org/index.php/for_patients_families/advance_care_planning

Sharing Your Wishes (Western and Central New York)
Increasing awareness of ACP and the importance of health care decision making for older adults; promotes local coalitions and provides a planning guide and a tool kit for community engagement.
 www.sharingyourwishes.org

Southern Tier End-of-Life Coalition (Binghamton)
Provides ACP workshops for religious, workplace, and social groups.
 www.steolc.org/index.html

North Carolina

End of Life Care Coalition (Greenville)
Presents ACP clinics and film series.
 www.endoflifecarecoalition.org/EOLCCEC/Home.html

North Carolina Medical Society
Video and other resources on ACP.
 www.ncmedsoc.org/pages/public_health_info/end_of_life.html

Project Compassion
Creates community and provides innovative support for people living with serious illness, caregiving, EOL, and grief; consult visits, workshops, and resources help people understand and communicate EOL care wishes; planning workbook *Getting It Together: Planning Ahead*.
 www.project-compassion.org/home

Ohio

Midwest Care Alliance

Ohio organization for hospice and palliative care. Provides ACP booklet, *Conversations That Light the Way*.

www.ohpco.org/aws/MCA/pt/sp/livingwills

Oklahoma

University of Oklahoma-Tulsa

ACP consultations through the University Center for Palliative Care.

www.ou.edu/content/tulsa/community_medicine/palliative-care/advance-care-planning.html

Oregon

Death With Dignity

Has led the legal defense and education of the Oregon Death with Dignity Law for nearly 20 years; links to ACP resources, including Alzheimer's and Dementia Mental Health Directive.

www.deathwithdignity.org

Pennsylvania

Coalition for Quality at the EOL

Engaging the community to build demand for better EOL care, building capacity among local health care institutions for the delivery of skilled and compassionate care, focusing attention on the regulatory and financial barriers to quality EOL care, and promulgating appropriate standards and measures; public awareness and educational campaigns.

www.dom.pitt.edu/dgim/iepc/cqel.html

Take Charge of Your Life Partnership

Educates, supports, and empowers people to deal with EOL issues through outreach to consumers, professionals, community organizations, and corporations. Site includes tool kits and *Just Talk About It* videos and discussion guides.

takechargeofyourlife.org

South Dakota

Life Circle of South Dakota (University of South Dakota)

Statewide collaboration of institutions, organizations, and people committed to improving EOL care; resources for community presentations on ACP, including EMT/EMS training for Comfort One (out-of-hospital DNR).

www.usd.edu/medical-school/life-circle-south-dakota/index.cfm

Tennessee

Tennessee End-of-Life Partnership
Encourages and supports local grassroots coalitions to improve EOL care; resources for community presentations on ACP.
   endoflifecaretn.org

Texas

The Y Collaborative
Provides EOL consulting services. Initiative of educator, leader, and life coach Dr. Susan Lieberman, with Nancy Rust in Houston, Texas; emphasizes conversation about ACP in advance of serious illness.
   www.ycollaborative.com/blog

Utah

End-of-Life Care Partnership of Utah
Coalition of individuals and member organization that promotes dialogue with professionals and the public to support practices that improve care for persons near the EOL and their families. Tool kit for ACP.
   carefordying.org

Vermont

Start the Conversation
Public education initiative on EOL planning by Vermont's nonprofit Visiting Nurses Association and Home Health and Hospice Agencies. In partnership with Vermont Ethics Network; education events and resources focused on conversation.
   www.starttheconversationvt.org

Washington

Center for Palliative Care Education
Curriculum to improve EOL care for persons with HIV/AIDS and applicable to other illnesses; includes module on ACP.
   depts.washington.edu/pallcare

Compassion and Choices of Washington
Assist with all aspects of EOL decision making; facilitate discussions about EOL choices between patients, physicians, and family members; includes Values Workshop to help explore EOL decisions and Alzheimer's Disease and Dementia Mental Health AD.
   compassionwa.org

West Virginia

West Virginia Center for End-of-Life Care
Sponsors Respecting Choices Facilitator Training to participants to assist patients and families with difficult EOL decisions and provides a method for converting patient's treatment preferences into medical orders that are recognized throughout the health care continuum; includes e-directory of ADs.
　　www.wvendoflife.org

Hospice of the Panhandle (Martinsburg)
Provides educational programs to the community about ACP.
　　www.hospiceotp.org/index

Wisconsin

Honoring Choices Wisconsin
Statewide initiative of the Wisconsin Medical Society to build system change, advocacy, and education around ACP; working to make ACP a standard element of patient care; training provided by Respecting Choices.
　　www.honoringchoiceswisconsin.org

Respecting Choices (Gundersen Health System, LaCrosse, Wisconsin)
Internationally recognized, evidence-based ACP program that has become the model for many other ACP initiatives. Provides assistance to other communities who want to transform how they provide EOL care. Uses a staged approach that is tailored to the individual's health status.
　　respectingchoices.org

Wyoming

Central Wyoming Hospice and Transitions (Casper)
Speakers bureau on issues of how to talk about death and dying and EOL decisions.
　　www.cwhp.org

PROFESSIONAL ASSOCIATIONS

American Academy on Communication in Healthcare

Provides education, research, and practice focusing on communication and relationships among patients, families, and health care teams.
　　www.aachonline.org

American Academy of Hospice and Palliative Medicine (AAHPM)

Professional organization for physicians specializing in hospice and palliative medicine.
www.aahpm.org

American Association of Critical Care Nurses

Education and resources for critical care nurses to help provide optimal care to critically ill patients.
www.aacn.org

American College of Health Care Administrators

Provides education and professional development for leaders in long-term care.
www.achca.org

American Hospital Association

Works to influence legislation and regulations related to health care and health care delivery.
www.aha.org

American Medical Directors Association

Professional association of medical directors, attending physicians, and others in the delivery of long-term care. Provides education, advocacy, information, and professional development.
www.amda.com

American Pain Society

Scientists, clinicians, and other professionals working to increase knowledge about pain and influence public policy and practice to reduce pain-related suffering.
www.ampainsoc.org

American Society of Bioethics & Humanities

Promotes the exchange of ideas and fosters multidisciplinary, interdisciplinary, and interprofessional scholarship, research, teaching, policy development, professional development, and collegiality among people engaged

in all endeavors related to clinical and academic bioethics and the health-related humanities.
    www.asbh.org

American Society of Law, Medicine & Ethics

Provides high-quality scholarship, debate, and critical thought to the community of professionals at the intersection of law, health care, policy, and ethics.
    www.aslme.org

American Society on Aging

Provides training and professional development for diverse individuals and organizations committed to promoting quality of life for older adults.
    www.asaging.org

Association for Death Education and Counseling

Multidisciplinary professional organization centered on death education, bereavement counseling, and care of the dying.
    www.adec.org

European Association for Palliative Care (EAPC)

Multidisciplinary organization that promotes collaboration, education, and research to promote palliative care in Europe.
    www.eapcnet.org

Gerontological Society of America

Research, education, and practice in the field of aging; disseminates information about aging among scientists, decision makers, and the general public. Includes Hospice, Palliative, and End-of-Life Care Interest Groups.
    www.geron.org

Hospice & Palliative Nurses Association (HPNA)

Palliative-specialty nursing organization providing evidence-based educational tools to assist members of the nursing team with ensuring quality nursing care delivery; managing complex symptoms along with grief and bereavement; having the difficult conversations; educating health care providers and family about the hospice or palliative care philosophy; and influencing palliative nursing through leadership and research.
    www.hpna.org

International Association for Hospice & Palliative Care (IAHPC)

Collaborates and works to improve the quality of life of patients with advanced life-threatening conditions and their families by advancing hospice and palliative care programs, education, research, and favorable policies around the world.

www.hospicecare.com

International Association for the Study of Pain (IASP)

Brings together scientists, clinicians, health care providers, and policy makers to stimulate and support the study of pain and to translate that knowledge into improved pain relief worldwide.

www.iasp-pain.org

National Council on Aging

Nonprofit service and advocacy organization; brings together nonprofit organizations, businesses, and government to develop creative solutions that improve the lives of all older adults.

www.ncoa.org

National Hospice and Palliative Care Organization (NHPCO)

Largest nonprofit membership organization representing hospice and palliative care programs and professionals in the United States; committed to improving EOL care and expanding access to hospice care with the goal of profoundly enhancing quality of life for people dying in America and their loved ones. Operates Caring Connections, national consumer and community engagement initiative.

www.nhpco.org

BOOKS

Atkinson, J. M. (2007). *Advance directives in mental health: Theory, practice and ethics*. London, UK: Jessica Kingsley.

Bruera, E., & Yennurajalingam, S. (2011). *Oxford American handbook of hospice and palliative medicine*. New York, NY: Oxford University Press.

Burgess, M., Cha, S., & Tung, E. E. (2011). *Advance care planning in the skilled nursing facility: What do we need for success?* Berwyn, PA: JTE Multimedia.

Byock, I. (1997). *Dying well: Peace and possibilities at the end of life*. New York, NY: Riverhead Books.

Byock, I. (2004). *The four things that matter most: A book about living.* New York, NY: Free Press.

Byock, I. (2012). *The best care possible: A physician's quest to transform care through the end of life.* New York, NY: Avery.

Chapple, H. S. (2010). *No place for dying: Hospitals and the ideology of rescue.* Walnut Creek, CA: Left Coast Press.

Connor, S. R. (2009). *Hospice and palliative care: The essential guide* (2nd ed.). New York, NY: Routledge.

Doka, K. J., Tucci, A. S., Corr, C. A., & Jennings, B. (2012). *End-of-life ethics: A case study approach.* Washington, DC: Hospice Foundation of America.

Dolan, S., & Vizzard, A. R. (2011). *The end of life advisor: Personal, legal, and medical considerations for a peaceful, dignified death.* New York, NY: Kaplan.

Doukas, D. J., & Reichel, W. (2007). *Planning for uncertainty: Living wills and other advance directives for you and your family.* Baltimore, MD: The Johns Hopkins University Press.

Hammes, B. J., & Briggs, L. (2000). *Respecting choices: Building a systems approach to advance care planning.* LaCrosse, WI: Gundersen Health Systems.

Hammes, B. J., Warner, M. R., & Leavitt, M. O. (Eds.). *Having your own say: Getting the right care when it matters most.* Washington, D.C.: CHT Press.

Holstein, M. B., Parks, M. B., & Waymack, M. H. (2011). *Ethics, aging, and society: The critical turn.* New York, NY: Springer.

Kaufman, S. R. (2005). *. . . And a time to die: How hospitals shape the end of life.* Chicago, IL: The University of Chicago Press.

Kellehear, A. (2005). *Compassionate cities.* New York, NY: Routledge.

Kellehear, A. (2007) *A social history of death.* New York, NY: Cambridge University Press.

Kiernan, S. P. (2007). *Last rights: Rescuing the end of life from the medical system.* New York, NY: St. Martin's Press.

Kinzbrunner, B., & Policzer, J. (2010). *End-of-life-care: A practical guide* (2nd ed.). New York, NY: McGraw-Hill Professional.

Kuebler, K. K., Heidrich, D. E., & Esper, P. (2006). *Palliative and end-of-life care: Clinical practice guidelines* (2nd ed.). Philadelphia, PA: Mosby.

Martensen, R. (2009). *A life worth living: A doctor's reflections on illness in a high-tech era.* New York, NY: Farrar, Straus and Giroux.

Meagher, D. K., & Balk, D. E. (Eds.). (2013). *Handbook of thanatology: The essential body of knowledge for the study of death, dying, and bereavement.* New York, NY: Routledge.

Meier, D. E., Isaacs, S. L., & Hughes, R. (Eds.) (2010). *Palliative care: Transforming the care of serious illness.* San Francisco, CA: Jossey-Bass.

Thomas, K., & Lobo, B. *Advance care planning in end of life care.* New York, NY: Oxford University Press.

JOURNALS

Advances in Social Work
journals.iupui.edu/index.php/advancesinsocialwork

American Journal of Hospital and Palliative Medicine
ajh.sagepub.com

American Journal of Law and Medicine
www.aslme.org/Back_Issues_And_Articles?journal=AJLM

Annals of Long-Term Care
www.annalsoflongtermcare.com

Anthropology and Medicine
www.tandfonline.com/toc/canm20/current

Bandolier: Evidence Based Thinking About Health Care
www.medicine.ox.ac.uk/bandolier

Bereavement Care
www.routledgementalhealth.com/journals/details/0268–2621/

British Medical Journal (on Palliative Care)
www.bmj.com/specialties/palliative-care

Clinical Gerontologist
www.tandfonline.com/loi/wcli20

Clinical Social Work Journal
www.springer.com/psychology/journal/10615

Death Studies
www.routledgementalhealth.com/journals/details/0748–1187

Educational Gerontology
www.tandfonline.com/loi/uedg20

The Forum: The Quarterly Publication of the Association for Death Education and Counseling
www.adec.org/The_Forum/4054.htm

Gerontology and Geriatrics Education
www.tandfonline.com/loi/wgge20

Health and Social Work
www.naswpress.org/publications/journals/hsw.html

Illness, Crisis and Loss
www.baywood.com/journals/PreviewJournals.asp?Id=1054–1373

Innovations in End-of-Life Care
Published 1999–2003; issues archived at: www2.edc.org/lastacts/issues.asp

International Journal of Aging and Human Development
baywood.com/journals/previewjournals.asp?id=0091–4150

Journal of Aging and Health
www.sagepub.com/journals/Journal200849

Journal of Aging and Social Policy
www.tandfonline.com/loi/wasp20

Journal of the American Geriatrics Society
onlinelibrary.wiley.com/journal/10.1111/%28ISSN%291532–5415

Journal of Applied Gerontology
jag.sagepub.com

Journal of Community Health
www.springer.com/public+health/journal/10900

Journal of Community Health Nursing
www.tandfonline.com/loi/hchn20

Journal of Gerontological Nursing
www.healio.com/journals/jgn

Journals of Gerontology
www.geron.org/Publications

Journal of Loss and Trauma: International Perspectives on Stress and Coping
www.routledgementalhealth.com/journals/details/1532–5024

Journal of Medical Ethics
jme.bmj.com

Journal of Palliative Care
www.criugm.qc.ca/journalofpalliativecare

Journal of Palliative Medicine
www.liebertpub.com/jpm

Journal of Pain and Symptom Management
www.aahpm.org/publications/default/journal.html

Journal of Social Work
jsw.sagepub.com

Journal of Social Work, Theory, and Practice
www.tandfonline.com/toc/cjsw20/current

Medical Anthropology
www.tandfonline.com/toc/gmea20/current

Omega—Journal of Death and Dying
baywood.com/journals/previewjournals.asp?id=0030–2228

Pain: Clinical Updates
www.iasp-pain.org/AM/Template.cfm?Section=PAIN_

Palliative Medicine
pmj.sagepub.com

Psychology and Aging
www.apa.org/pubs/journals/pag/index.aspx

OTHER

Agency for Healthcare Research and Quality (AHRQ)

Funds and disseminates research and collaborates with other institutions to promote the quality, safety, efficiency, and effectiveness of health care; administered by the U.S. Department of Health and Human Services.
www.ahrq.gov

Center for Practical Bioethics

Addresses bioethical issues related to aging and EOL care.
www.practicalbioethics.org

Dartmouth Atlas of Health Care

Provides data on health care resources throughout the country and state by state; includes research on EOL care.
www.dartmouthatlas.org

Dartmouth Biomedical Libraries

Portal for resources on life-threatening illness and EOL care.
www.dartmouth.edu/~library/biomed/guides/research/palliative.html

The Greenwall Foundation

Funding for bioethics research.
www.greenwall.org/index.php

The Growth House

Free access to over 4,000 pages of high-quality education materials about EOL care, palliative medicine, and hospice care, including the full text of several books; education for both the general public and health care professionals.
www.growthhouse.org

The Hastings Center

Research on bioethics, including books and articles on EOL care.
www.thehastingscenter.org/Issues/Default.aspx?v=244&gclid=CITmt
YHUjrUCFc6DQgodSgQAJw

Institute for Healthcare Improvement

Innovator in health and health care improvement; sponsors "Conversation Ready" initiative to give providers skills to communicate with patients and families about EOL preferences.
www.ihi.org

Robert Wood Johnson Foundation

History of funding for projects related to palliative and EOL care.
www.rwjf.org

Index